SEMANTIC PROCESSING *and* WORD FINDING DIFFICULTY ACROSS *the* LIFESPAN

A Practical Guide for Speech-Language Pathologists

SEMANTIC PROCESSING *and* WORD FINDING DIFFICULTY ACROSS *the* LIFESPAN

A Practical Guide for Speech-Language Pathologists

Pei-Fang Hung, PhD, CCC-SLP
Lei Sun, PhD, CCC-SLP

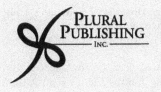

PLURAL
PUBLISHING
INC.

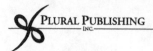

5521 Ruffin Road
San Diego, CA 92123

e-mail: information@pluralpublishing.com
Website: https://www.pluralpublishing.com

Library of Congress Cataloging-in-Publication Data:
Names: Hung, Pei-Fang, author. | Sun, Lei (Associate professor of
  speech-language pathology)
Title: Semantic processing and word finding difficulty across the lifespan
  : a practical guide for speech-language pathologists / Pei-Fang Hung,
  Lei Sun.
Description: San Diego, CA : Plural Publishing, Inc., [2022] | Includes
  bibliographical references and index.
Identifiers: LCCN 2021031205 (print) | LCCN 2021031206 (ebook) | ISBN
  9781635501940 (paperback) | ISBN 1635501946 (paperback) | ISBN
  9781635502190 (ebook)
Subjects: MESH: Language Disorders | Semantics | Phonetics | Verbal
  Learning | Speech-Language Pathology
Classification: LCC RC424.7 (print) | LCC RC424.7 (ebook) | NLM WL 340.2
  | DDC 616.85/5--dc23
LC record available at https://lccn.loc.gov/2021031205
LC ebook record available at https://lccn.loc.gov/2021031206

CONTENTS

PREFACE

The initial idea about writing this book was from several excited and heated discussions on a topic both of us are compassionate about: "Lexicon." Although we both are first-generation immigrants learning English as a second language, we have different personal experiences, training backgrounds, and research interests. It is not surprising that we have different views on lexical acquisition and disorders. However, after years of studying, teaching, and researching semantic processing and word-finding difficulty, we realized that we needed to take a step back and look at the bigger picture. In order to have a holistic understanding of semantic processing and word retrieval difficulty, this should be viewed on a continuum from both developmental and acquired perspectives.

We noticed that most clinical approaches addressing lexical deficits are based on the same theoretical foundations. Although clinical management strategies need to be tailored for individual needs or specific deficits, the fundamental concepts are similar. Hence, it makes sense to review the conceptual frameworks and theoretical principles through an integrated approach and compare the similarities and differences among different types of semantic-related language disorders across the lifespan.

We start the book by providing readers with a review of the fundamental basis and research evidence related to semantic processing and word retrieval difficulty. We review the related research studies from different disciplines, including speech-language pathology, linguistics, psychology, neuroscience, and education, to help readers understand lexical processing and retrieval from a different but holistic viewpoint. We also try to interpret the relevant research evidence from a clinical point of view and attempt to incorporate practical considerations into our discussion. Subsequently, readers can learn about the commonly implemented, evidence-based clinical approaches for addressing lexical deficits across the lifespan. As we aim to bridge the gap between research evidence and clinical practice, we add the section of clinical implications into our discussions along with providing sample therapy plans for the discussed treatment approaches.

While viewing developmental and acquired lexical deficits separately, we may miss out on the fundamental principles and theoretical frameworks and possibly overlook the connections between them. We hope readers can benefit from learning semantic processing and word retrieval difficulty from this nontraditional approach. This book is dedicated to practicing and future speech-language pathologists who provide valuable service to people who struggle with lexical learning and retrieval.

Pei-Fang Hung and Lei Sun
Long Beach, CA

ACKNOWLEDGMENTS

Our deep and sincere gratitude to all the contributing authors, including Dr. Kris Brock, Dr. Belinda Daughrity, Clair Small, and Sarah Larsen, for sharing their wisdom and outstanding work. It is our privilege to work with you, and we look forward to future collaborations.

We also want to thank our students and colleagues at the California State University, Long Beach, our clients with communication disorders, and their family members. We learn so much from working with you, from the conversations we engaged, and from the questions you posed.

We would like to thank our Project Editor, Christina Gunning, and the whole production team at Plural Publishing. They have worked dedicatedly on this project and provided us with tremendous support throughout the journey of writing this book.

Lastly, we want to thank our parents, siblings, and in-laws. Thank you for your love and continuous support.

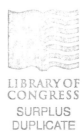

CONTRIBUTORS

Kris L. Brock, PhD, CCC-SLP
Assistant Professor
College of Rehabilitation and Communication Sciences
Department of Communication Science and Disorders
Idaho State University
Pocatello, Idaho
Chapter 5

Belinda Daughrity, PhD, CCC-SLP
Assistant Professor
California State University, Long Beach
Long Beach, California
Chapter 10

Sarah Larsen, MA
Speech-Language Pathologist
California State University, Long Beach
Long Beach, California
Appendices 8–1 and 9–1 through 9–7

Claire Small, MA, CF-SLP
Speech-Language Pathologist
Speech Pathology Group
Ojai, California
Appendices 8–1 and 9–1 through 9–7

REVIEWERS

Plural Publishing and the authors would like to thank the following reviewers for taking the time to provide their valuable feedback during the manuscript development process. Additional anonymous feedback was provided by other expert reviewers.

Ellayne S. Ganzfried, MS, CCC-SLP, ASHA Fellow, FNAP
Clinical Associate Professor
Pace University
New York, New York

Kristen Maul, PhD, SLP-CF
Speech-Language Pathology Program
Gallaudet University
Washington, D.C.

Laura Riddle, PhD, CCC-SLP
Associate Professor
Nazareth College of Rochester
Rochester, New York

1

INTRODUCTION TO LEXICON

Lei Sun

Chapter Objectives

1. Identify the essential elements needed for understanding and producing a linguistic message successfully.
2. Demonstrate the knowledge of the aspects of lexical competence.
3. Identify the relationships among lexicon (semantics), phonology and morphosyntax.

The Importance of Words

Words are essential to any kind of language-based processing and serve as the building blocks of the linguistic message people want to express to others. Words can convey verbal messages from speakers to listeners and convey written messages from writers to readers. Understanding and producing a linguistic message successfully requires several essential elements, inlcuding (1) good lexical knowledge (i.e., word knowledge), (2) good morphosyntactic knowledge (i.e., how the words are sequenced in a sentence), (3) paralinguistic features (e.g., intonation, pitch, volume), and (4) context (e.g., social and linguistic). The following two example sentences are used for our discussion.

(a) "The big dog angrily chases the little boy in the hallway."

(b) "The little boy angrily chases the big dog in the hallway."

Lexical Knowledge. Different lexical categories (i.e., classes of words) are required to constitute a linguistic message. Content words, words that have semantic content, play a vital role in a sentence because of the rich messages they carry. The content words in the aforementioned example sentences include nouns (dog, boy, hallway), verbs (chase), adjectives (big, little), and adverbs (angrily). Not knowing the meaning of content words can significantly affect the listener's understanding of the intended message. On the other hand, although function words, such as articles (the) and prepositions (in), do not carry the key meaning, these words are needed to form a complete, syntactically correct sentence.

Morphosyntactic Knowledge. Both example sentences contain the same number of words and morphemes; however, they convey very different messages because of the different word order. In other words, switching the subject (person or animal performs the action) and object (person or animal receives the action) in a sentence can create different meanings. The listener has to understand the meanings of words as well as sentence structure in order to comprehend the message correctly. Therefore, both lexical and morphosyntactic knowledge is essential for correctly understanding and constructing the intended meaning.

Paralinguistic Features. Paralinguistic features include intonation, stress, pitch, volume, speech rate, modulation, and fluency, and these features can also affect the meaning of the words and sentence. For example, the intended meaning can be changed and modified when a speaker alters the intonation. The speaker can say "The little boy angrily chases the big dog in the hallway." with a rising tone to express the disbelief of this observation or with a falling tone to just give information about the observation. Furthermore, changing the stress pattern within a word can alter the meaning entirely. For instance, the word class and meaning of the word "record" change when the stress is moved from the first syllable ([REcord]: noun.) to the second syllable ([reCORD]: verb).

Context. The meaning of a word may also change depending on the social and linguistic contexts. Social context means how people use language, and linguistic context refers to the surrounding words that can help determine word meaning and interpretation. For example, the phrase "kick the bucket" can be interpreted both literally and figuratively. When it is interpreted figuratively, all three words must be interpreted together because an idiom phrase is considered a giant lexical unit (Nippold, 1985).

Similarly, words with multiple meanings also make the process of understanding word meanings challenging. For example, the word "arm" presents very different meanings in the following two sentences: (1) "I have a mosquito bite on my *arm*" versus (2) "It's important to *arm* yourself with knowledge." Therefore, speakers must know not only the word meaning and word class but also the appropriate context to use the word. In the next section, we will attempt to answer a seemingly simple question that remains difficult to answer: What is lexicon?

What Is Lexicon?

Lexicon, also known as vocabulary, means a broader understanding of words, including usage, categorization, and the association between words and phrases. Lexicon is a broad, complex, and multifaceted concept. In this book, we use the terms *lexicon* and *vocabulary* interchangeably. Words are learned when both form (phonological representations) and meaning (semantic representations) are acquired and accessible to the person (Swingley, 2009). More specifically, *lexical learning* refers to the ability to acquire phonological representations (e.g., /kæt/ for the word "cat") and semantic representations (e.g., color, shape, pattern, and animacy) of a word (Nation, 2014). The learning process begins by recognizing the word and then mapping it to the conceptual referent. The word meaning is continuously refined based on linguistic context (other words that surrounding the intended word can help determine its interpretation) and social context (how people use the word in a given language) (He & Arunachalam, 2017). Learners use the information gained from linguistic and social contexts to gradually derive the meaning. The elaborated discussion about the process of mapping concepts to word form and meaning is in Chapter 3. Once a word is learned, it is stored in long-term memory and becomes part of one's mental lexicon for later use.

Mental lexicon is a mental dictionary that contains information about the meaning, pronunciation, usage, and grammatical features of a word. The structure of the mental lexicon is more complex than a physical dictionary because it is not organized in alphabetic order like a typical dictionary. Instead, words in the mental dictionary are interconnected and categorized like a spider web-like network without following a predetermined set of rules (Aitchison,1994). Additionally, how a word is related to other words and how frequently a word is used can impact how well the word is stored. The frequency of a word is being retrieved (used) can enhance the storage power of the word. *Lexical storage* and *lexical retrieval* influence each other because how well words are stored in long-term memory will have an impact on how easily the words can be retrieved.

Lexical access, the act of **lexical retrieval**, is the ability to access the mental lexicon. Specifically, it involves the selection of semantically-specified and syntactically-specified lexical representations and the corresponding phonological representations (Caramazza, 1997). For example, when retrieving the word "dog," several features can be activated, such as basic semantic features (e.g., fur, bark, four legs), superordinate features (e.g., animal, mammal), subordinate features (e.g., golden retriever), phonological representations (/dɔg/), and orthographic structures (d-o-g). A detailed discussion of lexical processing models that involves the different levels of lexical selection is presented in Chapter 2.

How words are stored, organized, and retrieved has been discussed extensively in the literature of neuroscience, linguistics, and psychology. Word learning is a continuous process throughout the lifespan as we continue to add new words to our mental lexicon through experiences. In the next section, we provide an overview on how someone develops lexical knowledge and how to evaluate lexical competence.

Lexical Knowledge and Lexical Competence

Lexical (word) knowledge is acquired through three processes proposed by Aitchison (1994), including labeling/mapping, packaging, and network building. The *labeling/mapping process* is the first step in developing word knowledge. People connect the new word to its referent or concept by matching the sounds to the referent. Children first link a specific sound combination to the referent and then gradually change the sound sequence to an adult form. Similarly, adults learn new words by going through the same mapping process, including connecting the new word to its concept, sound sequence, and print. The second process is *packaging* which refers to knowing different meanings of a word. Depending on the grammatical class, a word may have different meanings and pronunciations. For example, when using the word "produce" as a noun, it means the product of gardening (i.e., fruits and vegetables). However, when using "produce" as a verb, it means to create, to make, or to manufacture. The packaging process requires people to have a more extensive understanding of the word meaning than merely linking the word to the concept or referent. The third process is *"network building,"* which refers to the process of discovering the semantic relations among words.

Lexical competence is competence in understanding words, and it is a reflection on how good someone's word (lexical) knowledge is. Henriksen (1999) proposed three closely interrelated dimensions that should be considered when evaluating lexical competence, including receptive-expressive knowledge, depth of knowledge, and partial-precise knowledge.

Receptive-Expressive Vocabulary Knowledge

Receptive vocabulary knowledge means that someone understands the meaning of the word when he/she hears or reads it. Expressive vocabulary knowledge means someone uses the word either in speaking or writing. Receptive lexical knowledge (comprehension) development usually precedes expressive lexical acquisition. According to the normative data of the MacArthur-Bates Communicative Development Inventories, Second Edition (MB-CDI 2nd edition; Fenson et al., 2007), it shows that at the age of 8 months, infants understand an average of 42 words, and this number steadily increases to more than 200 words at the age of 17 and 18 months. On the other hand, at the age of 8 months, infants produce only 1 to 10 words, and the average number of vocabulary production does not exceed 20 words until the age of 14 months. Receptive and expressive vocabulary continues to expand over time across the lifespan, but receptive vocabulary is still about twice the size of expressive vocabulary. For instance, the receptive vocabulary is estimated to be 8,000 to 14,000 words and about 2,600 expressive words for average first graders. This receptive-expressive gap continues into adulthood, and the size is still about twice in receptive vocabulary than expressive vocabulary (McDaniel et al., 2019).

Partial-Precise Knowledge

Lexical knowledge develops on a continuum from no word knowledge to partial word knowledge to precise word knowledge. Henriksen (1999) indicates that we may not have a full understanding of words because we can use inferential strategies and contextual cues to close the gaps in lexical knowledge. Also, our understanding of words changes over time based on the expansion of world knowledge and continuous language development. Therefore, it is important to keep in mind that word knowledge is not all or none but rather a continuous development process.

It is also crucial not to assume that a person who can produce a word successfully has a complete understanding of the word meaning. It is possible that word production may occur without full comprehension of the word (Singleton & Shulman, 2002). For example, children may start using some rote phrases (e.g., a piece of cake) without fully understanding the meaning of each word and the inferential meaning of the word combination. Along the same vein, a person who doesn't use the word may have some knowledge about the word meaning.

Receptive vocabulary tests (or known as recognition tests) are commonly administered to evaluate someone' lexical knowledge. The procedure of the receptive tests is asking examinees to point to the picture that matches the target word. However, examinees may correctly select the target word based on partial knowledge or using test taking strategies (e.g., elimination). This means that the receptive vocabulary tests are not sensitive enough to successfully differentiate the words with partial knowledge from the words with precise knowledge. Clinicians can also utilize expressive vocabulary tests to evaluate lexical knowledge which requires the examinees to produce the target word. However, it should be noted that someone may be able to successfully say a word with partial knowledge but might misuse the word in wrong contexts due to incomplete lexical understanding. For example, it is not uncommon to see a child who can label an object but is unable to use the word beyond the immediate environment.

Depth of Knowledge

The third dimension to be considered is the depth of knowledge. The depth of knowledge is defined as "the quality of the person's vocabulary knowledge" (Henriksen, 1999, p. 305). It is essentially what the person knows about the word. Word knowledge changes over time, depending on the relationships between words and continuous exposure in various contexts. According to Henriksen (1999), rich meaning representation encompasses not only the knowledge of the relationship between the concept and the referent but also relations with other words in the vocabulary. In addition, the knowledge about syntactic and morphological features of the word is crucial to word knowledge. Knowing a word should include the knowledge of meaning, lexical organization, spelling, sound structure, syntax, and context (Qian, 2002).

In summary, it is important to keep in mind that estimating a client's lexical competence is related to how lexical knowledge is evaluated. When evaluating a client's word knowledge, it is necessary to administer both receptive and expressive lexical assessments at different levels. Because lexical knowledge acquisition is a dynamic and evolving process, it is essential to conduct the evaluation at different points of time. For example, through repeated exposures and support of contexts, a child can associate the meaning to the referents and further consolidate the word meaning to be used beyond the referent. The child may hear the word "sloth" several times before she/he can correctly use "sloth" to label the animal. Once the child further learns about the extended meaning of sloth, the child may use it in an analogy such as "you are slow like a sloth."

The Relationships Among Language Domains

Bloom and Lahey (1978) explained the relationships among five language domains by categorizing them into three conceptual groups, including (1) "Form" (phonology, syntax, morphology), (2) "Content" (semantics), and (3) "Use" (pragmatics). Bloom and Tinker (2001) further elaborated this concept by adding engagement (social and emotional development) and effort (cognitive development) to it. Similarly, other researchers also capitalize the importance of context and social functions in the language learning process and highlight how use of language can promote language acquisition and development (Bates, Thal, & Mac-Whinney, 1991, p. 134). Ruben (1999) further stated that phonology, semantics, and syntax are developmentally interdependent with different critical periods and constraints. While expanding vocabulary is crucial to lexical development, phonological, syntactic, and morphological information also plays a vital role in word acquisition. Figure 1–1 illustrates the relationships among these language domains. In this section, we briefly review the lexical-phonological and lexical-morphosyntactic relationships.

Lexicon and Phonology

Words are the building blocks of language, whereas sounds are the building blocks of words. Hence, phonological development plays a critically important role in lexical development; a new word has to be perceived and decoded correctly in order to link the sound pattern to its meaning. In other words, having the ability to associate a label (word/sound pattern) to its referent (concept/meaning) is essential for lexical development. Additionally, rich linguistic input (e.g., social interactions in daily communications) and repetitive exposures are required to strengthen the association between labels and referents and to facilitate forming strong mental representations. Infants are able to link what they hear (word/sound pattern) to the object (referent) and form a tentative association through just a few exposures (Kemp, Scott, Bernhardt, Johnson, Siegel, & Werker, 2017). Thus,

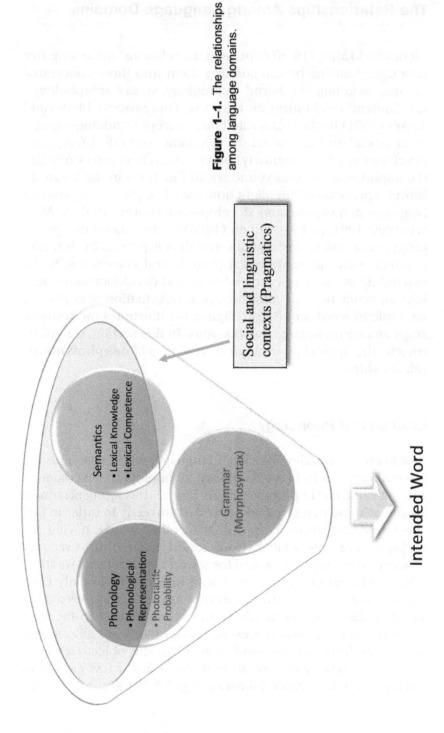

Figure 1–1. The relationships among language domains.

it is not surprising that the early developing words are mostly words that used frequently in daily life, such as mommy, bye, hi, and no.

Furthermore, the early developing words are not only correlated to the frequency of environmental input but also the sounds and sound patterns that acquired early in life (Stoel-Gammon, 2011). The early developing words often contain sounds or the syllable patterns that children are able to produce or ready to use, such as consonant-vowel (CV, e.g., hi, bye, no, go, me), vowel-consonant (VC, e.g., up, out), consonant-vowel-consonant-vowel (CVCV, e.g., mama, dada, nigh-nigh, boo-boo), consonant-vowel-consonant (CVC, e.g., cat, dog, bike, cup). Many factors can have an impact on phonological development; we highlight the two key factors that are associated with lexical and phonological development, including phonological representation and phonotactic probability.

Phonological Representation

Phonological representation provides the foundation for spoken words, and it means "abstract phonological information stored in long term memory" (Sutherland & Gillon, 2005, p. 295). The phonological representation can be presented either as a word unit (e.g., /dɔg/) or sound segments of a word (e.g., /d//ɔ//g/). Phonological representations are established and then gradually shaped through repetitive exposures and social contexts. Research has shown a strong correlation between phonological and lexical developments, and there is a bidirectional activation between lexical and phonological representations (Sosa & Stoel-Gammon, 2012; Storkel & Morrisette, 2002).

For adults with well-established phonological representations, words can be organized based on phonological similarity, which creates a *phonological neighborhood*. The words within the same phonological neighborhood usually differ by one phoneme. However, not all words have the same amount of phonological neighbors. For example, the word "hat" has many phonological neighbors (e.g., bat, cat, rat, fat, kat, pat, sat, ham, etc.) whereas the word "these" has fewer neighbors (e.g., tease, peace, cheese). Words that have ten or more phonologically similar words are considered words with high phonological neighborhood density. Words with high neighborhood density have an advantage in word production because it is easier to learn other words in the same phonological neighborhood. However, the disadvantage is that phonologically similar words can create a competition and result in speech errors (Sosa & Stoel-Gammon, 2012; Storkel, Armbruster, & Hogan, 2006; Storkel & Morrisette, 2002; Vitevitch, 2002). Fortunately, young children, at least before age of 7 years old, do not experience much lexical competition like adults because the size of their vocabulary repertoire is still relatively small. Lexical competition increases when neighborhood density grows and sufficient words are added to the repertoire (Sosa & Stoel-Gammon, 2012).

Additionally, young children do not process unfamiliar words by analyzing individual phonemes like adults; instead, they learn words as whole. The ability to process phonemic information does not emerge until children have more mature phonological representation and an understanding of phonemic features, which occurs during preschool years. It is around the same time when phonological awareness, a metalinguistic ability important to literacy development, starts to develop (Storkel & Morrisette, 2002; Sutherland & Gillon, 2005). If the reader is interested to see more examples, please visit Dr. Caroline Bowen's website (https://www.speech-language-therapy.com).

Phonotactic Probability

Another important factor associated with lexical processing is *phonotactic probability*. **Phonotactic probability** refers to the frequency of sounds and sound patterns in a language (Sosa & Stoel-Gammon, 2012; Storkel & Morrisette, 2002). Both children and adults recognize and produce *common* sound sequences (e.g., sit) faster and more accurately than *rare* sound sequences (e.g., these). This is because common sound sequences have stronger facilitatory connections with each other that increase the speed of threshold activation during word recognition and production (Aslin, Saffran, & Newport, 1998; Sosa & Stoel-Gammon, 2012; Storkel & Morrisette, 2002). In other words, rare sound sequences have few neighbors while common sound sequences have more neighbors (Storkel & Hoover, 2010, p. 3). Infants as young as 8 months old are sensitive to phonotactic information as they are exposed to words that comprise common sound sequences. Infants start learning about phonotactic rules in a given language around 9 months old (Owens, 2012) and show the ability to form new links between an object and its sound pattern as early as 15 months old (Shafer & Plumkett, 1998 as cited in Nazzi & Bertoncini, 2003). Moreover, words with high phonological neighborhood density are usually composed of common sound sequences.

In summary, because semantics and phonology are strongly correlated, it is critically important for clinicians to consider all related factors that can influence lexical acquisition and word retrieval, such as word frequency, neighborhood density, and phonotactic probability. For instance, high-frequency words and words with high phonological neighborhood density could facilitate lexical acquisition and word production. Paying attention to these factors and considering how words may compete with each other could help speech-language pathologists make clinical decisions. Thus, clinicians should consider selecting target words that can promote the development in both domains, such as words that are frequently used in a client's environment, words that contain sounds in a child's phonetic inventory (sounds that are correctly produced independently at least two times), and words that have common sound sequences. To strengthen the link between sounds, labels, and mental representations, it is also a good idea to provide clients with frequent exposure to target words and opportunities to use these words in a meaningful context. When working with children with developmental speech and language disorders, it is also important to expand their existing phonetic inventory and sound sequences to facilitate lexical development. For example, for young children or children with limited verbal output, adding high frequency words containing early developing or common sounds in spoken English (e.g., n, t, s, d) may promote their vocabulary development. However, it should be noted that the possibility of competition from phonologically similar words may increase while using words with high phonological neighborhood density in therapy.

Lexicon and Morphosyntax

There is also a strong correlation between semantics and morphosyntax because words are essential for forming phrases and sentences. The size of vocabulary repertoire is essential to the success of phrase and sentence building, as well as morphological application. Additionally, learning words involves learning the grammatical features of the word, such as the role the word plays in a syntactically correct sentence and the use of inflectional morphemes (Dixon & Marchman, 2007).

Understanding how verbs are acquired can help us understand how lexical development interacts with morphosyntactic development. Vocabulary is acquired in a sequential manner, starting with learning early developing words (mostly nouns) around the first birthday and combining words into phrases/ sentences around two years of age. Learning verbs requires more than simply mapping labels to the referents because learning verbs requires making an association between the role of the subject (person or animal performs the action) and object (person or animal receives the action), as well as the relationship between argument structure of a verb (i.e., subject and object) (Fisher et al., 2010). Gleitman and Gleitman (1992) reviewed a series of studies on the role of morphosyntax in vocabulary acquisition and concluded that children may understand the semantic relationship between the subject and object of a verb before they use it. Additionally, children are able to analyze the sentence structure and understand the role of argument structure as young as 16 months old.

Understanding morphosyntactic information is required for verb acquisition (Gleitman & Gleitman,1992). For example, children begin to understand the role of function words (e.g., "a" and "on") during the first year of life and start using the syntactic information to infer the meaning of unknown content words during the second year of life (Christophe et al., 2008). In other words, young children are able to understand syntactic information and use it to derive the meaning and syntactic categories of unknown words.

Syntactical bootstrapping is a term that describes a child's ability to use syntactic information to guide and facilitate verb learning (Fisher et al., 2010). Because verb learning takes more than simply associating (mapping) a verb to the action, there are additional factors to be considered, such as the number of argument structure, thematic role, transitivity, and nonaction verbs (e.g., mental verbs). These factors can further complicate the verb acquisition process. In order to figure out the meaning of a verb, learners have to identify the number of participants involved and the role that each participant plays. For instance, the sentence "The dog barks," has only one participant which indicates the use of an intransitive verb. On the other hand, the sentence "The dog chases the boy," involves two participants which indicates the use of a transitive verb. Besides knowing the number of participants and transitivity of the verb, learners must understand the word meaning of the verb (e.g., bark, chase) (Fisher et al., 2010). Amazingly, toddlers are able to use syntactic information to infer the participant's role and transitivity of the verb. Additionally, toddlers can use syntactic information, such as word order, to learn new verbs.

In conclusion, language domains are intertwined and interconnected. Difficulty in one language domain may lead to problems in another. It is important to understand the factors that may contribute to a client's word access and retrieval difficulty. For example, based on the developmental data, it is understandable that verbs are more challenging to acquire than nouns, especially for children with developmental language disorders. Because of the unique nature of verbs, people with acquired language disorders can experience increased difficulty retrieving verbs than nouns. Hence, it is critical for clinicians to keep in mind that certain types of words may be more difficult to access and retrieve after brain damage. Clinicians should consider implementing different techniques to help clients overcome the challenge with lexical acquisition and/or word retrieval.

Impact of Language Disorders on Lexicon: An Overview

Lexicon is essential to communication. Someone's lexical knowledge and lexical competency significantly affect their ability to understand and convey a message. As discussed above, successfully conveying a meaningful message requires essential lexical knowledge, correct morphosyntactic structure, appropriate paralinguistic features, and proper pragmatic skills that reflect the context. Successfully producing an intended word is a complex and multifaceted process that requires linguistic, cognitive, and motor functions. Therefore, an interruption resulted from communication disorders may cause a breakdown at any point in the lexical retrieval process. People with communication disorders can have difficulty with lexical acquisition or word retrieval. For example, children with developmental language disorder or a concomitant language disorder (e.g., autism spectrum disorder) can struggle with lexical development. They tend to learn new words slowly, have difficulty associating sounds with its meanings/concepts, and struggle with retaining the newly learned words. They may not only have a small existing vocabulary repertoire but also have a hard time consolidating the newly learned words by making an association with the existing vocabulary. Due to immature lexical knowledge, the chances for making errors in these children increase because the words with similar meaning and sounds can compete with the intended word during the lexical retrieval process.

Similarly, people with acquired, neurogenic language disorders (e.g., aphasia) can also struggle with word finding due to damaging or interrupting the lexical access process. Several lexical access models have been developed based on identifying and investigating the speech errors made by people with aphasia during their word retrieval process. These theoretical models can provide a framework for clinicians to understand how words can be produced successfully and to reveal the possible locus of interruption during the word production process. Additionally, these models offer a starting point for us to discuss lexical access and retrieval difficulty from both developmental and neurogenic perspectives. A more detailed discussion of lexical retrieval models is presented in Chapter 2, and how different types of communication disorders may affect lexical acquisition and retrieval processes is discussed in Chapter 6.

The purpose of this book is to help speech-language pathologists and other related professionals gain knowledge in semantic processing and then develop an appropriate and effective clinical intervention program for managing lexical acquisition and word retrieval difficulty. It is important to know the root causes of word access and retrieval difficulty. Therefore, we will review several lexical process models, key concepts related to lexical acquisition, and variables that may contribute to word storage and retrieval process in Chapters 2 to 5. After reviewing the theoretical basis, we will then discuss word access and retrieval difficulties from developmental and acquired perspectives, assessment considerations, and evidence-based lexical treatment intervention options in Chapter 6 to 10.

Discussion Questions

1. What does the word "lexicon" mean to you? Based on your word learning experience (e.g., learning a second language, learning a new word in your primary language), how would you describe the process of lexicon storage, organization, and retrieval?
2. Discuss the three dimensions of lexical competence proposed by Henriksen (1999) and their clinical implications in vocabulary assessment and intervention.
3. Describe the relationships between lexicon and phonology as well as lexicon and morphosyntax.
4. Explain the required functions that are needed for producing an intended word or conveying a message successfully.

References

Aitchison, J. (1994). *Words in the mind: An introduction to the mental lexicon* (2nd ed.). Wiley-Blackwell.

Aslin, R., Saffran, J., & Newport, E. (1998). Computation of conditional probability statistics by 8-month-old infants. *Psychological Science*, 9(4), 321–324. https://doi.org/10.1111/1467-9280.00063

Bates E., Thal D., & MacWhinney B. (1991) A functionalist approach to language and its implications for assessment and intervention. In T. M. Gallagher (Ed.), *Pragmatics of Language*. Springer. https://doi.org/10.1007/978-1-4899-7156-2_5

Bloom, L. & Lahey, M. (1978). *Language development and language disorders*. Wiley.

Bloom, L., & Tinker, E. (2001). The intentionality model and language acquisition: Engagement, effort, and the essential tension in development. *Monographs of the Society for Research in Child Development, 66*(4, Serial No., 267).

Bowen, C. (2011). *Neighborhood density and "Jack" -Considering lexical properties in target selection.* https://www.speech-language-therapy.com

Caramazza, A. (1997). How many levels of processing are there in lexical access? *Cognitive Neuropsychology, 14*(1), 177–208. https://doi.org/10.1080/026432997381664

Christophe, A., Millotte, S., Bernal, S., & Lidz, J. (2008). Bootstrapping lexical and syntactic acquisition. *Language and Speech, 51*(Pt. 1–2), 61–75. https://doi.org/10.1177/00238309080510010501

Dixon, J., & Marchman, V. (2007). Grammar and the lexicon: Developmental ordering in language acquisition. *Child Development, 78*(1), 190–212. https://doi.org/10.1111/j.1467-8624.2007.00992.x

Fenson, L., Marchman, V. A., Thal, D. J., Dale, P. S., Reznick, J. S., & Bates, E. (2007). *MacArthur-Bates Communicative Development Inventories: User's guide and technical manual* (2nd ed.). Brookes.

Fisher, C., Gertner, Y., Scott, R., & Yuan, S. (2010). Syntactic bootstrapping. Wiley Interdisciplinary Reviews: *Cognitive Science, 1*(2), 143–149. https://doi.org/10.1002/wcs.17

Gaskell, M. G., & Ellis, A. W. (2009). Word learning and lexical development. *Philosophical Transactions of the Royal Society, 364,* 3607–3615. https://doi.org/10.1098/rstb.2009.0213

Gleitman, L., & Gleitman, H. (1992). A picture is worth a thousand words, but that's the problem: The role of syntax in language acquisition. *Current Directions in Psychological Science, 1*(1), 31–35. https://doi.org/10.1111/1467–8721.ep10767853

He, A., & Arunachalam, S., (2017). Word learning mechanisms. *WIREs Cognitive Science, 8*(4), e1435. https://doi.org/10.1002/wcs.1435

Henriksen, B. (1999). Three dimensions of vocabulary development. *Studies in Second Language Acquisition, 21*(2), 303–317. https://doi.org/10.1017/S0272263199002089

Kemp, N., Scott, J., Bernhardt, B.M., Johnson, C., Siegel, L., & Werker, J. (2017). Minimal pair word learning and vocabulary size: Links with later language skills. *Applied Psycholinguistics, 38,* 289–314. https://doi.org/10.1017/S0142716416000199

McDaniel, J., Yoder, P. J., Woynaroski, T., & Watson, L. R. (2019). Predicting receptive-expressive vocabulary discrepancies in preschool children with autism spectrum disorder. *Journal of Speech, Language, and Hearing Research, 61*(6), 1426–1439. https://doi.org/10.1044/2018_JSLHR-L-17-0101

Nation, K. (2014). Lexical learning and lexical processing in children with developmental language impairments. *Philosophical Transactions of the Royal Society B, 369*(1634), 20120387. http://doi.org/10.1098/rstb.2012.0387

Nazzi, T., & Bertoncini, J. (2003). Before and after the vocabulary spurt: Two modes of word acquisition. *Developmental Science, 6*(2), 136–142. https://doi.org/10.1111/1467-7687.00263

Nippold, M. A. (1985). Comprehension of figurative language in youth. *Topics in Language Disorders, 5*(3), 1–20. https://doi.org/10.1097/00011363-198506000-00004

Nippold, M. (2009). School age children talk about chess: Does knowledge drive syntactic complexity? *Journal of Speech, Language, and Hearing Research, 52*(4), 856–871. https://doi.org/10.1044/1092-4388(2009/08-0094)

Owens, R. (2012). *Language development: An introduction* (8th ed.). Pearson.

Qian, D. (2002). Investigating the relationship between vocabulary knowledge and academic reading performance: An assessment perspective. *Language Learning, 52*(3), 513–536. https://doi.org/10.1111/1467-9922.00193

Ruben, B. (1999). Simulations, games, and experience-based learning: The quest for a new paradigm for teaching and learning. *Simulation & Gaming, 30*(4), 498–505. https://doi.org/10.1177/104687819903000409

Shafer, G., & Plunkett, K. (1998). Rapid word learning by fifteen-month-olds under tightly controlled conditions. *Child Development, 69*, 309–320.

Singleton, N., & Shulman, B. (2002). *Language development: Foundations, processes and clinical applications* (2nd ed.). Jones & Bartlett Learning.

Sosa, A., & Stoel-Gammon, C. (2012). Lexical and phonological effects in early word production. *Journal of Speech Language, and Hearing Research, 55*(2), 596–608. https://doi.org/10.1044/1092-4388(2011/10-0113)

Stoel-Gammon, C. (2011). Relationships between lexical and phonological development. *Journal of Child Language, 38*(1), 1–34. https://doi.org/10.1017/S0305000910000425

Storkel, H., Armbruster, J., & Hogan, T. (2006) Differentiating phonotactic probability and neighborhood density in adult word learning. *Journal of Speech, Language, and Hearing Research, 49*(6), 1175–1192. https://doi.org/10.1044/1092-4388(2006/085)

Storkel, H., & Hoover, J. (2010). Word learning by children with phonological delays: Differentiating effects of phonotactic probability and neighborhood density. *Journal of Communication Disorders, 43*(2), 105–119.

Storkel, H., & Morrisette, M. (2002). The lexicon and phonology. *Language, Speech, and Hearing Services in Schools, 33*(1), 24–37. https://doi.org/10.1044/0161-1461(2002/003)

Sutherland, D., & Gillon, G. (2005). Assessment of phonological representations in children with speech impairment. *Language, Speech, and Hearing Services in Schools, 36*(4), 294–307. https://doi.org/10.1044/0161-1461(2005/030)

Swingley, D. (2009). Contributions of infant word learning to language development. *Philosophical Transactions of the Royal Society B, 364*(1536), 3617–3632. https://doi.org/10.1098/rstb.2009.0107

Vitevitch, M. (2002). Naturalistic and experimental analyses of word frequency and neighborhood density effects in slips of the ear. *Language and Speech, 45*(4), 407–434. https://doi.org/10.1177/002383 09020450040501

2

INTRODUCTION TO LEXICAL PRODUCTION MODELS AND RELATED NEURAL NETWORKS

Pei-Fang Hung

Chapter Objectives

---

1. Describe the different levels of lexical processing based on the theoretical framework.
2. Explain the involvement of left and right cerebral hemispheres in lexical processing.
3. Discuss the clinical applications of the theoretical lexical production models and cortical organization of lexical processing.

Lexical Production Models

Word production is a high-speed, multifaceted, and complex process that involves many steps before the correct and intended word can be successfully uttered. Since the 19th century, numerous psychologists and linguists, such as Meringer and Mayer (1895), Cutler (1982), Cohen (1966), and so forth, have been trying to understand the processes of word production. Consequently, there are several theoretical models that have been developed to conceptualize the processes of spoken word production. All of these theoretical models can be categorized into two major types. The first type of theoretical models is known as "chronometric models," which was developed based on the measurement of response latencies (response time) in naming tasks, such as Levelt's (1989) Speech Production model. The second type is known as "speech error models," which was developed based on the analysis of spontaneous or induced word finding errors, such as Interactive Two-Step Model.

A detailed review of all word production models is outside the scope of this book. In this section, we provide a brief overview of few lexical production models to guide our discussion on lexical development and word production difficulty. It is beneficial to understand the theoretical frameworks before further discussing why lexical access/ production difficulty may occur. The highlighted lexical processing models in this section are Levelt's Speech Production model (1989), WEAVER++ model (1992), and

Dell's two-step interactive model (1986). These models have been applied prevalently in different disciplines, such as psychology, education, linguistics, and speech-language pathology.

Levelt's Speech Production Model

Levelt's Speech Production Model (1989) is one of the chronometric models introduced by Willem Levelt to conceptualize spoken word production. The stages include conceptualization, linguistic formulation, and articulation stages. According to Levelt's model, word production starts with the first stage called *"Conceptualizer"* (i.e., *conceptual representations*). It is initiated by the speakers' knowledge about an object or an idea that they intend to express; a lexical concept is created at this stage. Although this stage is a preverbal stage, it is activated in a language-specific manner (Hartsuiker & Vigliocco, 2009). For example, when speakers try to say or name the word "cat," they often start by thinking about what a cat looks like and its associated features (e.g., whiskers, purrs, meows, catches mice, etc.). Because of the shared semantic network, additional features that are associated with the target word can also be activated, such as animal, furry, pet, and four legs.

The lexical concept (conceptual representation) then triggers the next stage called *"Formulator."* Each lexical concept is connected to a lemma, which is further connected to grammatical properties (i.e., syntactic properties) of the word, such as grammatical class (e.g., nouns, verbs), number, mass or count for nouns, semantic arguments for verbs (e.g., transitive vs. intransitive), or grammatical gender for a gendered language. In other words, this lexical selection stage involves grammatical encoding, which is a process of adding appropriate grammatical information to form lexical-syntactic information. Only a lemma that receives the most activation will be selected for the next level of processing (Caramazza, 1997; Hartsuiker & Vigliocco, 2009; Levelt, 1999). Continuing the same example, the target word "cat" will be activated because its distinguishing semantic features (e.g., purrs and meows) and syntactic properties (e.g., count noun and singular) make the target lemma (i.e., cat) stand out from the other competing lemmas (e.g., dog, turtle, fish). Therefore, the selection of lemma is the selection of the syntactic and semantic information that defines the word (Caramazza, 1997).

After grammatical coding is completed and lemma is selected, it progresses to the next stage called "*phonological (morphophonological) encoding.*" The morphological and phonological information of the word can be accessed (Levelt, 1999, p. 88). During the phonological encoding stage, the selected lemma activates its phonological codes that contain sound sequences. Then, the last stage is called "*Articulator*"; this is where the phonetic plan is executed. Each phonological syllable is prepared for phonetic encoding that gets ready for articulation. This last stage also involves motor programming, planning, and execution (Levelt, 1999). Figure 2–1 is the illustration of Levelt's speech production model using the word "cat." The one directional arrow from top to bottom means that speech production is a sequential process. The activation can only flow from lemma level to lexeme (word form) level, and lemma selection takes place before phonological encoding.

WEAVER++ Model

The WEAVER++ (Word-form Encoding by Activation and VERification) is another chronometric model introduced by Ardi Roelofs in 1992 and then modified in 1997. This model is also based on the results of response-time studies similar to Levelt's model. The WEAVER++ model suggests that word retrieval is a process of spreading activation from conceptual preparation to phonological encoding. The main difference between this model and Levelt's model is that the WEAVER++ model further emphasizes that lemma access and word-form encoding are two discrete and separated steps. Additionally, the word form encoding level (stage) is further divided into three levels: morphological encoding, phonological encoding, and phonetic encoding (Dell & Cholin, 2012).

According to the WEAVER++ model, competitions happen at the lemma level. The target concept (e.g., "*cat*") also activates semantically related concepts and lemmas (e.g., "*dog*" and "*bird*"). The selection of target lemma is based on the competition with other activated nontarget lemmas, and a verifica-

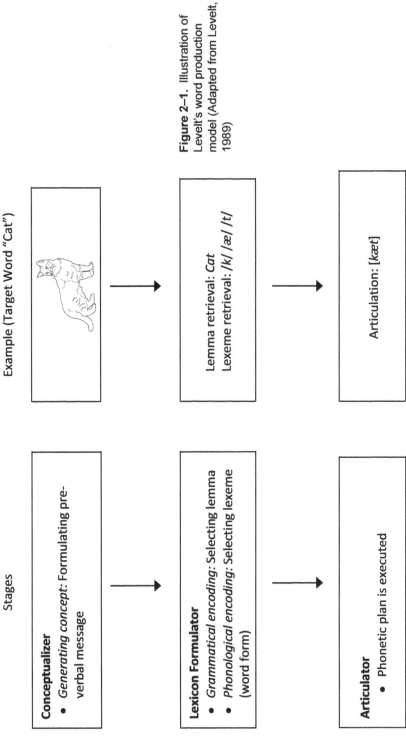

Stages

Conceptualizer
- *Generating concept:* Formulating pre-verbal message

Lexicon Formulator
- *Grammatical encoding:* Selecting lemma
- *Phonological encoding:* Selecting lexeme (word form)

Articulator
- Phonetic plan is executed

Example (Target Word "Cat")

Lemma retrieval: *Cat*
Lexeme retrieval: /k/ /æ/ /t/

Articulation: [kæt]

Figure 2–1. Illustration of Levelt's word production model (Adapted from Levelt, 1989)

tion process is operated by the production rule. The production rule verifies the link between the activated lemma and the appropriate concept. After the lemma is selected, the corresponding word form (i.e., lexeme) will then be activated. Figure 2–2 illustrates the WEAVER++ model using the target word "cat" as an example. In Figure 2–2, only the word form of lemma "cat" will be activated while the word form for "dog" and "bird" will remain inactivated. For readers who would like to learn more about

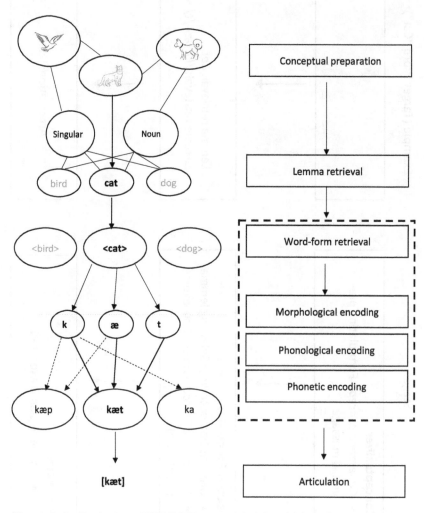

Figure 2–2. Illustration of WEAVER++ model (Adapted from Roelofs, 1992)

the WEAVER++ model, please refer to Dell and Cholin's (2012) chapter.

Interactive Two-Step Model of Lexical Access

The interactive two-step model proposed by Dell (1986) was developed based on speech errors as these errors help researchers understand the breakdown of the speech production process. A key difference between Levelt's model and the interactive two-step model is how the activation flows from one level to another. In Levelt's model, the spreading activation is in a top-down, one-way sequential hierarchy. On the other hand, in Dell et al.'s model, the spreading activation between the layers (levels) are bidirectional and interactive, meaning that activation can flow downward (i.e., from semantic to lexical to phonological levels) or upward (i.e., from phonological to lexical levels). In Levelt's model, phonological representation cannot be activated until the target lemma (lexical node) is selected. However, Dell et al.'s model proposes the interactive nature of these processes and suggests that the phonological level can be activated before the lexical selection is complete (Morsella & Miozzo, 2002). Based on the interactive model, the target lemma receives an additional boost from phonological level to gain greater activation because several lexical nodes simultaneously activate their corresponding phonological units. In other words, Levelt's model emphasizes the concept of lexical selection whereas Dell et al.'s interactive model focuses on the concept of lexical activation.

The interactive two-step model proposes that nodes representing distinct units of speech (e.g., concepts, phonemes, etc.) are interconnected and interact in any direction among different levels. This model proposes two clear levels, including word retrieval level and phonological retrieval level. At the word retrieval level, the lemma (word) is selected based on the most activated semantic features. Then, at the phonological retrieval level, corresponding phonemes are selected from three separate pools, including *onsets*, *vowels*, and *codas*. Figure 2–3 illustrates how the target word "*cat*" is selected through the competition with other words and other competing phonemes based on this model (Dell, Chang, & Griffin, 1999).

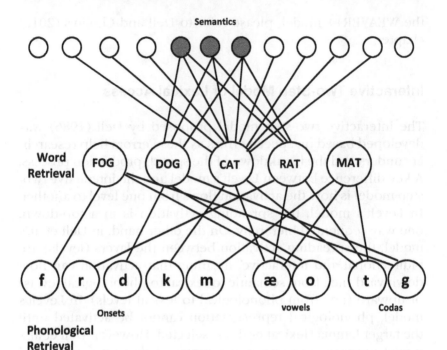

Figure 2–3. Illustration of interactive two-step model (Adapted from Dell, Schwartz, Martin, Saffran, & Gagnon, 1997)

Based on the interactive two-step model, lexical errors can happen due to the breakdowns at the word retrieval level, phonological encoding level, or both levels. The different types of errors are listed below.

- Semantic errors. A nontarget word "dog" is produced instead of the target ("cat") because the competing semantic features were activated. Wrong lexicons are activated because of incorrect feedback from the level of semantic processing.
- Phonological/phonemic errors. An unintended word "mat" is produced instead of the target ("cat") because the competing phonemic features were activated. Wrong lexicons are activated because of incorrect feedback from the level of phonological decoding. This bottom-up, interactive flow of activation between lexical and phoneme

levels is unique to Dell et al.'s model. An incorrect selection of phoneme will result in one or more phoneme substitutions or omissions, which leads to phonological errors. For example, "*dat*" or "*at*" may be activated (for the word [cat]) because of the result of incorrect phoneme selection or missing phoneme.

■ Mixed semantic-phonological errors. An unintended word "rat" is produced instead of the target ("cat") because "rat" shares semantic features and syntactic properties (e.g., animal, four legs, noun) and phonemes (e.g., /æ/ and /t/) with the target word (Dell, Chang, & Griffin, 1999; Foygel & Dell, 2000; Morsella & Miozzo, 2002).

■ Unrelated errors. An unintended word "fog" is produced instead of the target ("cat") because of the stronger activation of unintended phonemes or the combination of inaccurate semantic processing and phonological encoding.

There are similarities and differences in the models we just reviewed. Debate still exists in how spreading activation flows from one level to another. Although there are several different variations of lexical processing models, we list several major levels of representation below.

■ *Conceptual Preparation Level:* Formulating concepts or general knowledge about what to be expressed
■ *Lemma Level:* Selecting semantically and syntactically specified lexical nodes (i.e., lemma) based on concepts
■ *Lexeme Level:* Selecting the corresponding phonological representation or word form (i.e., lexeme) based on the activated lexical representation
■ *Articulation Level:* Executing the phonetic plan

Clinical Implications of Lexical Production Models

Lexical production difficulty can happen to everyone occasionally. However, when the frequency of word finding difficulty is beyond typical, it is considered a deficit and can significantly affect the effectiveness of everyday communication. The aforementioned theoretical lexical processing models contribute to our understanding of word production and provide a practical framework for speech-language pathologists to manage lexical production difficulty. Based on lexical processing models, different stages (levels) of the word production process are activated from conceptual formation to phonological encoding in a sequential manner. Correct word production relies on adequate representations at all levels and strong connections between the levels to facilitate correct selection and sufficient spreading activation. Generally speaking, word production difficulty and speech errors can be the result of *a weak activation of the intended concept, an inaccurate selection of lemma, an incorrect sound sequence*, or *a combination of all*. Lexical processing models can provide the foundation for identifying the root of the deficit because different types of speech errors may reflect different causes and loci of word production difficulty.

Conceptual representations may be well preserved or fragile. For example, people with certain types of aphasia still have well-preserved conceptual formation. On the other hand, children with developmental language delay may have a weak activation of the intended concept due to lack of exposure, insufficient practice, or inadequate development of conceptual knowledge. The underdeveloped conceptual representations can affect the activation of lemmas and corresponding lexemes. Moreover, these children tend to have an impoverished phonological short-term memory, which is essential for the development of receptive vocabulary (Gray, 2006) and early expressive vocabulary (Newbury et al., 2015). Thus, when conducting assessment on lexical production, clinicians should start with evaluating conceptual formation to rule out if speech errors are due to a weak activation of the intended concept. Conceptual structures and semantic access can be evaluated via standardized tests, for example the Pyramid and Palm Trees Test, or nonstandardized tests, such as picture association tasks. Individuals with a deficit at the conceptual level often struggle with picture association tasks and cannot successfully identify if two pictures are related.

By conducting error analysis, clinicians can identify the types of speech errors and their frequency of occurrence. For example, based on Levelt's model, semantic errors can also result from the competition of semantically related lemmas or weak semantic relations of words. Individuals with preserved phonological encoding ability may only make semantic errors but barely make any phonological errors (Friedmann et al., 2013). Semantic speech errors (e.g., saying "*dog*" for the target word [cat]) can be the result of a weak connection between conceptual and lexical levels, which hinders the effectiveness of word retrieval. In addition, through error analysis, clinician can better understand the nature of a client's word production difficulty. For example, clients may have no problem with naming items that are commonly seen in daily life (or have high imageability), but show difficulty when naming less common items or items that have low imageability. Furthermore, some individuals may only experience word production difficulty when naming words in a certain category. Because the semantic-conceptual system is organized in a domain-specific manner (Caramazza & Shelton, 1998), it is not uncommon that clients may only have naming difficulty in a specific category but not others.

Individuals with preserved semantic concepts and lexical representations may only make phonological or phonemic errors (e.g., saying "*mat*" for the word [cat]), and have difficulty selecting the correct word form (i.e., phonological representation or sound sequence) (Hartsuiker & Vigliocco, 2009). For example, children with phonological disorders without language impairments can have well-developed conceptual and lexical representations. However, their underdeveloped phonological representations limit adequate speech sound development, affecting their speech intelligibility. In other words, phonological errors can be the result of a breakdown at the lexeme/phoneme level (phonological encoding) due to weak activation of a corresponding sound sequence of the intended word, or a more robust activation of the competing phonemes.

Theoretical frameworks and research evidence can guide clinical practice and help speech-language pathologists make clinical decisions. Clinicians should make their decisions based on a comprehensive understanding of theoretical frameworks, the analysis of the client's speech errors, other related clinical characteristics, and a complete review of relevant and current research evidence that supports a specific treatment approach. For example, phonological-based treatment approaches may be more effective for some individuals because the intervention directly addresses phonological encoding. On the other hand, semantic-based interventions may be beneficial to those individuals who produce semantic errors predominantly because developing and strengthening semantic-conceptual representations can facilitate retrieving target words successfully. Strengthening the connection between conceptual representations and lemmas can be accomplished by providing meaningful exposures to vocabulary that is important to daily communication, and by offering opportunities for using newly learned words across different contexts. Additionally, lemmas are connected to grammatical properties of the word, such as grammatical class, mass or count (for nouns), and semantic arguments (for verbs). Thus, retrieval of verbs may require a different intervention approach than nouns because the inclusion of arguments may facilitate retrieval of verbs. For example, the Verb Network Strengthening Program (VNeST; Edmonds et al., 2009) is a semantic-based treatment that aims to improve retrieval of verbs and related nouns. Because syntactic information is connected to lemmas, working on the lexical-syntactic connection may also facilitate the selection of correct lemma.

Understanding the lexical processing models provides readers with a foundation before discussing vocabulary development, lexical access and word production difficulty, assessment approaches, and treatment intervention found later in this book. Detailed information about individuals who have difficulty with developing and accessing lexicon will be elaborated in Chapter 6. Information for vocabulary assessment and intervention is discussed in Chapters 7, 8 and 9.

The Involvement of Cerebral Hemispheres in the Word Retrieval Process

In this section, we quickly review neurological evidence regarding the involvement of both cerebral hemispheres in the lexical production process. A detailed discussion of specific brain areas based on their roles in lexical processing is beyond the scope of this book. Instead, we will briefly summarize the findings of related studies and discuss the implications of the findings in clinical practice.

The Role of the Left Hemisphere in Lexical Processing

The left cerebral hemisphere plays a primary role in speech and language processing. More specifically, the left inferior frontal gyrus (IFG), also known as *Broca's area* or Brodmann Area (BA) 44/45, is critical for speech production. The left IFG is highly active during semantic processing. Kiran et al., (2019) stated that most neuroimaging findings supported the correlation between left IFG and semantic processing. Specifically, the left posterior IFG (BA 44) is vital to phonological processing, and the left pars triangularis (BA 45) plays an important role in lexical-semantic control and retrieval process (Marcotte et al., 2012). Additionally, the left anterior IFG (BA 47) is involved in semantic working memory, search, and comparison. Although specific brain regions have been identified for processing specific linguistic information, these cortical areas are interconnected. When processing related linguistic tasks, these nearby cortical regions can co-activate concurrently. For example, phonological processing tasks may activate multiple areas within IFG, not just posterior IFG (BA 44). Therefore, damage to one of these regions can affect the whole Broca's area because the regions within IFG are highly connected.

The left posterior superior temporal gyrus (STG), also known as *Wernicke's area* or BA 22, supports language comprehension. The left posterior STG is involved in processing auditory short-term memory and speech comprehension, and accessing word derivation and compounding (Graves et al., 2008). According to neuroimaging studies, both anterior and posterior STG are involved in the processing of word meanings (Leff et al., 2009). Specifically, the left temporal lobe is specialized for incorporating distinctive semantic features for connecting concepts to words during the lemma selection process (Schwartz et al., 2009). Therefore, damage to the left temporal lobe could compromise the function of semantic differentiation, which in turn increases the competition of semantically similar words and further results in naming errors. Lastly, the left posterior temporal regions, including the middle temporal gyrus (MTG) and the inferior temporal gyrus (ITG), are also associated with word retrieval (Ries et al., 2016).

The semantic-conceptual system is organized in a domain-specific manner; different concepts activate different cortical areas for lexical processing. Some findings of neuroimaging studies show that semantic information may be stored in different brain areas based on the type of semantic categories (Caramazza & Shelton, 1998; Damasio et al., 1996). In addition, studies show that a more specific and refined category seems to be associated with a more precise cortical area (Bookheimer, 2002; Ursino et al., 2011). For example, words for nonliving things, such as tools, specifically activate the areas near left BA 45, 46, 20, and 21, whereas words for animals strongly activate the left fusiform gyrus (also known as *occipitotemporal gyrus*). An individual with word finding difficulty (WFD) may only have difficulty with naming nonliving things (e.g., *chair*), but not living things (e.g., *fish*) (Friedmann et al., 2013). This may be because naming living things links to the lateral fusiform gyrus and superior temporal sulcus regions, whereas naming nonliving things involves the left medial fusiform gyrus.

Naming nouns and verbs can activate different cortical areas in the brain as this reflects the different brain organization for nouns and verbs (Ardila, 2012; Damasio et at., 1996). Verbal production of nouns is associated more with the left temporal lobe, whereas verbal production of verbs involves more cortical areas in the left frontal lobe, especially the left prefrontal/premotor region. Research findings also show that lesions in the left posterior perisylvian regions are correlated with noun retrieval difficulty, whereas verb impairments are associated with lesions in the left anterior perisylvian regions, such as Broca's area (Kambanaros, 2010). However, Bookheimer (2002) suggested that there is no single brain area for category-specific representations because semantic information may be organized based on the perceptual and functional features in multiple but nonoverlapping brain areas.

According to Ries et al. (2016), left temporal regions are associated with lexical activation, whereas left lateral and medial frontal regions are more active during lexical selection. Specific brain locations within the left temporal and frontal regions and their correlations with lexical selection and activation have been identified in multiple studies (for detailed reviews, see Ries et al., 2016). Figure 2–4 illustrates the cortical areas that are involved in lexical production based on the study of Indefrey (2011).

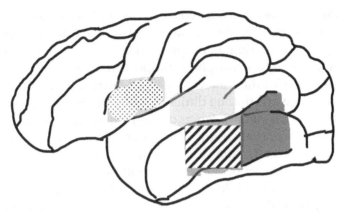

Figure 2–4. The cortical areas in the left hemisphere that are involved in lexical production (Adapted from Indefrey, 2011). *Light gray area:* Processing auditory short-term memory and word meanings (left posterior superior temporal gyrus). *Diagonal stripe area:* Lemma retrieval and selection (left middle temporal gyrus). *Dark gray area:* Phonological retrieval (left posterior middle temporal gyrus). *Dotted area:* Articulation and phonological processing (left inferior frontal gyrus).

The Role of the Right Hemisphere in Lexical Processing

The involvement of the right hemisphere in lexical production is indirect, instead of direct, in processing lexical information. The role of the right cerebral hemisphere in lexical processing comes from the involvement of areas that are homologous to the left perisylvian regions (language areas) (Vigneau et al., 2010). Although the right cerebral hemisphere does not play a primary role in lexical production, it can be involved in certain aspects of lexical processing. For example, the right occipital and temporal-occipital cortices are actively involved in processing visually complex objects in all categories (Bookheimer, 2002). Additionally, the right cerebral hemisphere is involved in processing context and paralinguistic features, but does not have phonological and syntactic functions (Vigneau et al., 2010).

The right hemisphere is actively involved in the cognitive control needed for successful lexical processing, and it becomes increasingly important when word retrieval becomes a challenge (Ries et al., 2016). Extensive bilateral activation reflects increased retrieval effort needed for word access and retrieval. In other words, the more difficult lexical tasks become, the more activation appears in the right hemisphere (Perani et al., 2003). Studies show that the right hemisphere supports naming in older adults to compensate for their increasing word retrieval difficulty. When experiencing word-finding difficulty, older adults have more activation in the left perisylvian and mid-frontal regions, as well as the counterparts in the right hemisphere (Obler et al., 2010). In addition, more activation of the right hemisphere during word retrieval has been reported in adults with word finding difficulty than with healthy adults in the study of Ries and colleagues (2016). Specifically, activation of the right frontal and temporal regions were noted when word retrieval becomes increasingly difficult. Other brain regions, such as the left and right hippocampi, also showed robust activation in adults with word retrieval difficulty. In other words, the right hemisphere may be involved in word retrieval when word retrieval becomes effortful. However, the involvement and efficacy in lexical processing of the right hemisphere is less robust than the left hemisphere.

Injury-Induced Neuroplasticity

Studies in neuroplasticity can help researchers and practitioners understand the role and involvement of both hemispheres in lexical processing and post-injury recovery. Most research studies support the involvement of bilateral hemispheres during language recovery (Heiss & Thiel, 2006; Thompson, 2000). The recruitment and involvement of the right hemisphere after brain damage (e.g., stroke) to compensate for language functions has been widely studied. Neuroplasticity refers to the changes or modifications of brain structure and function in response to changes in the environment. This change of neural circuits happens during development throughout a lifetime based on experiences, as well as after brain damage, by either modifying the existing neural circuits or generating new neural circuits (Fridriksson & Smith, 2016; Marcotte et al., 2012).

The postinjury changes are specifically referred to as *injury-induced neuroplasticity*. In order to restore and reestablish the lost function after brain injury (e.g., stroke), the brain undergoes *functional reactivation* and *functional reorganization*. Functional reactivation primarily relies on expanding language-related cortical areas (e.g., preserved linguistic neural circuits and regions adjacent to the lesion) to restore and regain speech and language functions. Functional reorganization is accomplished via recruiting nonlanguage areas, including other undamaged areas in the left hemisphere (which are responsible for other nonlinguistic functions) and homologous area adaptation (also known as *right hemisphere compensation*) (Fridriksson & Smith, 2016; Marcotte & Ansaldo, 2010). The brain engages in a spontaneous recovery within the first few weeks during tissue reperfusion after the left hemisphere damage. During the reorganization phase, it was noted that the activities of the homologous areas in the right hemisphere had been increased (Kiran et al., 2019). In other words, the improvement from poststroke aphasia may reflect the brain's functional reorganization; it involves both undamaged language regions in the left hemisphere and homologous areas in the right hemisphere.

Regardless of the language recovery phase, the extent of unimpaired cortical areas in the left hemisphere plays a critical role in the prognosis and outcome of recovery (Heiss & Thiel, 2006; Kiran et al., 2019). In other words, preserved left hemisphere regions, as well as spared tissues in the left hemisphere, play an essential role in the recovery process. Heiss and Thiel (2006) proposed three possible types of poststroke language recovery. First, the lesion is small, so a complete language recovery and restoration is highly expected and may be achieved by reorganizing the partially affected language network in the left hemisphere. Second, an incomplete but satisfactory recovery may be achieved by reactivating the perilesional regions (i.e., the nearby cortical areas that are responsible for nonlinguistic functions) in the left hemisphere. Lastly, if the lesion in the left hemisphere is extensive and the language network is severely damaged, the language function may be compensated by shifting to the undamaged right hemisphere. In other words, the prognosis of language recovery is usually poor in severe aphasia if caused by a massive lesion in the left hemisphere because function reorganization solely relies on the compensation from the homologous regions in the right hemisphere (Kiran et al., 2019; Marcotte & Ansaldo, 2010). Additionally, when the damage to the left hemisphere is extensive, increased activation may also extend to the domain-general regions that commonly engage in cognitive control. The increased activation in domain-general regions seems to indicate that additional cognitive efforts are needed to perform language tasks.

Ries et al. (2016) indicate that several factors can influence the recruitment of the right hemisphere in language recovery, such as the location and size of the lesion, time after the injury, and age of onset. It should be noted that the right hemisphere cannot fully compensate for the impaired language functions resulting from lesions in left hemisphere because the key function of the right hemisphere is not language processing. Generally speaking, individuals who had smaller lesions, higher integrity of white matter tracts, and normal-like connections between brain regions tend to show better improvement (Kiran et al., 2019).

Treatment-Induced Neuroplasticity

Brain structural change and functional reorganization can be achieved and facilitated via well-planned therapy programs. Intensive and systemic practice and repetition are key to all kinds of learning and relearning. The association between practice and changes in brain activity has been evident in healthy adults during various language tasks (Kurland et al., 2018). Thus, therapy-induced neuroplasticity may be achieved by intensive, repetitive, and effective speech-language treatment programs even in individuals at the chronic stage of recovery (Jokel et al., 2016; Mohr, 2017).

Therapy-induced neuroplasticity and functional reorganization can be facilitated and promoted via treatment approaches that specifically target lexical production (Kelly & Garavan, 2005). For example, the perilesional areas in the left hemisphere (e.g., left supramarginal gyrus and left inferior parietal lobule) and right front-temporal regions have been recruited after therapy, and the activation of these areas is associated with better language recovery (Marcotte et al., 2012, van Hees et al., 2014). van Hees et al. (2014) reported that the left caudate nucleus (subcortical structure, part of basal ganglia) became more actively involved in monitoring semantic competition after treatment. Additionally, increased neural activities in the left supramarginal gyrus (SMG) were also observed. In their study, Johnson et al. (2019) investigated treatment-related neural changes after a semantic-based lexical therapy in 26 individuals with chronic aphasia. Their study results support the improvement in naming accuracy and increased bilateral cortical activation after therapy.

Marcotte and Ansaldo (2010) compared behavioral improvement and changes in brain activities before and after semantic-based lexical treatment (i.e., semantic feature analysis) in two individuals with chronic and severe aphasia due to different etiologies: one is poststroke aphasia and the other is progressive aphasia. The results showed that even though changes in neural networks were different due to distinct etiologies, both participants showed bilateral activations after therapy. Marcotte and Ansaldo (2010) indicated that similar behavioral improvement may result from different therapy-induced brain plasticity, and brain plasticity may still happen to individuals who are in the chronic stage of recovery (e.g., several years post stroke). Vitali et al. (2007) also provided more neuroimaging evidence by comparing the naming performance before and after phonological cues training. Their findings showed the reactivation of left perilesional regions is correlated with better naming performance in the participant with smaller lesion sizes. On the other hand, the participant with more extensive damage to the language areas showed more activation in the right frontal regions after treatment.

Clinical Implications of Neuroplasticity in Language Recovery

Kiran and Thompson (2019) proposed several tips/principles for promoting treatment-induced neuroplasticity in individuals with neurogenic speech and language disorders.

1. *Selecting treatment approaches that directly address lexical processing and word production.* Impairment-based treatment approaches typically target specific language processes, so these treatment approaches aim to rebuild and reorganize the targeted language neural networks. For example, the impairment-based lexical treatment approaches aim to strengthen specific language processes

involved in word retrieval, and it may, in turn, rebuild language networks. Treatment approaches focusing on a specific impaired language process (e.g., word retrieval, auditory comprehension) may facilitate recovery of the underlying neural network associated with the specific process.

2. *Incorporating individual-relevant treatment materials.* The use of individual-relevant contexts and personal experience may enhance motivation and attention that promotes language encoding. Kiran et al. (2019) indicated that activation in domain-general regions (essential for cognitive functions) may be associated with therapy-induced neuroplasticity because additional cognitive engagement is required and is essential for processing language tasks.

3. *Repetition and treatment intensity.* Intensive treatment sessions and repetitive practice can facilitate neuroplasticity and promote the posttreatment therapy gain and generalization.

4. *Promote generalization.* Assigning untrained items as homework can be a good starting point for promoting generalization. Clinicians can start first by introducing words that share linguistic features with the trained targets (e.g., in a same or similar semantic category, sound patterns, sentence structures). Kendall et al. (2019) reported that the effect of two treatment approaches (i.e., semantic feature analysis and phonomotor treatment) were successfully generalized to untrained words that shared linguistic features with the trained words. On the other hand, generalization of treatment effects was not found in words that do not share features (semantic features or phonological sequence) with trained words.

5. *Incorporating complex words as treatment materials.* Training complex structures may promote learning and generalization. The treatment efficacy of using complexity approach can be found in other language domains, such as phonology. Drs. Lyn Williams and Adele Miccio have been advocating the use of complex and later developing speech sounds to treat phonological disorders because acquiring difficulty sounds may promote a system-wide

phonology change. Along the same vein, Kiran and Thompson (2019) suggested that training complex words (e.g., abstract nouns) and sentence structures (e.g., transitive verbs like "*She broke the window*") may generalize to less complex words (e.g., concrete nouns) and sentence structures (e.g., intransitive verbs like "*Mom is cooking*").

These are tips and recommendations suggested by research. We discuss commonly implemented treatment approaches to management of word production difficulty in detail in Chapters 8 and 9.

Chapter Summary

In this chapter, we briefly reviewed three lexical production models, including Levelt's speech production model, the WEAVER++ Model, and the interactive two-step model of lexical access. Although these models propose different levels of lexical processing and address speech production from different perspectives, they all propose several common processing stages (levels), including conceptual, semantic, lexical, and phonological levels. The conceptual level is where the preverbal conceptual message is formed. The semantic level is typically "*modality-neutral*" meaning it can contribute to both spoken and written word production. At the semantic level, the semantic nodes are activated based on the conceptual message. At the lexical level, the lemma (lexical node) is selected based on the activated semantic nodes. At the phonological level, the corresponding phonemes (i.e., word forms) are retrieved and further processed with syllabic encoding and stress information. Lastly, the phonetic plan is sent to articulators for speech production.

Based on the related neuroimaging studies, it is known that both cerebral hemispheres are involved in lexical production. First, word production is a complex process that can involve more than one cortical area or one cerebral hemisphere; it depends on the complexity of the target word or context. The role of the left inferior frontal gyrus (Broca's area) and the left posterior superior temporal gyrus (Wernicke's area) in lexical production and comprehension has been supported by evidence (Kiran et al., 2019). Depending on the complexity of the lexical item, the right hemisphere may also be involved in the process of word production, such as when cognitive demands increase. There are also other factors that can affect the involvement of the cortical areas and right hemisphere, such as the type of stimulus (e.g., nouns, verbs), the complexity of words (e.g., frequency, imaginability), and categorical information (e.g., living vs. nonliving). Secondly, based on neuroplasticity studies, it is difficult to predict how or when the right cerebral hemisphere would compensate for the impaired language functions after left hemisphere damage. It was observed that the right homologous regions may become more active than usual after the left language areas were damaged. However, it should be noted that the right hemisphere may have limited contribution in directly processing linguistic information and may not be able to fully compensate for the lost linguistic function. Despite the inconclusive results on the involvement of the right hemisphere in the recovery process, speech-language pathologists should consider promoting therapy-induced neuroplasticity to facilitate language recovery. Based on the study of Kiran et al. (2019), brain reorganization and the increased brain activities significantly correlate with speech-language therapy. In addition, neuroimaging studies and clinical data support the effects of lexical production treatments. Therefore, when planning treatment programs for word retrieval and production, speech-language pathologists should consider the tips and principles proposed by Kiran and Thompson (2019) to promote neuroplasticity in language recovery and generalization of treatment gains.

Discussion Questions

1. What are the stages (levels) of word production in the lexical production process?
2. What are the similarities and differences between Levelt's speech production model (1989) and Dell's interactive two-step model (1986)?
3. What are the cortical areas that are directly involved in lexical processing?

4. What is the role of the right cerebral hemisphere in spoken word production?
5. What can speech-language pathologists do to promote treatment-induced neuroplasticity?

References

Ardila, A. (2012). Interaction between lexical and grammatical language systems in the brain. *Physics of Life Reviews*, *9*(2), 198–214. https://doi.org/10.1016/j.plrev.2012.05.001

Bookheimer, S. (2002). Functional MRI of language: New approaches to understanding the cortical organization of semantic processing. *Annual Review of Neuroscience*, *25*, 151–188. https://doi.org/10.1146/annurev.neuro.25.112701.142946

Caramazza, A. (1997). How many levels of processing are there are lexical access. *Cognitive Neuropsychology*, *14*(1), 177–208. https://doi.org/10.1080/026432997381664

Caramazza, A., & Shelton, J. (1998). Domain-specific knowledge systems in the brain: The animate-inanimate distinction. *Journal of Cognitive Neuroscience*, *10*(1), 1–34. https://doi.org/10.1162/089892998563752

Damasio, H., Grabowski, T., Tranel, D., Hichwa, R., & Damasio, A. (1996). A neural basis for lexical retrieval. *Nature* 380, 499–505. https://doi.org/10.1038/380499a0

Dell, G. (1986). A spreading activation theory of retrieval and sentence production. *Psychological Review*, *93*, 283–321.

Dell, G., Chang, F., & Griffin, Z. (1999). Connectionist models of language production: Lexical access and grammatical encoding. *Cognitive Science*, *23*(4), 517–542. https://doi.org/10.1207/s15516709cog2304_6

Dell, G. S., & Cholin, J. (2012). Language production: Computational models. In M. J. Spivey, K. McRae, & M. F. Joanisse (Eds.), *Cambridge handbooks in psychology. The Cambridge handbook of psycholinguistics* (pp. 426–442). Cambridge University Press. https://doi.org/10.1017/CBO9781139029377.029

Dell, G. S., Schwartz, M. F., Martin, N., Saffran, E. M., & Gagnon, D. A. (1997). Lexical access in aphasic and nonaphasic speakers. *Psychological Review*, *104*(4), 801–838. https://doi.org/10.1037/0033-295X.104.4.801

Edmonds, L.A., Nadeau, S. E., & Kiran, S. (2009). Effect of verb network strengthening training (VNeST) on lexical retrieval of content words in sentences in persons with aphasia. *Aphasiology*, *23*(3), 402–424. https://doi.org/10.1080/02687030802291339

Foygel, D., & Dell, G. S. (2000). Models of impaired lexical access in speech production. *Journal of Memory and Language*, *43*(2), 182–216. https://doi.org/10.1006/jmla.2000.2716

Fridriksson, J., & Smith, K. (2016). Neuroplasticity associated with treated aphasia recovery. In G. Hickok & S. Small (Eds.), *Neurobiology of Language* (pp. 1007–1013). Academic Press.

Friedmann, N., Biran, M., & Dotan, D. (2013). Lexical retrieval and its breakdown in aphasia and developmental language impairment. In C. Boeckx & K. K. Grohmann (Eds.), *The Cambridge handbook of biolinguistics*. Cambridge University Press.

Graves, W. W., Grabowski, T. J., Mehta, S., & Gupta, P. (2008). The left posterior superior temporal gyrus participates specifically in accessing lexical phonology. *Journal of Cognitive Neuroscience*, *20*(9), 1698–1710. https://doi.org/10.1162/jocn.2008.20113

Gray, S. (2006). The relationship between phonological memory, receptive vocabulary, and fast mapping in young children with specific language impairment. *Journal of Speech, Language and Hearing Research*, *49*(5), 955–969. https://doi.org/10.1044/1092-4388(2006/069)

Hartsuiker, R., & Vigliocco, G. (2009). Word production. In L. R. Squire (Ed.), *Encyclopedia of neuroscience* (pp. 509–516). Academic Press.

Heiss, W., & Thiel, A. (2006). A proposed regional hierarchy in recovery of post-stroke aphasia. *Brain and Language*, *98*(1), 118–123. https://doi.org/10.1016/j.bandl.2006.02.002

Indefrey, P. (2011). The spatial and temporal signatures of word production components: a critical update. *Frontiers in Psychology*, *2*, 255. https://doi.org/10.3389/fpsyg.2011.00255

Johnson, J., Meier, E., Pan, Y., & Kiran, S. (2019). Treatment related changes in neural activation vary according to treatment response and extent of spared tissue in patients with chronic aphasia. *Cortex*, *212*, 147–168. https://doi.org/10.1016/j.cortex.2019.08.016

Jokel, R., Kielar, A., Anderson, N., Black, S., Rochon, E., Graham, S., . . . Wai, D. (2016). Behavioural and neuroimaging changes after naming therapy for semantic variant primary progressive aphasia. *Neuropsychologia*, *89*, 191–216. https://doi.org/10.1016/j.neuropsychologia.2016.06.009

Kambanaros, M. (2010). Action and object naming versus verb and noun retrieval in connected speech: Comparisons late bilingual Greek-English anomic speakers. *Aphasiology*, *24*(2), 210–230. https://doi.org/10.1080/02687030902958332

Kelly, A., & Garavan, H. (2005). Human functional neuroimaging of brain changes associated with practice. *Cerebral Cortex*, *15*(8), 1089–1102. https://doi.org/10.1093/cercor/bhi005

Kendall, D., Moldestad, M., Allen, W., Torrence, J., & Nadeau, S. (2019). Phonomotor versus semantic feature analysis treatment for anomia in 58 persons with aphasia: A randomized controlled trial. *Journal of Speech, Language, and Hearing Research*, *62*(12), 4464–4482. https://doi.org/10.1044/2019_JSLHR-L-18-0257

Kiran, S., Meier, E., & Johnson, J. (2019). Neuroplasticity in aphasia: A proposed framework of language recovery. *Journal of Speech, Language, and Hearing Research*, *62*(11), 3973–3985. https://doi.org/10.1044/2019_JSLHR-L-RSNP-19-0054

Kiran, S., & Thompson, C. (2019). Neuroplasticity of language networks in aphasia: Advances, updates, and future challenges. *Frontiers in Neurology*, *10*(295), 1–15. https://doi.org/10.3389/fneur.2019.00295

Kurland, J., Liu, A., & Stokes, P. (2018). Effects of a tablet based home practice program with telepractice on treatment outcomes in chronic aphasia. *Journal of Speech, Language, and Hearing Research*, *61*(5), 1140–1156. https://doi.org/10.1044/2018_JSLHR-L-17-0277

Leff, A. P., Schofield, T. M., Crinion, J. T., Seghier, M. L., Grogan, A., Green, D. W., & Price, C. J. (2009). The left superior temporal gyrus is a shared substrate for auditory short-term memory and speech comprehension: Evidence from 210 patients with stroke. *Brain: Journal of Neurology*, *132*(Pt. 12), 3401–3410. https://doi.org/10.1093/brain/awp273

Levelt, W. J. (1989). *Speaking: From intention to articulation*. MIT press.

Levelt, W. J. (1999). A Blueprint of the speaker. In C. Brown & P. Hagoort (Eds.), *The neurocognition of language* (pp. 83–122). Oxford Press.

Marcotte, K., Adrover-Roig, D., Damien, B., de Préumont, M., Généreux, S., Hubert, M., Ansaldo, A. (2012). Therapy induced neuroplasticity in chronic aphasia. *Neuropsychologia*, *50*(8), 1776–1786. https://doi.org/10.1016/j.neuropsychologia.2012.04.001

Marcotte, K., & Ansaldo, A. (2010). The neural correlates of semantic feature analysis in chronic aphasia: Discordant patterns according to the etiology. *Seminars in Speech and Language*, *31*(1), 52–63. https://doi.org/10.1055/s-0029-1244953

Mohr, B. (2017). Neuroplasticity and functional recovery after intensive language therapy in chronic post stroke aphasia: Which factors are relevant? *Frontiers in Human Neuroscience*, *11*(332), 1–5. https://doi.org/10.3389/fnhum.2017.00332

Morsella, E., & Miozzo, M. (2002). Evidence for a cascade model of lexical access in speech production. *Journal of Experimental Psychology: Learning, Memory, and Cognition*, *28*(3), 555–563. https://doi.org/10.1037/0278-7393.28.3.555

Newbury, J., Klee, T., Stokes, S., & Moran, C. (2015). Exploring expressive vocabulary variability in two year olds: The role of working memory. *Journal of Speech, Language, and Hearing Research*, *58*(6), 1761–1772. https://doi.org/10.1044/2015_JSLHR-L-15-0018

Obler, L., Rykhlevskaia, E., Schnyer, D., Clark-Cotton, M., Spiro III, A., Hyun, J., Kim, D., Goral, M., & Albert, M. (2010). Bilateral brain regions associated with naming in older adults. *Brain and Language, 113*(3), 113–123. https://doi.org/10.1016/j.bandl.2010.03.001

Perani, D., Cappa, S., Tettamanti, M., Rosa, M., Scifo, P., Miozzo, A., . . . Fazio, F. (2003). A fMRI study of word retrieval in aphasia. *Brain and Language, 85*(3), 357–368. https://doi.org/10.1016/S0093-934 X(02)00561-8

Ries, S., Dronkers, N., & Knight, R. (2016). Choosing words: Left hemisphere, right hemisphere or both? Perspective on the lateralization of word retrieval. *Annals of the New York Academy of Science, 1369*(1), 111–131. https://doi.org/10.1111/nyas.12993

Roelofs, A. (1997). The WEAVER model of word-form encoding in speech production. *Cognition, 64*(3), 249–284. https://doi.org/10.1016/S00 10-0277(97)00027-9

Schwartz, M., Kimberg, D., Walker, G., Faseyitan, O., Brecher, A., Dell, G., & Coslett, H. (2009). Anterior temporal involvement in semantic word retrieval: Voxel-based lesion-symptom mapping evidence from aphasia. *Brain, 132*(12), 3411–3427. https://doi.org/10.1093/brain/awp284

Thompson, C. K. (2000). Neuroplasticity: Evidence from aphasia. *Journal of Communication Disorders, 33*(4), 357–366. https://doi.org/10.1016/s0021-9924(00)00031-9

Ursino, M., Cuppini, C., & Magosso, E. (2011). An integrated neural model of semantic memory, lexical retrieval and category formation, based on a distributed feature representation. *Cognitive Neurodynamics, 5*, 183–207. https://doi.org/10.1007/s11571-011-9154-0

van Hees, S., McMahon, K., Angwin, A., de Zubicaray, G., Read, S., & Copland, D. A. (2014). A functional MRI study of the relationship between naming treatment outcomes and resting state functional connectivity in post-stroke aphasia. *Human Brain Mapping, 35*, 3919–3931. https://doi.org/10.1002/hbm.22448

Vigneau, M., Beaucousin, V., Hervé, P., Jobard, G., Petit, L., Crivello, F., . . . Tzourio-Mazoyer, N. (2010). What is right-hemisphere contribution to phonological, lexico-semantic, and sentence processing?: Insights from a meta-analysis. *NeuroImage, 54*(1), 577–593. https://doi.org/10.1016/j.neuroimage.2010.07.036

Vitali, P., Abutalebi, J., Tettamanti, M., Danna, M., Ansaldo, A.-I., Perani, D., . . . Cappa, S. F. (2007). Training-Induced brain remapping in chronic aphasia: A pilot study. *Neurorehabilitation and Neural Repair, 21*(2), 152–160. https://doi.org/10.1177/1545968306294735

3

EARLY LEXICAL DEVELOPMENT: FROM PRELINGUISTIC STAGE TO TODDLER

Lei Sun

> ## Chapter Objectives
>
> 1. Explain the correlation between concept formation and lexical development.
> 2. Discuss the role of gesture and babbling in early lexical development.
> 3. Recognize the cognitive and linguistic processes needed for word learning.

What Comes Before Words Are Produced?

As children acquire language, babbling, facial expressions, vocalizations, and gestures are used before true words are uttered around the first birthday. Does it mean that the concepts of words are formed before words are spoken? Does a child already form the concept of "cup" when she/he points to the cup? Based on the studies done by psychologists and linguists, we can better understand the relationships between vocabulary and conceptual development, between gesture and language development, and among different language domains. In this section, we will discuss the relationship between concept formation and lexical development, theories related to early lexical acquisition, and factors related to learning new words during the prelinguistic stage.

Concept Formation and Lexical Development

What is a concept? According to Merriam-Webster dictionary, a concept is an abstract idea or a general notion. For example, concepts about "dog," can include facts related to it, such as its features and superordinate categories (e.g., pet, animal, mammal). A concept can be something unobservable and abstract, such as an emotion or state of mind. When we communicate, we convey the intended concepts using precise words and form based on the perceived message and context. How do we know what words to use when conveying a concept? How early can a child form different and correct concepts? According to Westermann and Mareschal (2013), infants as young as two months can form perceptual categories at basic (e.g., dogs, cats) and global levels (e.g., animals) for commonly seen objects. Interestingly, these categories are formed based on the infant's home environment, which indicates the importance of familiarity in concept learning. For example, infants may not know what a cat or a dog is if they have no prior exposure to these animals.

Dr. Sandra Waxman, one of the leading researchers who studies conceptual and language development, emphasized that "word learning requires coordination between linguistic and conceptual systems" (Arunachalam & Waxman, 2010, p. 548). Conceptual representations, as well as the object categories, are refined over the course of development. During the first year of life, the development of categorization and concepts are facilitated by simply exposing infants to language (Balaban & Waxman, 1997). Perceptual categories may be developed as early as four months, and object categories may also appear before 12-months-old. The ability to form mental representations of objects and events is correlated with cognitive development. Furthermore, forming categories and categorizing objects also involves cognitive processes. For example, infants must understand object permanence (understanding that things and people continue to exist even though they cannot be seen or heard) and means-end behavior (the ability to carry out a sequence of steps to achieve a goal) before they acquire object names (Barrett, 2017). Therefore, word learning is not only a process of linguistic development as it requires an appropriate level of cognitive development to form mental representations and categories that the words can be mapped onto. Waxman and Gelman (2009) also suggested that when new words are presented in a social and communicative context, infants are more likely to make the association between words and objects. According to Ferguson, Havy, and Waxman (2015), infants who have formed more precise associations between the labels and categories can comprehend and produce more words than infants who only form broad connections. It is amazing that by 12 months, infants can pair words to objects and become increasingly sensitive to the features of the objects, which facilitates categorization

(Arunachalam & Waxman, 2010; Ferguson et al., 2015; Westermann & Mareschal, 2013). By the end of the first year, most
infants can not only link labels to objects but also demonstrate
the ability to label new objects in the same category. Additionally, 10-month-olds can learn new label-object mapping and generalize new labels to new exemplars of the same category after a
short period of intensive training (Taxitari et al., 2019; Twomey
& Westermann, 2018). Children continue to expand their sensitivity to the concepts beyond common objects to other related
concepts, such as color, temperature, texture, and even mental
states, during their second year of life. The range of concepts and
rich representations provide children with a good foundation for
word learning (Arunachalam & Waxman, 2010).

Theories for Early Lexical Development

This subsection provides only a brief overview of the key lexical
development theories. Readers are encouraged to read Barrett's
chapter titled, "Early Lexical Development" (2017) which provides a very detailed and thorough review of the theories that
explain early lexical development. The first theory, *semantic
feature theory*, was proposed by Clark (1973). The core idea
of the theory is that the words share a set of semantic features
such as size and shape. Children first acquire general features
and then learn the features specific to the concept over time
by adding and deleting features. Both general and specific features are critically important for mapping the word to the object.
For example, children learn about the word "dog" through first
acquiring general features (e.g., animals, four legs) and then
learning and adding specific features (e.g., bark, fetch).

The second theory is called the *prototype theory*. It claims
that words are learned through prototypical referents for a target
word, not through semantic features or contrasts. Prototypes
are defined as "holistic mental representations of individual
referential exemplars that the child has encountered (Barrett,
2017, p. 379)." These representations are further divided into
perceptual and functional features. When the referents share
many features in common with the prototype, these referents
are considered highly typical referents of the word. For example,

chair, sofa, desk, table are considered highly typical referents for "furniture," but television, refrigerator are the least typical referents. The idea of this theory is that all referents share some common features with the prototype. However, each referent does not have to share common features with other referents. The difference between the semantic feature and prototype theory lies in deciding whether referents share common features with other referents. These prototypes are important to explain how the child expands their vocabulary because typical referents will be included first, then followed by the least typical referents (Barrett, 2017). The prototype theory can explain the two behaviors commonly observed in young children: under-extension (e.g., only use "dog" for family dog but not other dogs) and overextension (e.g., all men are "daddy"), whereas semantic feature theory cannot.

The third theory, ***event representation theory***, proposed by Nelson (1983), began to consider context and social interaction. This theory suggested that children establish knowledge of events that frequently occur in routine and daily social interaction before they acquire their first word. Because word learning is context-bound, the first words can typically be found in daily routines, such as play and mealtime. During the first year of life, children learn the event concepts and form mental representation holistically. By two years of age, children are able to analyze the event representations into constituents based on people, objects, actions, and relations involved in the event. Children can later use those words that share similar concepts beyond context to refer to other people, objects, actions, and relations.

The last theory is the ***multi-route model*** proposed by Barrett (1991). Two routes are proposed to explain the mapping between words and mental representations. The first route processes context-bound and social-pragmatic words. Similar to the event representation theory, these words are connected to event representations. The second route is for the mapping of referential words. Similar to the prototype theory, these words are used to refer to objects, actions, and states. These properties are mapped onto prototypical referents to examine how closely the referent resembles the prototype. Therefore, how the word is connected to the representation depends on the nature of the referent.

Although each theory has its limitations, it is clear that lexical development involves not only mapping the word onto the mental representations or prototypes, but also observing related factors such as context and events, as well as the nature of the referent. Lexical knowledge develops on a continuum from unstable and limited mental representations to enriched representations over time and is based on the child's experience and exposure to the concepts. The richness of the mental representation further influences word retrieval, word knowledge, and vocabulary expansion (Capone, 2007; Capone & McGregor, 2005).

Learning Nouns Versus Verbs

As we learn from the above lexical development theories, different mapping takes different routes of processing. Additionally, word learning requires more than mapping the word to the concept or object. Learning different types of words requires different types of information (Arunachalam & Waxman, 2010; Ferguson, Havy, & Waxman, 2015). In order to learn a word, infants need to integrate information from different sources and pay attention to surrounding linguistic elements related to the word, including syntactic, morphological, and prosodic elements (Arunachalam & Waxman, 2010; Westermann & Mareschal, 2013). Empirical data supports different lexical developmental trajectories across different word classes. Fenson et al. (1993) reported that more than 50% of the first 100 words are nouns. The development of verbs and adjectives emerges when the overall size of their vocabulary is between 50 to 100 words. Noun development is typically preceding the acquisition of other word classes (i.e., verbs, adjectives), and the acquisition of nouns provides a good foundation for association-making and categorization, which facilitates the acquisition of other types of words.

Verb acquisition takes longer than learning nouns because verbs are used to describe a dynamic process and must be interpreted both semantically and syntactically. Children have to figure out thematic roles that each word plays in order to understand the verb meaning. In other words, children have to identify "who" is "doing what" on "whom." For example, in order to understand the meaning of the verb in the sentence "the dog chases the boy," children need to identify the subject (i.e., "dog" the animal performs the action), object (i.e., "boy" the person receives the action), and verb ("chase" the action word that used to describe the event). Additionally, children also need to know the nouns in the sentence before they can make an association between the action and its referents.

Golinkoff and Hirsh-Pasek (2008) provided a thorough review of verb learning which highlighted the need to map verbs to events during the verb learning process. Unlike nouns, the referents for verbs are not perceptual and salient. Even though some verbs are more imaginable, such as action verbs (e.g., run, open), the meaning of a verb may receive less attention than the subject and object involved in the event. Golinkoff and Hirsh-Pasek (2008) indicated that several factors are crucial in verb mapping, including the property of the referent (e.g., imaginability and accessibility), the conceptual and semantic components from experience and social interactions (Genter, 2006), and linguistic cues. The accessibility of conceptual information along with the easiness of labeling a dynamic event can impact verb acquisition and explain variations within the verb acquisition. For example, the verbs "give, want" are acquired earlier than the verbs "sell, borrow."

The phenomenon "noun advantage" means learning nouns before other types of words. This advantage exists because, (1) concepts of objects are generally more stable and easily acquired than concepts of actions or events, and (2) nouns with high imageability make the concepts more concrete and accessible (Waxman et al., 2013). Additionally, children need to develop fundamental knowledge of certain nouns before they can readily acquire verbs. They also need to develop the ability to identify the relation between nouns, such as "subject" performs the action while "object" receives the action. Therefore, in order to derive the meaning of an unknown verb, children need to have lexical knowledge of surrounding nouns, positions of nouns, and the relation between the nouns. When social and other linguistic information is not accessible for the child, the verb meaning cannot be obtained. All this information makes learning verbs less straightforward than learning noun-object relations. Figure 3–1, adapted from Golinkoff and Hirsh-Pasek's article (2008), shows readers the role of individualization, concreteness, and imaginability in noun and verb acquisition. As shown in the figure, concrete and proper nouns have the advantage because of clear individualized referents, high imageability, and concreteness.

Is learning verbs more difficult than learning nouns across different languages? Waxman and colleagues (2013) examined the early noun advantage (i.e., learning nouns before verbs) in other languages, especially in verb-friendly languages (e.g., Mandarin Chinese, Japanese, and Korean). They concluded that young children, in general, can easily map nouns to objects but not verbs to actions although some cases of verb advantage have been reported in verb-friendly languages. Some verbs may be produced earlier in verb-friendly languages because these are frequently used in early parent-child interaction. However, because there are different rules involved in using verbs, nouns are still considered easier to acquire than verbs in verb-friendly languages. By the age of 24 months, toddlers, regardless of their primary language, can successfully map nouns to objects and verbs to actions. Representations of concepts are usually formed before words can be readily acquired, regardless of the type of word (Waxman et al., 2013).

Clinical Implications

What does the research tell us in clinical practice?

1. *Concepts and mental representations are crucial for developing lexical knowledge.* A rich pool of representations must be established for the mapping process to happen. The representations may be developed through events, routines, exposure, and experience. This highlights the importance of environmental input and cognitive readiness in the process of word learning. Intentionality, joint attention (share the focus on something with someone else), object permanence, means-end behavior, and symbolic play all play an important role in language development. It should be noted that cognitive and linguistic functions develop in parallel but are tightly

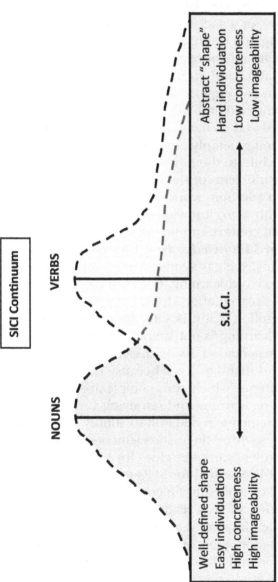

Figure 3-1. Reprinted from *Trends in Cognitive Sciences*, 12(10), Golinkoff, R. and Hirsh-Pasek, K., How toddlers begin to learn verbs, 397–403, Copyright 2008, with permission from Elsevier.

correlated. When conducting assessments, it is important for SLPs to test beyond labeling and evaluating if the child has established a stable connection between underlying concepts and labels. Also, different descriptions and pictures should be used to stimulate or examine different representations. For example, mental representations may be different for a concrete object (e.g., cake), a mental state (e.g., happy), or a social event (e.g., birthday). Making the strong and stable mapping between the word and its representation is necessary for word acquisition and word retrieval. In addition, encouraging the child to use, talk about, and explore the new word in various contexts can strengthen and enhance the connection between the word and its mental representations which consolidates learning. Simply labeling an object or action or exposing the child to the new word a few times without elaboration is insufficient for the child to learn and retain the new word. In addition, world knowledge should develop along with word knowledge while considering each child's social context and life experience.

2. ***Considering word knowledge in a linguistic context.*** Linguistic elements, such as syntactic information, may also contribute to word learning. For example, when an unknown word is placed after "drink," the listener can make the presumption that it is something liquid and drinkable. Word learning is not simply mapping the word to its mental representation. As discussed above, verbs are considered more difficult to learn because of how they are used in a sentence which adds complexity to verb learning. Therefore, learning and retrieving verbs requires other linguistic elements in addition to simply labeling the referents, and these other linguistic elements (e.g., subject, object, thematic roles) can offer clues for learning the verb meaning. Thus, it is essential for SLPs to expose children to a good variety of words in the environment through interactive activities, such as reading books and symbolic and sociodramatic play, based on a child's present level. SLPs can also promote their lexical learning and retention through discussion and elaboration. For example, SLPs can present three land animals and three sea animals and then discuss what they eat, what they do, how they

are similar, and how they are different from each other. Children can learn about categories, different semantic and phonological features, and word associations. Verbs can be introduced through modeling the actions on different, known objects by using self-talk (e.g., SLP describes what she or he is doing, seeing, and thinking), parallel talk (e.g., SLP describes what the child is seeing, doing, and thinking), and other indirect language stimulation (e.g., expansion, extension, etc.). SLPs can also introduce new verbs to describe what the different animals can do and how different word order and verbs may change the meaning of the sentence. When describing the subject, action, and object, the target words should be highlighted by alternating intonation and manipulating referents accordingly. When working with children with limited words and unstable mental representations, repeated exposure of referents and discussion of events is essential. SLPs can also teach different concepts by keeping the same sentence structure and only manipulating actions and/or referents to avoid cognitive overload, such as "the boy throws the ball," "the girl catches the ball," and "the cat chases the dog."

3. *Considering word knowledge in a social context.* Lexical development and language development occur in social contexts and interactions. Daily routines and social interactions provide rich contexts for children to develop event representations, as well as social pragmatic words, such as "bye, hi, no." Early developing words include the words used in daily activities, such as games (e.g., peekaboo), routines (e.g., mealtime), and shared book reading. This highlights the importance of constant exposure and structured activities (e.g., routines) in the word learning process. There is no doubt that lexical knowledge development requires more than exposure to labels and making associations between labels and concepts. The learning process also requires the social context, knowledge of different linguistic elements, ability to integrate information from multiple sources (e.g., sensory domains and experiences), and repeated word usage to refine and advance word knowledge and enrich mental representations. It involves not only cognitive

processes and multiple sensory sources but also social contexts, experiences, and meaningful environment input while learning new words. As clinicians, SLPs are encouraged to capitalize on social interactions, routines, and contexts while helping children advance and expand their word knowledge (Crais, 2011). SLPs can help parents understand the power of learning new words from daily routines (e.g., mealtime, bath time, brush teeth) and through connecting words to the child's personal experiences (e.g., making friends, reading books, fun trips). Based on the child's present level and progress, gradually adding new words can avoid cognitive overload and promote a positive learning experience.

Gestures and Early Lexical Development

Gestures are defined as actions produced with the intent to communicate through using fingers, hands, arms, and sometimes, facial expressions (Iverson & Thal, 1998). Words and gestures both serve crucial communicative functions for young children, and gestures have been studied broadly as a method to assist communication across the lifespan. In this subsection, we briefly discuss the relationship between gestures and early lexical development.

Gestures, language, and speech are strongly correlated in their development, and seem to share common cognitive processes. Neuroimaging studies suggested that comprehension of symbolic gestures and spoken language may be supported by largely overlapping brain regions; this supports the developments of symbolic gestures and spoken language are closely related, yet parallel (Xu et al., 2009). Gestures and spoken language are both symbolic, so the same brain regions may be activated when forming an expression. Besides the overlapping brain areas for processing gestures and language, parental responsiveness and environmental input also play an essential role. When gestures are used by the child, adults tend to respond with eye gaze, gestures, or words to facilitate the child's learning of new concepts or words. When parents respond to the child's gesture with labeling, the connection between the referent and label becomes clear and reinforced, which in turn facilitates the child's word learning. Additionally, Goldin-Meadow and Wagner (2005) reported a positive correlation between the frequency of parental gesture use and the size of gesture and vocabulary in the children at 14 months old. Rowe et al. (2008) further indicated that the types of gesture use at 14 months may reliably predict the child's vocabulary size two years later.

Gestures usually emerge about three months before the words are initially produced. Iverson and Goldin-Meadow (2005) claimed that gesturing provides children the opportunity to practice the word meaning, which further sets up a foundation for word production. A simple explanation is that using gestures is less cognitively demanding than using words while infants are still in the process of developing speech and language. Goldin-Meadow and Wagner (2005) emphasized that gestures can present the intended idea holistically and efficiently with less cognitive effort than formulating speech; the use of gestures can also facilitate lexical learning when the representation is unstable or limited. Also, pairing gesturing while speaking can free up some cognitive resources and enable the child to focus on processing words (Iverson & Goldin-Meadow, 2005; Wagner et al., 2004). It is evident that gestures found in the child's communication typically appear in the child's lexicon months later. The same observation can also be found in the gesture-word combination that precedes the use of two-word combinations such as "mommy + point to the ball" as indicating "play with the ball." Therefore, it suggests that mental representations of an object (e.g., ball) and its semantic relations (e.g., ask mommy to roll the ball) have been formed before the words are verbally produced (Capone, 2007; Iverson & Goldin-Meadow, 2005). Infants typically start to gesture before 9 months old (Crais et al., 2009; Iverson & Goldin-Meadow, 2005); 8-month-olds produce an average of 10.7 gestures according to the MacArthur-Bates Communicative Development Inventories-Second Edition (MB-CDIs 2nd edition; Fenson, et al., 2007). The number of gestures increases to around 50 gestures by 18 months.

Among the different types of gestures, **deictic gestures** and **representational gestures** are both reported to enhance word learning (McGregor, 2008). **Deictic gestures** typically emerge between 7 to 12 months and are used to "indicate referents in the immediate environment" (Iverson & Goldin-Meadow, 2005, p. 368). Depending on the involvement of direct contact with the object, deictic gestures can be further divided into two subtypes, including *contact gestures* (for the purpose of showing and giving) and *distal gestures* (for the purpose of commenting). Deictic gestures are more strongly related to word comprehension than production. Additionally, the use of deictic gestures can predict the size of a child's vocabulary development (Capone & McGregor, 2005; Fenson et al., 2007). A new word can be better learned when the referent is pointed out, labeled, and manipulated along with repeated exposure. Object labeling through pointing is common in early child-adult interaction, which explains the phenomenon of noun advantage in early lexical development. Let's think about how parents teach their baby a new word. The parents may point to the bubbles when popping them and simultaneously say, "pop bubbles." A simple action like this can be repeated more than a dozen times while blowing and popping bubbles in the park. This modeling and repeated exposure can provide the child the learning opportunity to map the word "bubbles" to the action "pop." When children use gestures correctly, the parents also respond positively to facilitate learning and the use of gestures. Thus, the use of gestures from both children and adults creates a rich context for language development and word learning (Goldin-Meadow & Singer, 2003; Iverson & Goldin-Meadow, 2005).

Common gestures used by 9-month-old children are mostly for requesting (e.g., grab the pacifier) and protesting (e.g., push a toy away). **Representational gestures** appear around 12 months of age and are used to symbolize referents with no context bounding (Capone & McGregor, 2005; Crais, Watson, & Baranek, 2009; McGregor, 2008), such as putting the index finger in front of lips (to ask people to be quiet), flapping arms (to indicate a bird), waving hands (to say goodbye), or holding something close to the ear (to pretend to speak on the phone during play). These gestures are developed through imitation, daily routines, social games, and parent-child interactions; therefore, gesture use may be affected by social context and cultural background (Crais, Watson, & Baranek, 2009).

Crais, Watson, and Baranek (2009) summarized three major roles of gestural use in communication, including (1) behavior regulation (e.g., protesting and requesting), (2) social interaction (e.g., the use of representational gestures, such as blow kisses, waving bye, and gestures used in symbolic play), and (3) joint attention (e.g., making comments to supply or request information, such as pointing to mother when being asked where mommy is, pointing to a picture in the book for further explanation). Children typically use the combination of gestures and speech rather than gestures alone. Gesture-word combinations are commonly used to *enhance* (e.g., raising a hand to the cheek when saying, "call"), *complement* (e.g., pointing to a flying balloon when saying, "fly") or *supplement* (e.g., pointing to a cookie jar when saying "cookie" to indicate wanting a cookie) the intended message. The most frequently used combinations by 20-month-old children are for supplementary purposes (Capone & McGregor, 2005). The use of gestures decreases over time when children increase verbal production, but gestures continue to be used to aid and enhance communication effectiveness in adulthood. After 20 or 24 months of age, toddlers primarily use spoken words. Table 3–1 is the timeline of gesture development discussed in the article of Capone and McGregor (2005).

Clinical Implications

Capone (2007) claimed that the use of gestures may provide a window to examine a child's lexical knowledge and mental representations during the transition from vocalization to two-word combinations. The use of deictic and representational gestures facilitates the development of both receptive and expressive language which include word learning. Gestures serve as a window to look into the child's cognitive development and formation of mental representations. Additionally, the use of gestures, especially pointing, is one of the reliable indicators to differentiate late talkers from late bloomers, as well as assist with identification of autism spectrum disorders. Moreover, gesture use not only reveals a child's mental representations and category formation, but also reinforces the word learning by strengthening the referent-label association, as well as enriching the mental representation. Because gesturing is less cognitively demanding

Table 3–1. A Timeline of Gesture Development

10–13 Months	12–13 Months	15–16 Months	18–20 Months	2–5 Years	School Age
Showing Giving Pointing Ritualized Request	Representational gestures, play Schemes	Gesture or vocal preference	Spoken word preference, gesture + spoken combinations	Speech-gesture integration, beat gestures emerge	Mismatched gesture + spoken combinations
POINT predicts First words	First words emerge		Significant increase in words (types, tokens)	Gesture scaffolds spoken expression and comprehension	Mismatches indexes the transitional knowledge state
Other prelinguistic behaviors include eye contact, joint attention, and turn-taking	Gesture serves a complementary function to spoken forms		Increased pointing in combination with spoken words	Transition from BPO to IO gestures	Gesture aids in the transition to concept acquisition
			Transition to empty-handed play schemes	Iconic and beat gestures accompany longer utterances	

Note. BPO = body part as object; IO= imaginary object.

Source: Capone, N., & McGregor, K. (2005). The effect of semantic representation on toddlers' word retrieval. *Journal of Speech, Language and Hearing Research, 48*(6), 1468–1480. https://doi.org/10.1044/1092-4388(2005/102) Used with permission from ASHA.

and shares some similar cognitive processes and brain regions with language development, the use of gestures in communication should be promoted. When a child's speech production is limited, parents are encouraged to pair gestures with verbal modeling to facilitate language development. Parental input and social contexts play an important role in gesture and lexical development. When caregivers model gestures and respond to the child's gestures more frequently in a meaningful way, it facilitates gesture, word, and language development.

Crais, Watson, and Baranek (2009) emphasized the importance of considering frequency, variety, and communicative function of gesture use when evaluating communication effectiveness in young children, children with limited verbal output, and children with suspected language delays. When a child shows delays in gesture use, as well as comprehension and production of spoken language, the child may be at risk for having a language impairment. For detailed information on how to evaluate gesture use in infants and toddlers, readers are encouraged to review the studies done by Crais (2011) and Crais, Watson, and Baranek (2009).

Gestures are naturally used in daily life to facilitate thought process, word retrieval, and communication. Gestures are used across cultural and linguistic backgrounds to convey messages. As gesture use is a reliable predictor of vocabulary and language development, gesture use should be included in assessment and intervention to examine the child's development of mental representation, object categorization, and receptive vocabulary. Gestures are included in a few standardized tests such as the MacArthur-Bates Communicative Development Inventories (MB-CDIs) (Fenson et al., 2007), Rossetti Infant-Toddler Language Scale (Rossetti, 2006), and Communication and Symbolic Behavior Scale (CSBS) (Wetherby & Prizant, 1993).

SLPs should consider incorporating gesture use in clinical management when working with young children. Collaborating with psychologists and early interventionists to identify the frequency, variety, and function of gesture use may provide a good picture of a child's current communication effectiveness and language development. The child's hand movements may reveal what they know and what the next step would be in the developmental process. When working with children with limited verbal output, gesture use should be encouraged to lessen the cognitive demands while facilitating the word learning or word retrieval process. When working with children with limited mental representations and perceptual categories, adults can use gestures to enhance label-referent connection and to promote learning words. It is clear that both parent and child gesture use may assist word learning, and child gesture use can be encouraged by adult gesture use. When working with children who struggle with word combinations, word-gesture combinations should be introduced to facilitate the development of word combinations. Also, adults' responsiveness to the child's communicative intent, despite modalities, is vital to the child's language development and word learning.

From Babbling to Protowords and True Words

During the first year of life, infants learn to segment words in continuous speech and gradually fine tune phonological contrasts specific to their primary language (Gaskell & Ellis, 2009). Word learning requires not just mapping words to concepts but also mapping sounds to meanings. However, mapping sound to meaning is a challenging task because words may be produced in different ways (e.g., vary in loudness and pitch) and have to be segmented from continuous speech stream first (Christophe et al., 1997). Infants can learn language features specific to their primary languages, such as phonological contrasts, sound patterns, phonotactic constraints, and syntactic rules during the first year of life. **Phonological bootstrapping** is the ability to use phonological analysis to acquire lexicon that emerges early in life. In other words, infants can use phonological information to learn word forms in their primary language. (Christophe et al., 1997; Morgan & Demuth, 1996). Aside from mapping the sounds to words, vocalization and babbling reflect the process of acquiring specific sounds and sound patterns. Stoel-Gammon (2011) claimed that the more often babies practice the sounds and syllable shapes when they vocalize, the easier and more automatic the movements become when verbalizing these sounds. Because babies can make the association between articulatory movements and vocal productions through an auditory-articulatory feedback loop, it lays the foundation for word production. Vihman

(1992) claimed that meaning can be more easily attached to a large repertoire of practiced syllables. Stoel-Gammon (2011) also suggested that, "babbling provides more practice for the development of early spoken words" (p. 9). The importance of babbling to language development is unquestionable. There is continuity in speech sound development from reduplicated babbling, emerging around 6 months, to variegated babbling that appears around 9 months. Through an auditory-articulatory feedback loop, babies continue to learn phonological contrasts and expand on the repertoire of speech sounds and syllable shapes to be ready for word production.

Protowords are used before true words and are learned by "associating the phonetically underspecified sound patterns to specific objects" through repeated exposure (Nazzi & Bertoncini, 2003, p. 137). For instance, a child consistently points to water while saying "gaga" is an example of using protowords. Although "gaga" is not a real word and does not sound like the target word (water), the child has learned to use a sound pattern (i.e., /gaga/) consistently to refer to a specific object (i.e., water). True words are the words that sound similar to the adult form and can be consistently used by a child to refer to a specific refer-ent in a specific context. In other words, the use of true words indicates attaching phonetically specified sound patterns directly to its referent rather than a specific object. For example, "wawa" refers to not only wanting the water bottle but also indicating water in the pool. Also, the use of true words reflects the infant's ability to use language to represent the world and the "beginning of the referential use of language" that goes beyond immedi-ate context (i.e., decontextualization) (Nazzi & Bertoncini, 2003, p. 136). Turnbull and Justice (2012) laid out three key features that distinguish true words from protowords. First, true words are used to refer to people or objects in the immediate environ-ment. Second, true words have recognizable speech patterns similar to adult forms. Third, true words are used consistently in a specific context and can be extended beyond the original text.

It is not surprising that a child's productive phonology is correlated with lexical development, as evident in the sounds and sound patterns used in babbling and true words. Sounds (e.g., nasals, stops, and glides) and syllable shapes (e.g., consonant-vowel [CV] and consonant-vowel-consonant-vowel [CVCV]) commonly used in babbling are also observed in true words. Children tend to produce words with the consonants in their phonetic inventory (i.e., the sounds that a child can consistently produce correctly), which further supports the influence of productive phonology on early lexical development (Stoel-Gammon, 2011). In addition to a child's ability to acquire speech sounds from auditory input and feedback, the support from adult-child interactions also facilitates the use of specific sounds and syllable shapes in the child's verbal production. Tamis-LeMonda et al. (2003) reported that parental responses to infants' vocalization, such as imitation, expansion, naming, and acknowledgment, predicted the acquisition of their first 50 words.

Clinical Implications

Going from the coo and goo stage to producing first words requires a child's cognitive and linguistic abilities as well as social context and adult-child interactions. Good varieties in consonants and vowels along with sufficient syllable shapes are the building blocks for spoken word production. Lack of canonical babbling and limited speech sounds may put a child at risk of delays in language and lexical development. Stoel-Gammon (2011) indicated that phonological development has a significant influence on lexical development, especially from birth to two and a half years old. Children with a large vocabulary often have more advanced phonological development than children with a small vocabulary; this supports the relationship between lexical and phonological development. In other words, small phonetic inventory may limit lexical growth because sufficient sounds and syllable shapes are needed for word production.

It is important to keep in mind that speech sounds, syllable shapes, and lexical development are closely correlated. A thorough inventory of a child's productive phonology and word production should be evaluated when conducting language assessments. It is essential to accurately identify a child's *present level* and then to determine the *zone of proximal development* (i.e., the child's ability to perform target behavior with some support) by considering the child's linguistic background, cognitive development, and learning ability. Children with speech delays, regardless of etiologies, have been shown to follow the developmental sequence that is similar to their typically developing peers, but at a slower pace. Therefore, it is essential to evaluate the child's productive phonology, including consonants, vowels, and syllable shapes through language samples, clinical observation, and parent interviews.

In regard to intervention planning, SLPs could focus on expanding the repertoire of speech sounds, syllable shapes, and words commonly used in the child's environment by carefully considering the child's phonetic restriction. Using early developing words as a starting point is recommended because most typically developing children acquire these words first. Paul and Norbury (2012) provided a list of words that clinicians may consider targeting first. For example,

"no, all gone, away" for rejection/disappearance;

"stop, all done" for cessation;

"more, again" for recurrence;

"get, eat, do, help, wash, bump, draw, do, sit, fall" for action;

"hi, bye, night-night" for social interaction;

"big, little, hot, dirty" for description;

"in, on, here, off, down, up" for preposition; and

"my, mine, want" for possession.

These words also serve various communication purposes and contain different word classes. Clinicians may want to consider other related factors, such as word frequency, phonotactic probability, and phonological neighborhood density, when selecting treatment words. A detailed discussion on the factors related to target word selection is in Chapter 5 and 8.

Fast and Slow Mapping

Words can be learned through different mechanisms (e.g., via listening or reading) at different points of time throughout life. Beginning around 18 months of age, children start producing up to nine words a day with an increasing speed; this phenomenon is known as **vocabulary spurt** (a.k.a., *word burst*) (Benedict, 1979). According to Lock (1980), vocabulary spurt represents the sudden growth in vocabulary and rapid acceleration in word learning emerging around 18 months. Nazzi and Bertoncini (2003) indicated that vocabulary spurt is associated with the development of object permanence and mental representations and the ability to categorize objects. However, Bloom (2004) reminded clinicains to be mindful not to overinterpret the observation of vocabulary spurt because it does not capture the full picture of a child's lexical development process. Word knowledge accumulates over time, and lexical development involves respective cognitive processes and the development of other language domains. For example, in order to learn the word "table," a child has to follow adults' gesture or eye gaze to associate the word (i.e., table) to its referent (i.e., the real object), sound sequence (i.e., /teɪbəl/), syntactic information (e.g., something you can put things on), and pragmatic use of the word in the context (e.g., clean the table, put the bottle on the table). Therefore, the development of several prerequisites has undergone prior to successfully saying the word.

Most children around eight months old can pick up new words after being exposed to them an average of 13 times and are able to retain these newly learned words for at least two weeks based on Jusczyk and Hohne's study (1997). Young children have the ability to associate sound patterns, concepts, and syntactic information to infer the word meaning. Amazingly, young children can form a hypothesis of the word meaning through just a few exposures. The term **fast mapping** is used to describe a child's ability to learn and retain new words for a short period of time and through only minimum exposure (Carey & Bartlett, 1978). When children encounter a new word, they have to create an initial phonological representation of the word and form a preliminary word meaning, and then connect these representations (Gray, 2006). Fast mapping in word learning is an ability commonly investigated by researchers, who found that older children and adults can fast map not only words but also novel facts (Bloom, 2004; Carey, 2010). Fast mapping ability has been found in typically developing children as young as 13 months as well as children with language deficits. The difference between typically developing children and children with language deficits lies in the number of words that can be fast mapped. (See Alt, Plante, & Creusere, 2004; Gershkoff-Stowe & Hahn, 2007 for a detailed review.) Studies have shown that children with language disorders can only fast-map fewer words than their typically developing peers. This means that these children need more time to make the initial mapping when encountering new words (Alt et al., 2004; Gray, 2006). Gray (2006) highlighted that the fast-mapping ability could further influence a child's overall lexical development because it is the "initial step in the word learning process" (p. 965).

However, fast mapping is a simplistic explanation of vocabulary spurt. It does not capture other factors related to vocabulary spurt, such as word meaning construction process, the development from fragile lexical representations to refined word knowledge, and decontextualized use of the word. Additionally, not all words can be learned from fast mapping. For example, verb acquisition requires the knowledge of other words in a sentence (e.g., nouns) and syntactic information associated with the word (Swingley, 2010). Also, the word learning process can vary significantly depending on the frequency of use (e.g., learning the word "dog" in an environment that has dogs), the complexity of the word (e.g., learning emotion words are more difficult than naming an object), the social and linguistic context (e.g., how the new word is used in the context), and how much effort the child requires to form the hypothesis of word meaning.

Word learning can be roughly divided into two phases, including fast mapping and slow mapping. The first phase, fast mapping, is linking a label to its referent in order to establish initial meaning. Based on McGregor, Friedman, Reilly, and Newman's study (2002), salient features, such as physical characteristics, functions, and movements, are usually first recognized by young children. However, without continued and repeated exposure along with meaningful association, newly learned words may decay due to unsuccessful storage in long-term memory. Therefore, **slow mapping** (a.k.a. extended mapping) is necessary for lexical development as the second phase. Extended mapping requires a child to strengthen the relationship between the words, referents, and concepts by updating and elaborating lexical representations. Lexical gaps and fragile lexical representations take months or years to be filled and consolidated through additional experience, and the process of consolidation depends on the complexity and frequency of the word (Gershkoff-Stowe & Hahn, 2007). It is not uncommon to observe overextensions (e.g., refering to all animals with four legs as dogs or all men as daddy) in toddlers because their lexical representations and knowledge are still limited. Children in preschool and early school years may also make similar overextensions or semantic errors due to incomplete word knowledge and fragile connections between the word, referent, concept, and sound sequence. McGregor and collegues (2002) claimed that the degree of lexical knowledge is also associated with word retrieval ability. Thus, semantic errors could be an indicator of those unstable and fragile lexical representations and show the need of extended mapping to refine the respective word knowledge.

Cognitive Factors That Are Related to Lexical Development

As discussed above, lexical development requires more than mapping a word to its referent. Knowing a word means that a person knows the meaning, semantic reference, sound pattern, and syntactic properties of the word (Swingley, 2009). Additionally, knowing a word means the person has sufficient word knowledge to understand and use the word in an appropriate context. Successful word learning requires adequate cognitive functions and linguistic processes. The underlying concepts and mental representations of the objects or events have to be acquired before words (i.e., labels) can be successfully produced. Bloom (2004) stated that learning words requires both adequate cognitive and linguistic abilities. It is because mental representations and underlying concepts have to be formed before words can be produced, such as knowing object categories (for learning object nouns) or event representations (for learning verbs). In other words, cognitive processes help create preliminary lexical representations for fast mapping, so new words can be mapped onto either existing cognitive structures or newly formed categories (Barrett, 2017).

Cognitive development and lexical acquisition support each other since young age. For example, the ability to form categories starts as young as three months old (Arunachalam & Waxman, 2010; Quinn & Johnson, 2000), and categorization provides the mechanism for grouping different properties, objects, and events (Gervits et al., 2016). On the other hand, the process of learning words (i.e., labeling) can facilitate the expansion and refinement of categories (e.g., semantic or phonological categories). In this section, we will discuss several key cognitive factors that are related to lexical development, including attention, working memory, speed of information processing, and long-term memory.

Attention and Social Experience

Word learning requires both adequate cognitive functions and linguistic input from the environment. Children's ability to follow eye gaze and pay attention to their communication partner's mouth and face during interaction is important to language development. Their attention to these cues can enhance the association between a word and its referent and also make the information about the word more salient, such as sound pattern and syntactic information (Tenenbaum et al., 2014). Along the same line, Tomasello (1995) claimed that young children learn words "when they understand that the adult is making that sound with the intention" (p. 101). Therefore, attention to word-object associations and the ability to access people's intentions through social interactions could contribute to word learning (Hollich et al., 2000; Parish-Morris et al., 2007).

Children use the information extracted from social interactions to guide their lexical learning (Baldwin & Moses, 2001). Social-pragmatic words (e.g., bye, hi, no) are among the early developing true words; these words support the importance of social context in lexical development. Adults usually respond positively to a child's vocalization and gestures by labeling, elaborating, and acknowledging using self-talk. Children develop language through overheard speech from the environment, social interactions, and daily routines regardless of whether the parent labels the referents or not. The concept "*abundant linguistic input"* means that young learners tend to pick up words that are frequently used in the linguistic input (Barrett, 2017). Hence, joint attention and the mutual engagement between a child and an adult play a vital role in language development. Tomasello (1995) proposed that mutual engagement by directing a child's focus to the referent can facilitate the mapping between a word and its referent. Additionally, mutual engagement may bring the child's attention to the adult's communicative cues, such as gesture and eye gaze, which assists in inferring word meaning (Shneidman et al., 2009). Children's attention to communication partners and their cues could facilitate the word learning process (Shneidman et al., 2009). In addition, children who actively observe people in the interactions are more likely to learn new words. In other words, the child's experience during interaction and attention to social cues facilitates word learning (Shneidman et al., 2009).

Working Memory

Working Memory (a.k.a. short-term memory), especially phonological short-term memory, plays an important role in word learning. When learning new words, it is critical to be able to temporarily process and retain phonological information of the new words (Gathercole & Braddeley, 1989). Let's briefly overview the working memory model proposed by a British cognitive psychologist, Alan D. Baddeley and his colleagues. This working memory model (Baddeley, 2000) is composed of four elements: the central executive, phonological loop, visual sketchpad, and episodic buffer. The *"central executive"* is the commander-in-chief that is responsible for allocating, coordinating, and controlling cognitive resources necessary to complete a task (e.g., naming a picture, telling a story). The central executive coordinates the information flow throughout the working memory system. The *"phonological loop"* is temporary storage for the initial process of verbal information, including encoding, rehearsal, and short-term retention. The *"visual sketchpad"* is related to visual (e.g., appearance) and spatial (e.g., location) information processing. Both phonology loop and visual sketchpad arc temporary, domain-specific storage systems. Children with language disorders tend to have a much better ability to process visual-spatial information than verbal information (Alt, 2013). Hence, clinicians could consider capitalizing the adequate visuospatial processing ability in children with language disorders by incorporating more images and visuals when making associations between words and referents. The fourth and last component of the model is the *"episodic buffer."* The episodic buffer is a limited capacity temporary storage that integrates information from various sources (e.g., phonology loop and visual sketchpad) (Gillam, 2002; Montgomery et al., 2010). The buffer combines the information from phonological loop and visual sketchpad as a sequence of events and coherent episodes. It serves as a temporary storing space before long term memory is formed (Baddeley, 2000; Montgomery et al., 2010; Newbury et al., 2015).

Many studies have shown that phonological short-term memory is strongly related to the development of receptive vocabulary (Gathercole, Hitch, Service, & Martine, 1997; Gray, 2006) and expressive vocabulary (Newbury et al., 2015). To successfully and accurately form the representation of a new word in long-term memory, the initial formation of short-term representation is crucial (Burgess & Hitch, 2005; Gaskell & Ellis, 2009; Jarrold et al., 2009). Children who have better ability to maintain new words in their phonological loop can form more accurate representations stored in long-term memory (Gathercole et al., 1997). In other words, the better a child can temporarily hold and process the new words in phonological short-term memory, the more stable and accurate phonological representations of the new words can be stored in long-term memory (Gillam, 2002; Jarrold et al., 2009). Unfortunately, children with language disorders generally do not have adequate phonological short-term memory, which prevents them from forming accurate representations.

Speed of Information Processing

Information processing speed refers to the "amount of information that can be processed in a given time" (Newbury et al., 2015, p. 1763). As a result of practice, information processing speed improves with age into adulthood. Slow processing speed may increase the risk of information decay, missing information, as well as creating a bottleneck for incoming information. For example, if linguistic information can not be efficiently processed, children may not be able to successfully map a new word to its referent. The result of a slow processing speed is that the child needs extra time and exposure to process and retain new information (Montgomery et al., 2010; Newbury et al., 2015). Working memory capacity and processing speed are strongly correlated when processing various types of information. Imagining working memory as a bucket, processing speed refers to how fast someone can empty the bucket (by processing the received information efficiently and effectively) in order to refill the bucket (to receive incoming information). The textbook written by Paul, Norbury, and Gosse (2017) highlights the role of processing speed and capacity in language development, as well as how breakdowns in these processes could hinder language development. Interested readers can refer to Paul et al.'s book (2017) for details.

Long-Term Memory

Working memory can only temporarily store, process, and manipulate information, so the perceived linguistic information has to be stored in long-term memory for future use (Lum et al., 2012; Lum & Kidd, 2012). Long-term memory can be divided into **declarative memory** (a.k.a., explicit memory) and **nondeclarative memory** (a.k.a., implicit memory). Declarative memory includes *semantic memory* (e.g., general facts and world knowledge) and *episodic memory* (e.g., personal facts and experiences); nondeclarative memory includes *procedural memory* (e.g., motor and automatic skills) and *priming*. Declarative memory is important for acquiring lexical knowledge, such as meaning, forms of words, and sound sequence. On the other hand, nondeclarative memory is responsible for unconscious and rule-governed procedural process learning, such as grammar. (Ullman, 2001). The difference between declarative and nondeclarative memory lies in not only the types of information but also the processes of learning. Declarative memory may be formed from a few exposures, but nondeclarative memory requires repeated practice to establish (Lum & Kidd, 2012). Therefore, in addition to processing the new words efficiently in the working memory system, it is also essential to have sufficient exposures and rehearsal in order to successfully consolidate and store the newly learned words in long-term memory for later retrieval.

Prior lexical knowledge is another factor that is related to word acquisition. When learning new words, the existing words in long-term memory that have similar sound patterns or meanings can be activated to assist recognition and facilitate learning the new words (Gathercole et al., 1997; Gillam, 2002; Gray, 2006). For example, learning the sound pattern of a new word can be aided by linking it to the existing words that have similar sound patterns. Because similar sounding words have been learned, it is easy for children to learn the new word (Gathercole et al.,1997). Thus, children with large vocabulary size have the advantage in word learning. Children with language disorders usually have fewer learned sound patterns and words stored in the long-term memory to draw from. They are less successful in making the associations to their prior lexical knowledge when learning new words.

Clinical Implications

Learning a new word is not a simple and static process. Instead, lexical learning involves numerous cognitive and linguistic processes. Fundamental cognitive processes (e.g., attention and memory) and social experiences (e.g., contexts) are required for successful lexical learning. Hence, when making clinical decisions, clinicians should take cognitive factors into considerations. Because cognitive functions play an important role in lexical development, it is important to evaluate a child's overall ability to attend, process, and retain both verbal and nonverbal information. For example, it is important to know if a child has limited phonological short-term memory or shows slow information processing speed. It is also essential to evaluate if a child could connect a word to its referent and sound sequence, and has ample exposures and opportunities to use the word.

Children with language disorders could have difficulty in encoding, retaining, and retrieving linguistic information. Thus, clinicians should consider implementing strategies to promote lexical learning and to accommodate the limitations in information processing speed, such as making the target word more salient or not including too many new words in one session. Also, adding pauses and carefully controlling the pace of clinical sessions would allow the child to more successfully process new information. Clinicians could also consider posing questions to probe the child's comprehension and promote learning. Additionally, SLPs could facilitate lexical learning by minimizing cognitive demands through embedding therapy goals in daily routines and repetitive contexts (e.g., sing songs, reading books). Capitalizing children's cognitive strengths could facilitate their overall language development. For example, if a child is good at processing visuospatial information, SLPs could frequently incorporate images (e.g., pictures or drawings) or visual aids (e.g., real objects or toys) to assist abstract lexical learning.

It takes time to consolidate and retain newly learned words and information, so it is beneficial to implement strategies, such as repeating the new information, making explicit associations, and maximizing the opportunity to use the newly learned words across different contexts. For example, when a 3-year-old is learning the word "bat," adults can talk about different meanings of it (e.g., *baseball bat* vs. *mammal bat*) and contexts that the word can be used in. Adults may use pictures, highlight context, and introduce other related words, such as discussing words related to baseball bats (e.g., pitch, throw, hit, coach) and words related to animal bats (e.g., coming out at night, can be found in caves). The child's personal experience can also be incorporated when discussing the target word, such as "do you remember watching yesterday's Dodger baseball game?" Follow-up activities, such as story retells or personal narratives, should be encouraged for practicing the use of the newly learned words. It is also essential to keep a child's cognitive limitations in mind. Adults and clinicians could introduce strategies and modifications to address the child's limitations in cognitive processes to promote lexical learning, such as carefully controlling the amount of new information, slow pace, repetitive practice, and eliminating distractions. It should be noted that these strategies and activities could benefit typically developing children as well as children with language disorders.

Chapter Summary

In this chapter, we review the theoretical models related to early lexical development. Additionally, we discuss the processes and factors related to learning new words during the prelinguistic stage, including the process of mapping between a label and its referent, mapping between a label and its sound sequences, and the underlying cognitive functions needed to support lexical development. It is important for clinicians to consider all the factors that are related to speech and language development and to carefully evaluate how these factors can impact lexical development. In order to have a good understanding of a child's lexical and language development, clinicians should take different prelinguistic and cognitive abilities into consideration, such as:

- Play skill development. Free and unstructured play is an important way for young children learn words. Readers are encouraged to read Dr. Carol Westby's (2000) chapter titled "A Scale for Assessing Development Children's Play" for a detailed review of how play and language development correlate.
- Communicative needs and intents
- Babbling and vocalization
- The use of gestures for communication
- Fast and slow mapping skills. The ability to fast map between a word and its referent and how much support a child needs to retain and use the newly learned word.
- Cognitive development, such as attention, working memory, and long-term memory

The information gathered can help clinicians get an idea of how a child learns and what support the child may need in order to better process and retain the newly learned words. Clinicians need to keep in mind that children with developmental language disorders follow the same developmental sequences as their typically developing peers. Thus, understanding normal cognitive and language development could help SLPs make clinical decisions based on the child's present level and make modifications on assessment and intervention plans accordingly. In the next chapter, we will discuss lexical development in school-age and older children.

Discussion Questions

1. Explain the role of gesture development in lexical development. Give an example of how a 10-month-old baby and a 15-month-old toddler may use gestures differently to support their lexical development.
2. Discuss how different cognitive functions may affect a young child's lexical development.
3. Explain the differences between and importance of fast mapping and slow mapping.
4. What aspects and factors should be considered when evaluating a young child's lexical development?

References

Alt, M. (2013). Visual fast mapping in school-aged children with specific language impairment. *Topics in Language Disorders, 33*(4), 328–346. https://doi.org/10.1097/01.TLD.0000437942.85989.73

Alt, M., Plante, E., & Creusere, M., (2004). Semantic features in fast mapping: Performance of preschoolers with specific language impairment versus preschoolers with normal language. *Journal of Speech, Language, and Hearing Research, 47*(2), 407–420. https://doi.org/10.1044/1092-4388(2004/033)

Arunachalam, S., & Waxman, S. (2010). Language and conceptual development. *WIREs Cognitive Science, 1*(4), 548–558. https://doi.org/10.1002/wcs.37

Baddeley, A (2000). The episodic buffer: A new component of working memory? *Trends in Cognitive Sciences, 4*(11), 417–423.

Balaban, M., & Waxman, S. (1997). Do words facilitate object categorization in 9-month-old infants? *Journal of Experimental Child Psychology, 64*, 3–26. https://doi.org/10.1006/jecp.1996.2332

Baldwin, D., & Moses, L. (2001). Links between social understanding and early word learning: Challenges to current accounts. *Social Development, 10*(3), 309–329. https://doi.org/10.1111/1467-9507.00168

Barrett, M. (1991). The multi-route model of early lexical development. *Anales de psicología, 7*(2), 123–136.

Barrett, (2017). Early lexical development. In P. Fletcher & B. MacWhinney (Eds.), *The handbook of child language* (pp. 361–392). Blackwell. https://doi.org/10.1111/b.9780631203124.1996.00015.x

Benedict, H. (1979). Early lexical development: Comprehension and production. *Journal of Child Language, 6*(2), 183–200. https://doi.org/10.1017/S0305000900002245

Bloom, P. (2004). Myths of word learning. In D. G. Hall & S. R. Waxman (Eds.), *Weaving a lexicon* (pp. 205–224). MIT Press.

Burgess, N., & Hitch, G. (2005). Computational models of working memory: Putting long-term memory into context. *Trends in Cognitive Sciences, 9*(11), 535–541. https://doi.org/10.1016/j.tics.2005.09.011

Capone, N. (2007). Tapping toddlers' evolving semantic representation via gesture. *Journal of Speech, Language, and Hearing Research, 50*(3), 732–745. https://doi.org/10.1044/1092-4388(2007/051)

Capone, N., & McGregor, K. (2005). The effect of semantic representation on toddlers' word retrieval. *Journal of Speech, Language, and Hearing Research, 48*(6), 1468–1480. https://doi.org/10.1044/1092-4388(2005/102)

Carey, S. (2010). Beyond fast mapping. *Language Learning and Development, 6*(3), 184–205. https://doi.org/10.1080/15475441.2010.484379

Carey, S., & Bartlett, E. (1978). Acquiring a single new word. *Papers and Reports on Child Language Development, 15*, 17–29. https://www.researchgate.net/publication/284657182

Clark, H. (1973). The language-as-fixed-effect fallacy: A critique of language statistics in psychological research. *Journal of Verbal Learning and Verbal Behavior, 12*(4), 335–359. https://doi.org/10.1016/S0022-5371(73)80014-3

Crais, E. R. (2011). Testing and beyond: Strategies and tools for evaluating and assessing infants and toddlers. *Language, Speech, and Hearing Services in Schools, 42*(3). 341–364. https://doi.org/10.1044/0161-1461(2010/09-0061)

Crais, E., Watson, L., & Baranek, G. (2009). Use of gesture development in profiling children's prelinguistic communication skills. *American Journal of Speech-Language Pathology, 1*(18), 95–108. https://doi.org/10.1044/1058-0360(2008/07-0041)

Christophe, A., Guasti, T., Nespor, M., Dupoux, E. & Van Ooyen, B. (1997). Reflections on phonological bootstrapping: Its role for lexical and syntactic acquisition. *Language and Cognitive Processes*, *12*(5–6), 585–612. https://doi.org/10.1080/016909697386637

Fenson, L., Dale, P., Reznick, J. S., Thal, D., Bates, E., Hartung, J., . . . Reilly, J. S. (1993). *The MacArthur Communicative Development Inventories: User's guide and technical manual.* Singular Publishing Group.

Fenson, L., Marchman, V. A., Thal, D. J., Dale, P. S., Reznick, J. S., & Bates, E. (2007). *MacArthur-Bates Communicative Development Inventories: User's guide and technical manual* (2nd ed.). Brookes.

Ferguson, B., Havy, M., & Waxman, S. (2015). The precision of 12-month-old infants' link between language and categorization predicts vocabulary size at 12 and 18 months. *Frontiers in Psychology*, *6*(1319), 1–6. https://doi.org/10.3389/fpsyg.2015.01319

Gaskell, M. G., & Ellis, A. W. (2009). Word learning and lexical development. *Philosophical Transactions of the Royal Society*, *364*, 3607–3615. https://doi.org/10.1098/rstb.2009.0213

Gathercole, S. E., & Baddeley, A. D. (1989). Evaluation of the role of phonological STM in the development of vocabulary in children: A longitudinal study. *Journal of Memory and Language*, *28*(2), 200–213. https://doi.org/10.1016/0749-596X(89)90044-2

Gathercole, S., Hitch, G., Service, E., & Martine, A. (1997). Phonological short-term memory and new word learning in children. *Developmental Psychology*, *33*(6), 966–979. https://doi.org/10.1037/0012-1649.33.6.966

Gentner, D. (2006). Why verbs are hard to learn. In K. Hirsh-Pasek & R. Golinkoff, (Eds.) *Action meets word: How children learn verbs* (pp. 544–564). Oxford University Press

Gershkoff-Stowe, L., & Hahn, E. (2007). Fast mapping skills in the developing lexicon. *Journal of Speech, Language, and Hearing Research*, *50*(3), 682–697. https://doi.org/10.1044/1092-4388(2007/048)

Gervits, F., Johanson, M., & Papafragou, A. (2016). Intentionality and the role of labels in categorization. *Cognitive Science Society*, 1146–1151. https://doi.org/10.1017/S1366728919000488

Gillam, R. (2002). The role of working memory in vocabulary development. *Perspectives on Language Learning and Education*, *9*(3), 7–11. https://doi.org/10.1044/lle9.3.7

Goldin-Meadow, S., & Singer, M. A. (2003). From children's hands to adults' ears: Gesture's role in the learning process. *Developmental Psychology*, *39*(3), 509–520. https://doi.org/10.1037/0012-1649.39.3.509

Goldin-Meadow, S., & Wagner, S. (2005). How our hands help us learn. *Trends in Cognitive Sciences*, *9*(5), 234–241. https://doi.org/10.1016/j.tics.2005.03.006

Golinkoff, R., & Hirsh-Pasek, K. (2008). How toddlers begin to learn verbs. *Trends in Cognitive Sciences, 12*(10), 397–403. https://doi.org/10.1016/j.tics.2008.07.003

Gray, S. (2006). The relationship between phonological memory, receptive vocabulary, and fast mapping in young children with specific language impairment. *Journal of Speech, Language, and Hearing Research, 49*(5), 955–969. https://doi.org/10.1044/1092-4388(2006/069)

Hansson, K., Forsberg, J., Lofqvist, A., Maki-Torkko, E., & Sahlen, B. (2004). Working memory and novel word learning in children with hearing impairment and children with specific language impairment. *International Journal of Language and Communication Disorders, 39*(3), 401–422. https://doi.org/10.1080/13682820410001669887

Hollich, G., Hirsh-Pasek, K., & Golinkoff, R. (2000). What does it take to learn a word? *Monographs of the Society for Research in Child Development, 65*(3), 1–16. https://doi.org/10.1111/1540-5834.00091

Iverson, J., & Goldin-Meadow, S. (2005). Gesture paves the way for language development. *Psychological Science, 16*(5), 367–371. https://doi.org/10.1111/j.0956-7976.2005.01542.x

Iverson, J., & Thal, D. (1998). Communicative transitions: There's more to the hand that meets the eye. In A. M. Wetherby, F. S. Warren, & J. Reichle (Eds.), *Transitions in prelinguistic communication* (pp. 59–86). Paul H. Brookes.

Jarrold, C., Thorn, A., & Stephens, E. (2009). The relationship among verbal short-term memory, phonological awareness, and new word learning: Evidence from typical development and down syndrome. *Journal of Experimental Child Psychology, 102*(2), 196–218. https://doi.org/10.1016/j.jecp.2008.07.001

Jusczyk, P. W., & Hohne, E. A. (1997). Infants' memory for spoken words. *Science, 277*(5334), 1984–1986. https://doi.org/10.1126/science.277.5334.1984

Lock, A. (1980). Language development, past, present and future. *Bulletin of the British Psychological Society, 33*, 5–8.

Lum, J., Conti-Ramsden, G., Page, D., & Ullman, M. (2012). Working, declarative and procedural memory in specific language impairment. *Cortex, 48*(9), 1138–1154. https://doi.org/10.1016/j.cortex.2011.06.001

Lum, J., & Kidd, E. (2012). An examination of the associations among multiple memory systems, past tense, and vocabulary in typically developing 5-year-old children. *Journal of Speech, Language, and Hearing Research, 55*(4), 989–1006. https://doi.org/10.1044/1092-4388(2011/10-0137)

McGregor, K. K. (2008). Gesture supports children's word learning. *International Journal of Speech-Language Pathology, 10*(3), 112–117. https://doi.org/10.1080/17549500801905622

McGregor, K., Friedman, R., Reilly, R., & Newman, R. (2002). Semantic representation and naming in young children. *Journal of Speech, Language, and Hearing Research*, *45*(2), 332–346. https://doi.org/10.1044/1092-4388(2002/026)

Montgomery, J., Magimairaj, B., & Finney, M. (2010). Working memory and specific language impairment: An update on the relation and perspectives on assessment and treatment. *American Journal of Speech-Language Pathology*, *19*(1), 78–94. https://doi.org/10.1044/1058-0360(2009/09-0028)

Morgan, J., & Demuth, K. (Eds.). (1996). Signal to syntax: *Bootstrapping from speech to grammar in early acquisition*. Psychology Press.

Nazzi, T., & Bertoncini, J. (2003). Before and after the vocabulary spurt: Two modes of word acquisition? *Developmental Science*, *6*(2), 136–142. https://doi.org/10.1111/1467-7687.00263

Nelson, K. (1983). The conceptual basis for language. In T. B. Seiler & W. Wannenmacher (Eds.), *Concept development and the development of word meaning. Springer Series in Language and Communication* (pp. 173–188). Springer.

Newbury, J., Klee, T., Stokes, S., & Moran, C. (2015). Exploring expressive vocabulary variability in two year olds: The role of working memory. *Journal of Speech, Language, and Hearing Research*, *58*(6), 1761–1772. https://doi.org/10.1044/2015_JSLHR-L-15-0018

Parish-Morris, J., Hennon, E., Hirsh-Pasek, K., Golinkoff, R., & Tager-Flusberg, H. (2007). Children with autism illuminate the role of social intention in word learning. *Child Development*, *78*(4), 1265–1287. https://doi.org/10.1111/j.1467-8624.2007.01065.x

Paul, R., & Norbury, C. (2012). *Language disorders from infancy to adolescence* (4th ed.). Elsevier.

Paul, R., Norbury, C., & Gosse, C. (2017). *Language disorders from infancy through adolescence: Listening, speaking, reading, writing, and communicating* (5th ed.). Elsevier.

Quinn, P., & Johnson, M. (2000). Global-before-basic object categorization in connectionist networks and 2-month-old infants. *Infancy*, *1*(1), 31–46. https://doi.org/10.1207/S15327078IN0101_04

Rowe, M., Qzcaliskan, S., & Goldin-Meadow, S. (2008). Learning words by hand: Gesture's role in predicting vocabulary development. *First Language*, *28*(2), 182–199. https://doi.org/10.1177/0142723707088310

Shneidman, L. A., Buresh, J. S., Shimpi, P. M., Knight-Schwarz, J., & Woodward, A. L. (2009). Social experience, social attention and word learning in an overhearing paradigm. *Language Learning and Development*, *5*(4), 266–281. https://doi.org/10.1080/15475440903001115

Stoel-Gammon, C. (2011). Relationships between lexical and phonological development. *Journal of Child Language*, *38*(1), 1–34. https://doi.org/10.1017/S0305000910000425

Swingley, D. (2009). Onsets and codas in 1.5-year-olds' word recognition. *Journal of Memory and Language, 60*(2), 252–269. https://doi .org/10.1016/j.jml.2008.11.003

Swingley, D. (2010). Fast mapping and slow mapping in children's word learning. *Language Learning and Development, 6,* 179–183. https://doi.org/10.1080/15475441.2010.484412

Tamis-LeMonda, C., Bornstein, M., & Baumwell, L. (2003). Maternal responsiveness and children's achievement of language milestones. *Child Development, 72*(3), 748–767. https://doi.org/0.1111/1467-8624.00313

Taxitari, L., Twomey, K., Westermann, G., & Mani, N. (2019). The limits of infant's early word learning. *Language Learning and Development, 16*(1), 1–21. https://doi.org/10.1080/15475441.2019.1670184

Tenenbaum, E., Amso, D., Abar, B., & Sheinkopf, S. (2014). Attention and word learning in autistic, language delayed and typically developing children. *Frontiers in Psychology, 5,* 490. https://doi.org/10.3389/fpsyg.2014.00490

Tomasello, M. (1995). Joint attention as social cognition. In C. Moore & P. J. Dunham (Eds.), *Joint attention: Its origins and role in development* (pp. 103–130). Lawrence Erlbaum Associates.

Turnbull, T., & Justice, L. (2012) *Language development from theory practice* (2nd ed.). Pearson.

Twomey, K., & Westermann, G. (2018). Curiosity-based learning in infants: A neurocomputational approach. *Developmental Science, 21*(4), 1–13. https://doi.org/10.1111/desc.12629

Ullman, M. T. (2001). The declarative/procedural model of lexicon and grammar. *Journal of Psycholinguistic Research, 30*(1), 37–69. https://doi.org/10.1023/A:1005204207369

Vihman, M. M. (1992). Early syllables and the construction of phonology. *Phonological development: Models, research, implications,* (pp. 393–422).

Wagner, S., Nusbaum, H., & Goldin-Meadow, S. (2004). Probing the mental representation of gesture: Is hand waving spatial? *Journal of Memory and Language, 50*(4), 395–407. https://doi.org/10.1016/j .jml.2004.01.002

Waxman, S., Fu, X., Aruachalam, S., Leddon, E., Geraghty, K., & Song, H. (2013). Are nouns learned before verbs? Infants provide insight into a long-standing debate. *Child Development Perspectives, 7*(3), 155–159. https://doi.org/10.1111/cdep.12032

Waxman, S., & Gelman, S. (2009). Early word-learning entails reference, not merely association. *Trends in Cognitive Science, 13*(6), 258–263. https://doi.org/10.1016/j.tics.2009.03.006

Westby, C. (2000). A scale for assessing children's play. In K. Gitlin-Weiner, A. Sandgrund, & C. Schaefer (Eds.), *Play diagnosis and assessment* (pp. 15–57). John Wiley & Sons.

Westermann, G., & Mareschal, D. (2013). From perceptual to language-mediated categorization. *Philosophical Transactions of the Royal Society, 369*(1634), 1–10. https://doi.org/10.1098/rstb.2012.0391

Wetherby, A. M., & Prizant, B. M. (1993). Profiling communication and symbolic abilities in young children. *Journal of Childhood Communication Disorders, 15*(1), 23–32. https://doi.org/10.1177/15257 4019301500105

Xu, J., Gannon, P., Emmorey, K., Smith, J., & Braun, A. (2009). Symbolic gestures and spoken language are processed by a common neural system. *Proceedings of the National Academy of Sciences, 106*(49), 20664–20669. https://doi.org/10.1073/pnas.0909197106

4

VOCABULARY EXPANSION FROM PRESCHOOL AND BEYOND

Lei Sun

> ## Chapter Objectives
>
> 1. Understand the connection between early and later lexical development.
> 2. Identify factors that facilitate vocabulary development in early school years.
> 3. Explain different methods that typically developing school-age children use to promote lexical expansion.

Introduction

The estimated number of English words known by young adults range from 9,800 to 215,000, depending on the definition of "word" and the tasks used by the researchers (Brysbaert et al., 2016). According to the authors, a 20-year-old native American English speaker knows about 42,000 root words (uninflected words), whereas Miller (1996) estimated 60,000 words known by a high school graduate, including proper names and idiomatic expressions, which equates to learning 10 new words a day. Nation and Waring (1997) reported a healthy native English speaker knows at least 20,000 words, including inflected and derived forms with a rate of 1,000 words per year starting from the age of 5. The estimated number of words learned by the time the individual reached early adulthood is inconclusive. Bloom (2004) challenged the simplicity of word calculation as word learning is not operating on an "all or none" basis, nor can it be calculated at a point in time. Bloom (2004) also questioned the use of the term "vocabulary spurt" (a rapid acceleration in word learning emerging around 18 months) specific to word learning at a young age, because not every child presents the phenomena of vocabulary spurt over the course of development. In addition, children significantly expand their vocabulary size when they start reading and utilizing morphological awareness and contextual cues to learn new words independently (Nippold, 2007). Therefore, the number is just a way to show that we continuously expand our vocabulary size throughout life. It does not represent how words are learned, how fast the new words are added to our lexicon, or how often we learn new words. Because of the exposure to new things (e.g., Google, Uber), new life experience (e.g., a new hobby, career), or new environment (e.g., moving to another country, learning a second language), we continue to add new words to our lexicon. The words we learn or use may shift depending on the contexts, experience, our world knowledge, and interests. Therefore, both the quantity and quality of the lexical knowledge should be considered rather than just a linear and straightforward calculation.

Beck, McKeown, and Kucan (2002) proposed three tiers of vocabulary. The first tier consists of basic and high-frequency words, such as happy, run, watch, dog, commonly used in conversation. Instruction is not necessary for Tier One vocabulary acquisition. The second tier comprises words that are frequently used by mature language users across different domains. These words may have multiple meanings and are usually learned from print and instruction. However, the lack of redundancy of Tier Two words makes learning these words challenging. The size of Tier Two vocabulary is a good indicator of the child's progress through school. Examples of Tier Two vocabulary include "fortunate, masterpiece, coincidence." Tier Three vocabulary are low-frequency, disciplinary-specific words. The size of Tier Three vocabulary is driven by the learner's interests and needs such as hobbies, academic field, occupation. These words are important when learning new concepts. Examples of Tier Three vocabulary include "amendment, peninsula, economics, isotope." Beck and colleagues (2002) estimated that Tier One has about 8,000 word families, and Tier Two contains about 7,000 word families. Therefore, for young children in early school years, the focus of word learning should be on Tier Two vocabulary. Stahl and Stahl (2012) referred to Tier Two words as Goldilocks words because "they are not too easy, not too difficult, but just right." (p. 76).

Vocabulary Development in Typically Developing Preschool Children

The development of Tier One vocabulary continues from the first birthday to preschool. Just like toddlers, preschool children make connections between concepts and words and among words to consolidate and retain new words. Through fast mapping, slow mapping, multiple exposures, and elaboration, typically developing (TD) young children quickly expand vocabulary by adding new words to existing word knowledge. It is like building a house. A good and solid foundation in lexicon and world knowledge is essential for lexical learning and information processing.

Shared Book Reading and Dialogic Reading

There is no doubt that young children learn their words primarily through linguistic input that occurs naturally from the environment, such as overhearing adult conversations, watching TV, playing with friends, and interacting with adults. Shared book reading may not be common in some cultures; however, research evidence supports the effects of book reading on promoting language development and school readiness (Ard & Beverly, 2004; Farrant & Zubrick, 2013; Mol et al., 2008; Wasik et al., 2016). Young children are not expected to learn words from reading books when they have not yet developed sufficient word recognition for reading. Therefore, shared book reading highlights the importance of the child's active participation in book reading while adults provide scaffolding during book reading. Shared book reading emphasizes the child's active participation by talking about pictures and adult's responsiveness through modeling, elaborating, and giving feedback. The main idea of shared book reading is to read with the child, not to the child (Fielding-Barnsley & Purdie, 2003; Mol et al., 2008). Ard and Beverly (2004) found that asking children questions and commenting throughout book reading facilitated expressive vocabulary, especially nouns, and commenting seemed to be more beneficial than asking questions. They also reported that shared book reading significantly improved receptive vocabulary more than expressive vocabulary. The finding is not surprising as the production of new words is more difficult than the comprehension of new words during fast mapping.

In a recent systematic review on vocabulary development and book reading done by Wasik et al. (2016), three factors important to word learning were described. These factors include (1) both explicit and implicit support provided to the child's word learning, such as definition, explanation, and association, (2) opportunities to process words for refining lexical representations, and (3) opportunities for the child to use words and to get feedback. Therefore, both systematic exposures and active processing of words are vital to word learning. Books provide a rich linguistic context for word learning. Wasik and colleagues (2016) also highlighted the benefit of learning words through book reading, including encountering a wide variety of words outside of daily conversation, increasing exposure to new words through the rereading of books, and offering opportunities for discussion of new words. In Mol et al.'s (2008) meta-analysis of dialogic book reading, the findings supported the importance of active adult involvement by posting open-ended questions and encouraging discussion during the book reading. They stressed that both the quantity and quality of the book reading are vital to language development. They also pointed out that dialogic reading is more beneficial to preschool-age children than kindergarten-age children as those school children might rely less on adult's facilitation during book reading. Pre-K children and kindergarteners may ask questions and request clarification when needed without the adult's prompting. We discuss the implementation of shared book reading and dialogic reading in detail in Chapter 8.

Based on the literature reviewed above, adult-child interaction during book reading is a natural and effective way to learn new words. Different strategies found to be effective in word learning through book reading include defining words, posting questions for elaboration and discussion, story retell, rereading, using props to elaborate on word meanings, and using follow-up activities after reading to discuss and explore new words. The combinations of these strategies are also commonly used by adults to promote learning new words and concepts.

In summary, shared book reading has been proved to be effective in promoting language development across language domains, including word knowledge. Book reading provides a rich, focused, interactive, and natural context for children to acquire new words and concepts. Additionally, because adults point out words and pictures throughout book reading, the structure facilitates the development of joint attention skills and vocabulary (Farrant & Zubrick, 2013). The key ingredient to effective book reading is to read "with" a child, especially with young children to highlight the "interactive" component. Even though repetitive book reading alone is sufficient for developing receptive vocabulary through multiple exposures, adult commenting during book reading is beneficial to the development of expressive vocabulary (Ard & Beverly, 2004). Stahl and Stahl (2012) suggested using picture talk and structured conversation to talk around words. Pictures can be previewed before reading as a foundation to discuss what the book is about and the new words. Pictures and discussions can help word learning in the story context, as well as post-reading activities to aid retention of the newly learned words. Farrant and Zubrick (2013) recommended that parents spend more than 10 minutes a day for shared book reading beginning early in a child's life until the early school years. It is essential to keep book reading as fun and as natural as possible to maintain the child's interest in book reading. Book reading should be enjoyable to the child, not an overwhelming experience. Using books based on a child's present level and within the child's zone of proximal development is recommended. Any books can be used to promote language development as long as adults use the right strategies with a manageable amount of new information during book reading.

From Semantic Network to Semantic Mapping

As discussed above, young learners acquire words through interaction with adults in conversation, play, and shared book reading. Furthermore, by actively listening and paying attention to social cues, young learners can form an initial mapping between the referent, sound pattern, and word with a shallow meaning. Even though it takes additional elaboration and exposure to further consolidate the word knowledge to retain in long-term memory, the initial word processing in short-term memory is vital. Depth of word knowledge accumulates over time, but how do children organize so many words? Why can some words be more easily retained than others?

Lexicon is organized much like a spider web, based on the semantic relations among the words. The words are like nodes, while the links indicate semantic relations connected between nodes (Beckage et al., 2010). Research has shown that late talkers learn words differently than typically developing peers in both quantitative and qualitative manners. Typically developing (TD) children are sensitive to connections between newly learned words and known words and acquire new words through the semantic association between new words and existing lexicon. Thus, TD children use known words to learn new words. On the other hand, late talkers seem to learn words slowly and in a less cohesive manner by simply adding new words to their lexicon without paying attention to semantic relations (Beckage et al., 2010). In general, new words are added based on the association between new words and existing known words. Or, when new words are more semantically related to the known words, they are more likely to enter the child's vocabulary (Hadley et al., 2018, p. 42; Hill et al., 2009;). Therefore, learning is facilitated by making an association between new words and existing known words, which also helps us develop vocabulary in a cohesive and organized manner. New words that have connections with existing words and categorical knowledge are more likely to be learned and retained than new words that have less semantic relations with prior knowledge (Borovsky et al., 2016; Hadley et al., 2018).

Hadley and colleagues (2018) suggested that dense semantic networks facilitate word processing and acquisition because preschoolers with rich vocabulary have more available "hooks" in the existing networks to acquire new words. Therefore, the depth of word knowledge can be achieved by creating more semantic relational connections that are conceptually linked. The finding of Hadley et al.'s (2018) study revealed that teaching words in a conceptually related fashion could deepen word knowledge. They recommended talking about "shared object function, perceptual and categorical features of words" to support the elaboration process because the shared information acts as a hook for new word learning (p. 55). Borovsky and colleagues' findings (2016) also supported that children even as young as two can more effectively recognize novel word meanings when they know more words in the same semantic category. Once again, children use their existing word knowledge to aid the acquisition of new words and vocabulary growth. Therefore, Borovsky et al. (2016) suggested that early word learning may be facilitated by using the semantic categories that the child has greater knowledge about (p. 16). For example, if the child is interested in transportation, new words such as motorcycle and scooter can easily be added to the child's existing repertoire because of the association between these two new words and bicycle, as well as other vehicles.

Our brief discussion on the semantic network assists readers in understanding how word knowledge grows and how new words are added to an existing repertoire. It also provides a good foundation for learning about a powerful vocabulary learning method, semantic mapping. Semantic mapping is defined as "a categorical structuring of information in the graphic form" (Johnson et al., 1986, p. 779). This teaching strategy is related to semantic networks because new words are learned through known words in semantically related networks. Semantic mapping uses graphic organizers to activate the child's existing knowledge about the word and visualize how concepts and words are related. Semantic mapping facilitates word acquisition by activating the child's prior knowledge and enhances retention by introducing the new words to existing semantic networks in a cohesive manner (Dilek & Yuruk, 2012; Stroller & Grabe, 1993). Different categories associated with the target word or concept are visually displayed to highlight the relationships among categories. Semantic mapping is used not only to facilitate vocabulary development, but also to support reading and studying skills (Dilek & Yuruk, 2012; Johnson et al., 1986). This method has been proved effective in teaching vocabulary and facilitating vocabulary learning through visualizing and highlighting the relationships between the words (Dilek & Yuruk, 2012; Saeidi & Atmani, 2010).

Semantic mapping has been commonly used in the classroom for different purposes, such as reading comprehension, word learning, across grades and contexts. It is a flexible and effective teaching method with one potential drawback. Baleghizadeh and Naeim (2011) suggested that semantic mapping may limit learners' mental ability to group related words if one fixed map is presented (p.13). One way to overcome this limitation is to change the map presentation and categories by relating words in different ways or adding new words to the map (Baleghizadeh & Naeim, 2011). For example, animals can be grouped based on where they live, what they eat, and how they look. Instead of grouping animals in a fixed category, children need to understand that animals can be grouped differently based on different features. Having flexible and expandable semantic maps help children to further refine and deepen their word knowledge. Another pitfall mentioned in Sokmen's article (1997) is that overusing semantic mapping may lead to cognitive overload due to the number of words introduced at once. Therefore, it is recommended that adults carefully control the number of words used in the map by assessing a child's current word knowledge. In addition, the maps should be incorporated into book reading and curriculum by providing multiple opportunities for review and expansion. Of course, the semantic mapping should be used according to a child's present level. Using both pictures and words for young learners is beneficial because pictures facilitate lexical development without creating too many cognitive demands. Two examples of semantic mapping, adapted from Stahl and Nagy (2006), Figures 4–1 and 4–2, are provided to be used with readers and pre-readers.

Clinical Implications

Most efficacy studies on semantic mapping are emphasized in the literature of teacher education, including teaching English language learners. As we learn from the research in semantic networks, the mental lexicon is organized like a spider web or library, and words are connected through semantic relations. Both semantic networks and semantic mapping capitalize on the importance of using existing word knowledge to facilitate the word learning process. Both methods highlight the importance of semantic relations in word acquisition and retention. The following steps are adapted from the general procedure of a semantic mapping lesson (Dilek & Yuruk, 2012; Johnson & Pearson, 1984; Johnson et al., 1986; Stahl & Nagy, 2006; Stahl & Stahl, 2012).

1. Choose a word and write on the whiteboard (can be a picture for pre-readers).
2. Encourage the child to brainstorm the words related to the keyword with other children and the clinician. The clinician leads the discussion and adds words with the explanation.

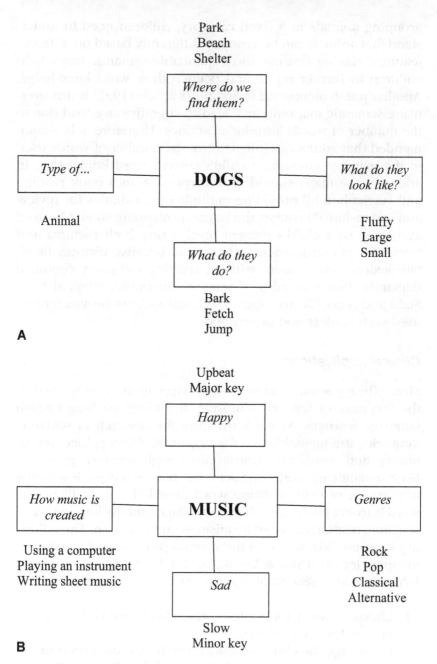

Figure 4–1. A. Semantic mapping using "dogs" as an example for readers. **B.** Semantic mapping using "music" as an example for readers (adapted from Stahl & Nagy, 2006).

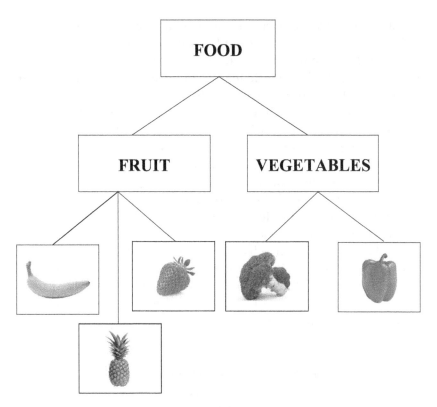

Figure 4–2. Semantic mapping using "food" as an example for nonreaders (adapted from Stahl & Nagy, 2006).

3. Ask each child to come up with a list of the words by category. Encourage the child to cluster words that they feel go together. All terms are drawn into a map on the whiteboard.
4. The clinician and the child discuss if new labels for categories are needed on the semantic map and why.
5. Engage in discussion with the child about the words on the map. Highlight the new words and how those new words are related to unknown words.

Better learning and retention can be achieved by deliberate learning with the opportunity to use a word with minimal assistance (Stahl & Nagy, 2006). Discussion is essential to using semantic mapping because it requires children to be active learners and enables children to connect new information to their existing word knowledge (Stahl & Vancil, 1986).

Another semantic elaboration technique related to semantic mapping is called semantic feature analysis and is mentioned in Sokmen (1997). Similar to semantic mapping, semantic feature analysis activates the child's prior knowledge to facilitate word retention and expand partial word knowledge through a discussion of common features. Again, discussions play an important role in both semantic elaboration techniques. However, semantic feature analysis may be appropriate for children with sufficient knowledge of most of the words listed in Table 4–1. As shown in the following example modified from Stahl (1999), the child is asked to use plus (+) and minus (–) sign to indicate the presence of semantic features listed on the top of the table. Table 4–1 shows an example of semantic feature analysis using Stahl and Nagy's template (2006, p. 93). Pictures paired with words can be used for pre-readers to promote lexical learning and bring the child's attention to print.

Table 4–1. Semantic Feature Analysis for Mammals

Mammals						
	Live in water	*Live on land*	*Able to fly*	*Have hooves*	*Have a pouch*	*Often live in trees*
Whales	+	–	–	–	–	–
Zebra	–	+	–	+	–	–
Bats	–	+	+	–	–	+
Elephants	–	+	–	–	–	–
Kangaroo	–	+	–	–	+	–
Sea Lion	+	–	–	–	–	–
Monkeys	–	+	–	–	–	+
Humans	–	+	–	–	–	–

Source: Adapted from Stahl & Nagy (2006, p. 93).

Lexical Development and Phonological Awareness

We reviewed the relationship between early phonological and lexical development in Chapter 1. As we discussed phonological short-term memory (PSTM) in Chapter 3, we also learn that PSTM is important in processing verbal information by encoding sound-based information for temporary storage. Children with good PSTM usually have good vocabulary knowledge. Gathercole and colleagues (1999) claimed that phonological memory skills were strongly related to vocabulary knowledge. Phonological awareness is defined as the ability to detect or manipulate sounds in spoken language (Lonigan, 2007). Phonological awareness is a set of metalinguistic skills and is related to phonological representations. These skills do not involve print and usually start to emerge around 3 years old. In addition, these skills develop in a sequence even though they may overlap (Schuele & Boudreau, 2008). How are phonological awareness and lexical development related?

Representations of words are more holistic in infants and toddlers and the representations become more "fine-grained and segmented" in preschool and school-age years (Lonigan, 2007, p. 24). As children learn more words, they start paying attention to the constituent parts. Therefore, lexical development not only "sets the stage for the development of phonological awareness" but also "predicts the growth of phonological awareness" (Lonigan, 2007, p. 24). In other words, children with larger vocabulary have lexicon presented segmentally, which facilitates the development of phonological awareness.

Metsala (1999) further discussed the process of segmental/phonemic restructuring of the lexicon. As the number of similar-sounding neighbors increases, children are under the pressure of developing more specific and distinct forms to store words in long-term memory. In other words, words in the dense neighborhood need more sophisticated phonological representations than words in the sparse neighborhood. For example, in order to differentiate between "bat" and its similar-sounding neighbors such as "bag," "cat," "hat," "bit," a more fine-grained representation is needed for "bat" to be stored for retrieval. This need drives the segmental/phonemic restructuring of lexical items.

Metsala (1999) claimed that early acquired, similar-sounding and highly familiar words have an advantage in the early restructuring process. Furthermore, her findings supported that the development of phonological awareness skills is correlated with vocabulary growth (Metsala, 1999, p. 17).

Because rhyming (words that end with identical sounds such as bat, cat, hat) and alliteration (words that share the same initial sound such as Mickey Mouse, pickled peppers, big black bug) are early developing phonological awareness skills, SLPs can work with preschool teachers to highlight the sounds shared by many words (rhymes) to enhance the connection between phonological and lexical representations. Taking advantage of words in the dense neighborhood (have many similar-sounding words) and high familiarity can facilitate the segmental restructuring process. As we know the importance of phonological awareness to literacy development, we want to highlight the connection between phonological awareness and vocabulary development. McBride-Chang et al. (2005) suggested that "phonological awareness becomes more distinct as vocabulary knowledge expands." Furthermore, the correlation between phonological processing and vocabulary development "is bidirectional and changes with development" (p. 428). Phonological awareness activities not only enhance phonological representations but also strengthen the connection between phonological and lexical representations. Using familiar and high-frequency words is a good starting point without cognitively burdening the child.

Vocabulary Expansion in Typically Developing School-Age Children and Adolescents

We have discussed children's amazing ability to learn words through fast mapping and extended mapping and from adult-child interaction to shared book reading. Anglin (1993) estimated that 4-year-olds know about 2,500 to 3,000 words, first graders know about 7,000 to 10,000 words, and fifth graders know 39,000 to 46,000 words. Nagy and Anderson (1984) estimated that by the end of 12th grade children are exposed to know roughly 88,700 words, and children typically learn 3,000 new words per year. How do children learn so many words in such a short time? We all know the answer is "reading." Books provide a rich context to learn words not commonly used in conversation, especially Tier Two vocabulary (Mol et al., 2008). Children learn to read beginning while very young when they hold and flip through a book and when they read with their parent. They develop print awareness by understanding that words and pictures are different, words run from left to right, and by holding the book in the right direction for reading. Preschoolers start to recognize letters, letter-sound correspondence, some sight words, as well as develop phonological awareness at the sentence, syllable, and word levels. Preschoolers are getting ready to learn to read by continuing advancement in oral language and developing their narrative skills (Justice et al., 2002). As illustrated in the reading rope by Scarborough (2001), it takes many skills to become a skilled reader. Reading is a multifaceted and complex learning process. The discussion of reading development is beyond the scope of this book. Even though we highlight the effect of reading on vocabulary development, readers need to keep in mind that other skills, such as word recognition, background knowledge, phonological awareness, and overall oral language development are equally important to written language development.

Vocabulary is the cornerstone of oral and written language development and the core of literacy. When we encounter too many unknown words in one paragraph, it affects our reading fluency and reading comprehension. Imagine reading a biochemical journal article or an article written in another language. Gambrell and colleagues (1981) found that fourth graders, with good reading skills, have one unknown word in every 100 words when reading a grade-level instructional material. On the other hand, poor readers encounter one unknown word in every 10 words read (Johnson and colleagues, 1986). The Matthew effect refers to the phenomenon "rich get richer while poor get poorer." It is a cumulative advantage that people who have more in the first place tend to acquire more. The Matthew effect has been used to explain the widening gap between good readers and poor readers over time because the reading performance is correlated to what the reader brings to the table, including vocabulary knowledge, background knowledge, reading fluency, and oral language skills (Stanovich, 1986). The Matthew effect can also be used to explain the semantic networks discussed earlier. Children who have less extensive vocabulary knowledge have fewer hooks to connect to the new words, which slows down their word acquisition process (Hadley et al., 2018).

Along the same line, Cain and Oakhill (2011) reported that children with reading difficulties have slower vocabulary growth. Both reading comprehension and reading experience were correlated with vocabulary development between the ages of 8 and 16. Similar to the fast mapping observed in young learners, older children learn new words through incidental exposure in reading. Wagovich et al. (2015) reported that both TD children and children with low language skills can acquire new words from the incidental reading experience. However, children with low language skills developed significantly less partial word knowledge than TD peers. Wagovich and colleagues (2015) suggested that children with low language skills were able to retain new words 2 to 3 days like their TD peers after several exposures in the same context. However, due to less partial word knowledge formed through incidental reading experience, these children need more exposures and additional support in acquiring new words. Verhoeven et al. (2011) examined vocabulary growth and reading development across the elementary school years. They suggested that continued vocabulary growth is crucial to word decoding and reading comprehension. The children's vocabulary in first grade predicted their second-grade reading comprehension, which in turn predicted their vocabulary in third grade (p. 19). Their findings indicated a reciprocal relationship between vocabulary growth and reading comprehension. In other words, children's early vocabulary knowledge assists children's early reading acquisition, and early reading skills, in turn, facilitates vocabulary expansion and advancement. Therefore, as children develop their vocabulary, their reading can also be promoted (p. 21). Given the importance of vocabulary knowledge to reading development, Verhoeven et al. (2011) advocated the pressing need for intensive vocabulary training throughout the elementary school years. In addition, children with limited language skills should be provided with abundant opportunities to develop vocabulary.

Wasik and colleagues (2016) reminded us that better word retention takes more than merely mapping the word to the referent. Active and deliberate learning of new words requires an understanding of the word meanings, multiple exposures to words in meaningful and diverse contexts, and opportunities to use words and get feedback from adults. Books not only offer a language-rich context to learn words outside of daily conversation, but also provide multiple exposures to the words in the same context through re-reading (Wasik et al., 2016). There is no doubt that vocabulary is essential to reading development, and reading, in turn, is needed for vocabulary expansion and advancement. Although children can gain partial word knowledge through incidental book reading without direct instruction, what else do children do to learn new words?

Changes From Early to Later Lexical Development

Word learning is a continuous and cumulative process, from partial word competence to more comprehensive word knowledge, and from Tier One to Tier Two and three vocabularies. Both internal factors such as cognitive and linguistic development and external factors such as a variety of resources for language learning contribute to later language and lexical development. Nippold (2007) pointed out four variables that make later language development different from early language development including, (1) increasing ability in abstract thinking, (2) the development of metalinguistic skills, (3) different sources for language learning, and (4) continued development in social perspective-taking and inference making.

Children's ability to think beyond the immediate context and make connections between words and intangible things (e.g., freedom, diversity) increases over time. Language development somehow parallels cognitive development. As we learned from Piaget's four stages of cognitive development, significant changes happen from the preoperational stage to the formal operational stage. During the formal operational stage, starting age 12, children are able to think abstractly and reason about hypothetical problems by using deductive and logical reasoning. Therefore, as children's cognitive abilities progress, they understand and think about abstract ideas, concepts, and situations without heavily relying on previous experience.

The second variable is the development of metalinguistic skills. Metalinguistic skills require children to reflect on, analyze, and manipulate language that is beyond meaning (Gombert, 1992). Essentially, metalinguistic competence enables children to consciously think about language and how language is used. For example, children start thinking about or playing with sound units when they have good phonological representations about the speech sounds. From sentence level to phoneme level sound manipulation, children gradually develop their ability to analyze syllables and sounds through different phonological awareness activities. Metalinguistic skills are required for children to define a word, to fix a grammatically incorrect sentence, to analyze word parts, and to develop written language and spelling skills.

The third variable that Nippold (2007) mentioned in her book is the sources of language learning. Schooling and the transition from "learning to read" to "reading to learn" enable children to expose to a wide variety of words across contexts and expand their word knowledge beyond direct instruction. Reading habits and experience are related to vocabulary development and reading comprehension (Cain & Oakhill, 2011). Books offer language-rich contexts for children to learn low frequency, abstract, and morphologically complex words. Nippold (2007) claimed that school-age children must understand later linguistic forms, including advanced adverbial conjuncts (e.g., *moreover*, *in contrast*), adverbs of likelihood and magnitude (e.g., *possibly*, *extremely*), technical terms related to curricular content (e.g., *bacteria, protein*), metalinguistic and metacognitive verbs (e.g., *imply*, *hypothesis*), words with multiple meanings (e.g., *strike, short*), and words with multiple grammatical functions (e.g., *hard, sweet*). Nippold (2018) referred to these later developing and advanced vocabularies as "literate lexicon." Literate lexicon is defined as "difficult words that occur in academic contexts, particularly middle and high school classes." (p. 211). Therefore, reading and schooling allow school-age children to expand both word and world knowledge beyond learning words through overhearing conversations between adult-child interactions commonly seen in preschool children.

The fourth variable is social perspective-taking and inference making. Perspective-taking and inference making are crucial for both oral and written language development because we always consider other people's perspectives and intentions when we communicate. Understanding that people have different beliefs, intentions, desires from ours is the development of Theory of Mind (ToM). Joint attention and intentionality are the precursors of ToM development. Therefore, the ability to put ourselves into someone's mental shoes starts to emerge around 13 to 15 months and continues to refine in adolescence (Korkmaz, 2011). Mental state words are used to monitor, interpret, and express internal states of people. The use of these terms is a key indicator of the development of ToM. Before age 3, children are able to talk about emotions (e.g., happy, sad), thoughts (e.g., know,) and beliefs (e.g., think) without a full comprehension of the mental implications of these words (Olson & Astington, 1993; Westby & Robinson, 2014). By age 5, preschoolers begin to understand that people have different beliefs, and these beliefs change depending on time, situation, and environment (Olson & Astington, 1993). The evidence of this improvement is that 5-year-olds consistently pass the first-order false belief tasks (realization of other's false beliefs about real events e.g., Sally-Anne task, smarties task). Researchers have advocated the discussion of different mental states with children to promote the awareness of their own and other people's desire (e.g., hope, need), cognition (e.g., believe, doubt), emotion (e.g., scare, surprise), perception (e.g., feel), and communication (e.g., admit, confirm) (Westby, 2013; Bang et al., 2013). Nippold (2007) also pointed out that school-age children encounter metalinguistic verbs, acts of speaking (e.g., predict, interpret, imply) and metacognitive verbs, acts of thinking (e.g., conclude, hypothesize, infer) frequently in oral and written language across settings. The ability to understand more advanced mental state terms indicates continued ToM development. Children age 6 to 8 years can understand what someone is thinking or feeling about what someone else is thinking and feeling. From age 8 and above, children begin understanding different types of figurative language, which requires continued development in ToM (Miller, 2009; Westby & Robinson, 2014, Westby, 2012). A thorough discussion of ToM and language is beyond the scope of this book. We want to include this piece of information because vocabulary has a wide variety of subtypes even within the same class, such as the difference between action verbs and mental state verbs. Different cognitive processes may underline different developmental sequences for different types of words. SLPs need to consider what abilities may be required for word learning when selecting words for therapy.

SLPs know well that children with language deficits show slow word learning process and difficulty with retention of new linguistic information. Children with language deficits have delayed development in abstract thinking, metalinguistic skills, perspective-taking, and written language development because of the limitations in language and cognitive processes. However, before we offer strategies to help children with language deficits, it is beneficial to learn how TD children expand and extend their vocabulary because children with language deficits still follow similar developmental sequences. Besides using the dictionary and direct teaching, Nagy and Scott (2000) suggested that typically developing school-age children often figure out the meaning of the new word through using context and morphology (word parts) (p. 275). Students are able to form an initial hypothesis of the word meaning through incidental learning by using both structure and context analysis (Carlisle, 2007). Therefore, we discuss both strategies commonly used by typically developing school-age children below in detail.

The Power of Context Clues

Context clues in a text may involve illustrations, examples, images, tables, or typographic information, such as bold and italic text. Context clues also include syntactic clues such as word order and the relation between words, as well as semantic clues such as synonyms, antonyms, definitions that offer meaning-based information (Baumann, Edwards, Boland, & Font, 2012, p. 146). According to Nagy and Herman (1987), children may learn 5% to 12% of the new words from a single exposure in the context. Graves (1986) estimated that children learn 1,000 to 5,000 new words from context during a school year, depending on the child's reading ability (Kuhn & Stahl, 1998). However, researchers have cautioned about the ineffectiveness of using context clues to aid word learning (Baumann, Edwards, Boland, & Font, 2012; Kuhn & Stahl, 1998; Schmitt & McCarthy, 1997; Spencer & Guillaume, 2006; Stahl & Nagy, 2006).

Using context clues for word learning has a long history in vocabulary instruction because it may facilitate reading comprehension. The literature on the effects of using context clues on word learning is limited and has conflicting results (Fukkink & de Glopper, 1998). In addition, context does not always reveal word meaning and may confuse readers when not used properly. In order to infer word meaning from the context successfully, children need to present sufficient background information about the topic, an understanding of meanings of other words in the context, an ability to use syntactic information from the sentence, and an awareness that meaning may go beyond the context (inference making). Without sufficient background knowledge, children cannot infer word meaning from context nor select an appropriate definition from the dictionary. Therefore, using context to infer new word meanings is not straightforward and involves many metalinguistic skills, including meta-semantics, meta-syntax, and meta-pragmatics (Nagy, 2007). Schmitt and McCarthy (1997) also added some challenges related to context use from the perspective of second language education. They pointed out that the guessing process of deriving meaning from the context is very slow, and sometimes context clues may be misleading. In addition, guessing from the context does not result in long-term retention. Monolingual-English speaking children with language deficits may encounter similar challenges to English language learners when using context clues to derive word meanings. As mentioned earlier, using context clues is essentially a metalinguistic ability. Metalinguistic skills require that children reflect on and consciously ponder about language and how language is used, as well as to develop the awareness of language components that go beyond the meaning. Unfortunately, children with language deficits usually fall behind in developing basic language skills and have even more difficulty with metalinguistic skills across the language domains.

Does it mean that using context clues should not be considered as an instructional strategy? Even though most research challenged the effectiveness of using context clues in inferring word meaning, it may be used with the support of discussion, feedback, and practice. Based on Fukkink's study (2005), children who start using contextual analysis may be good candidates for this method, and additional instruction on context use may improve the quality of learning word meanings from the context. Cain's findings (2007) suggested that asking children to further explain their reasoning behind definitions may facilitate children's ability to derive word meanings from the context. Also, adult's feedback on children's definitions and repeated practice improve their inferential skills and their meaning derivation process (Cain, 2007).

Clinical Implications

Many learning strategies used by school-age children require a good language foundation and adequate metalinguistic skills, which poses significant challenges to children with weak language skills and even more for children with language deficits. As Nagy (2007) mentioned in his article, the metalinguistic demands of word learning increase when a child moves to upper-grade levels. Therefore, school-based SLPs should carefully consider the cognitive and linguistic demands associated with a task, and what a child can bring to the table for learning new information. There is no best method. It is always about what works best for a child across settings while considering the child's zone of proximal development (ZPD). As we always do, incorporating modeling, discussion, and explanation into our therapy activities is necessary. Giving children plenty of opportunities to practice with our guidance and feedback is essential. Finally, carefully controlling the materials used in the session based on a child's ZPD to avoid cognitively burdening the child should always be considered. When teaching a new strategy such as using context clues, utilizing familiar passages that contain most of the known words would direct the child's attention to the strategy.

Beck and colleagues (1983) also supported that not every context can be used as effective instructional means for word learning. They recommended using pedagogical contexts specially designed for teaching unknown words, not natural contexts such as stories that do not necessarily provide cues for meaning derivation. They further suggested that effective vocabulary instruction should include pedagogical contexts with the discussion of the new word meanings. In addition, allowing children to use words in various contexts, making associations between newly learned words and known words, and comparing/contrasting differences in word meanings through discussion will facilitate word acquisition and retention.

Beck et al. (1983) and Stahl and Nagy (2006) claimed that context clues function on a continuum of effectiveness in natural contexts from directive (e.g., **Vulnerable** people are oftentimes *in need of protection under certain laws so others cannot take advantage of them.* [Example from http://www.teachthought. com]) to nondirective contexts (e.g., Freddie looked over the members of the team he'd been assigned. Each looked more **hapless** than the next.). Baumann, Font, Edwards, and Boland (2005) further specified five different types of directive context clues, as shown in Table 4–2. Please keep in mind that the examples used in therapy should be modified based on a child's current curriculum and present level. Since the content areas serve as a context for vocabulary development, school-based SLPs may collaborate with teachers to come up with examples

Table 4–2. Different Types of Directive Context Clues

Context Clues	
Context Clue Type	**Example**
1. **Definition:** the author explains the meaning of the word right in the sentence or selection.	The new neighbor was seen as **reclusive**, or *uninterested in the company of others*, and had only been seen peering out from behind his curtains.
2. **Synonym:** the author uses a word similar in meaning.	Lauren dribbled the ball down the court with unmatched **tenacity**. Her *persistence* did not go unnoticed by the coach.
3. **Antonym:** the author uses a word nearly opposite in meaning.	As a **frugal** spender himself, Andre could not understand Lacey's need for such *extravagance*.
4. **Example:** the author provides one or more example words or ideas.	**Amphibians** need a moist environment to survive. Because of this, you often find *frogs, toads, newts* and *salamanders* in swamps or rainforests.
5. **General:** the author provides several words or statements that give clues to the word's meaning.	She appeared rather **nonchalant** about the matter. While the patron yelled loudly, she observed *calmly* from the corner of the room, before she *shrugged* and sauntered away.

Source: Adapted from Baumann, Font, Edwards, & Boland (2005).

suitable for each child. Using a child's current curriculum not only minimizes the cognitive loads due to the child's familiarity with the materials, but also gives the child the opportunity for generalization of what the child has learned.

As Baumann, Edwards, Boland, and Font's (2012) work mentioned, context clues can be further categorized into syntactic cues and semantic cues. However, the literature on the discussion of context clues is sparse. Sinatra and Dowd (1991) specified six types of syntactic clues as listed in Table 4–3.

Sinatra and Dowd (1991) explained the key idea is to look at the overall idea within and between sentences of the semantic clues, not the grammatical structures (p. 226). Only some subtypes and examples are listed in Table 4–4 because other types of semantic context clues may overlap with Baumann, Font, Edwards, and Boland's (2005) five types of context clues listed above. The examples can be found in the content areas with some preparation by discussing with teachers about the examples used in the curriculum.

A typical lesson to teach context clues includes the following steps: (1) Pause when you find an unknown word; (2) Read the surrounding words and sentences to look for context clues; (3) Use the clues to infer the meaning of the unknown word; (4) Try out your inference to see if it makes sense (Graves et al., 2017, p. 537). Graves and colleagues (2017) suggested starting with definitions followed by synonyms, antonyms, and general clues when increasing the complexity of types of context clues the student has to deal with. The use of context clues is also highlighted in Common Core State Standards. For example, a second-grader is expected to use sentence-level context as a clue to derive the meaning of a word or phrase (CCSS.ELA-LITERACY.L.2.4.A), a fourth-grader is expected to use context (e.g., definitions, examples, or restatements in text) as a clue to derive the meaning of a word or phrase (CCSS.ELA-LITERACY .L.4.4.A), and a fifth-grader can use context (e.g., cause/effect relationships and comparisons in text) as a clue to derive the meaning of a word or phrase (CCSS.ELA-LITERACY.L.5.4.A). An example of a CCSS-oriented goal may be "the student will use context clues (e.g., syntactic information, synonyms, examples, word relations) to derive the meaning of the unknown

Table 4–3. Types, Definitions, and Examples of Syntactic Clues

Type	Definition	Examples
Predicate noun	The predicate noun can be equivalent to the subject noun or indicate an example.	That beautiful creature is a *flamingo*.
Coordinating conjunction	The coordinating conjunctions (and, but, or) link ideas of similar importance.	Last Saturday, Shelley parked her car near the junction, or intersection, of Gridley Creek and 25th Avenue.
Direct explanation	The word is directly defined in the sentence.	*Vulnerable* people are often in need of protection under certain laws, so others cannot take advantage of them.
Serial comma	Words in a particular category or with the same general meaning may be linked by serial comma.	• North American *predators* include grizzly bears, pumas, wolves, and foxes • The debris in the stadium stands included numerous paper cups, ticket stubs, sandwich wrappings, and cigarette butts.
Appositive structure	A noun or noun phrase immediately follows another noun to explain or identify it.	• *Discrimination*, the act of showing bias to one group, can have damaging effects.
Adjective structure	The adjective structure is located before or after the noun to modify it. These clauses are usually separated by commas.	• The *laptop*, dented from the fall, appeared to be broken beyond repair. • The *server*, who quickly took their order, returned momentarily with their beverages.

Sources: Adapted from Sinatra, R. and Dowd, C. (1991, pp. 226–227) and from Nippold, M. (2007, p. 31)

words." It is important to keep in mind that these standards are developed based on typically developing children. For children with language deficits, SLPs need to consider a child's present

Table 4–4. Types, Definitions, and Examples of Semantic Clues

Type	Definition	Example
Anaphoric relation	The meaning associations between words. Words in one sentence are used to replace other words.	The *veterinarian* was examining the puppy for fleas. She has been caring for animals in need for many years.
Restatement	The second sentence provides the meaning for the first sentence.	The first impression that crossed my mind was that the woman was *obese*. Her clothing was stretched across her vast surface of the skin like a lumpy balloon stretched to the bursting point.
Summary	The author makes a string of statements to help readers understand the word meaning.	Andrea was a very *impertinent* young lady; she was so rude that she talked while her teacher was explaining a lesson and showed no respect for other students. Her manners were very poor. Even her parents thought that Andrea was impolite.
Examples	Examples are provided to illustrate the meaning of the unknown word.	*Piscatorial* creatures, such as flounder, salmon, and trout, live in the coldest parts of the ocean. (https://www.mdc.edu/kendall/collegeprep/documents2/context%20cluesrev8192.pdf)
Figure of speech	The authors try to make abstract ideas more concrete by using simile, metaphor, and so forth.	• Alveoli are tiny balloon shaped structures and are the smallest passageway in the respiratory system. (simile) • White blood cells protect the body against both infectious disease and foreign invaders. (metaphor)
Comparison/ Contrast	The clues that tell the reader what the word does not mean.	The conversation with his boss regarding his resignation was not unpleasant but *cordial*.

Table 4–4. *continued*

Type	Definition	Example
Cause/ Effect	Use cause effect relationship to predict the word meaning. Signal words may include because, since, so, thus, and so forth.	She wanted to impress all her dinner guests with the food she served, so she carefully studied the necessary *culinary* arts. (https://www. mdc.edu/kendall/collegeprep/ documents2/context%20 cluesrev8192.pdf)
Mood	The meaning can be inferred from the overall tone that the writer tries to convey.	The doctor's office was so clean and shiny that Merton thought even the chairs must be *sterile*. (https://resources .readingvine.com/what-are- the-different-types-of-context- clues/)

Source: Adapted from Sinatra, R. and Dowd, C. (1991, pp. 226–227) and from Nippold, M. (2007, p. 31)

level and baseline data when developing the goals. Thus, a sixth-grader with language deficits may have a goal comparable to second-grade standards. Progress tracking may require data collection from both therapy sessions and learning in class. SLPs can also train a child with some self-monitoring strategies when the child becomes more independent in using context clues. Some self-monitoring questions may include, "What kind of clues did I use?" "Did the context clues help? Why? Why not?" Details in implementing context clues are discussed in Chapter 8.

Morphological Structure Awareness/Word Part Analysis

When context clues are clear, the need for using word part analysis may not be always necessary. As we learned from the literature, context analysis may not always work. Thus, we next discuss morphological structure awareness, which is an ability to use word parts to derive word meanings. A morpheme is the smallest unit of meaning in a given language. Free morphemes (e.g., cat, tree) can stand alone and refer to their semantic meanings whereas bound morphemes (e.g., -s, -ing, -ness) have to attach to free morphemes to function and carry syntactic purposes. There are two types of bound morphemes. Inflectional morphemes indicate the grammatical function of a word, such as plurality, verb tense, or procession. These are usually developed and mastered much earlier than derivational morphemes. Derivational morphemes, affixes attached before or after the word, are used to create new words or a new form of an existing word by changing the grammatical class. For example, the word "happy" (adjective) can be changed to "unhappy" (adjective) "happiness" (noun). Compound words are created by combining two free morphemes into one word, such as "cowboy," "toothbrush." Similar to using context clues, analyzing word parts is a metalinguistic skill that requires a child to think about the component morphemes consciously. McBride-Chang et al. (2005) reported that both morpheme identification and morphological structure awareness are important to fostering word learning. In other words, the ability to analyze the word parts makes it easier to learn new words and generalize these morphemes to new contexts. Similar to phonological awareness mentioned earlier, the larger vocabulary repertoire a child has, the more examples of morphologically related words a child can draw from when learning new words. It helps a child to become more aware of morphological relationships between the words, which in turn facilitates the use of word part knowledge to infer the meanings of unknown words (Carlisle, 2007; Nagy, 2007).

Why Teach Word Parts?

Anglin (1993) suggested that children learn newly derived words at a rate of more than three times that of learning new root words. Furthermore, students learn 4,000 root words, but 14,000 derived words between first and fifth grade. Nagy and Anderson (1984) claimed that about 60% of unfamiliar words students encounter in texts are derived words whose meanings can be figured out by analyzing word parts (Carlisle, 2007). Kirby and

Bowers (2012) also estimated one to three additional morphological related words can be easily understood for every word we learn. For example, words that can be elicited from the root word "nat (birth, born)" include native, innate, nation, prenatal, and so forth. People can infer the meaning of these derived words from the root word, which allows for vocabulary extension and expansion (Schmitt & McCarthy, 1997). Nippold (2007) claimed that morphological awareness skills increase significantly from 4th grade to 8th grade and continue to develop into adulthood. Along the same vein, Nagy, Diakidoy, and Anderson (1993) recommended that teaching morphological analysis may be appropriate from 4th grade and above.

Morphology is crucial to vocabulary acquisition and reading. Working on morphological awareness can also improve orthography and phonological awareness. For example, the word "uncomfortable" can be pronounced by breaking the word into component morphemes as un-comfort-able, which also helps with how the word is written. Children with language deficits have difficulty using word part analysis because they may have a limited size of root words and affixes to infer the meaning and limited morphological related words to draw from. These limitations prevent children with language deficits from using this powerful strategy effectively, which in turn makes their vocabulary expansion much slower than their peers (Kirby & Bowers, 2012; Wolter & Green, 2013). Kirby and Bowers (2012) recommended that morphological instruction is more effective for children in early grades (Pre-K to second grade) and children with underdeveloped language skills. Because morphological analysis involves phonology, orthography, and semantics, it should be used in conjunction with other curriculum-based learning activities such as spelling and word association. Beck, McKeown, and Kucan (2002) reminded us that emphasizing relationships among words is important to word learning because words are organized like a network. Therefore, these connections serve as entry points to access word knowledge and build new words upon existing words. Children can generalize what they have learned about affixes to infer the meanings of new words, such as from neighborhood to brotherhood, or motherhood.

What Word Parts to Teach?

Children learn most inflectional morphemes during the preschool years, including some early developing derivational suffixes such as -er (e.g., teacher) and -y (e.g., cheesy). As children move to upper-grade levels, they continue to expand their Tier Two words and encounter more Tier Three, low-frequency words in textbooks across content areas. White, Sowell, and Yanagihara (1989) reported that 20 prefixes accounted for 97% of prefixed words in printed school English, and the top nine prefixes accounted for 79% of the prefixed words. The nine prefixes should be included in instruction are un-, re-, in-/im-/il-/ir- (not), dis, en-/em-, non-,in-/im-(in), over-, mis- (Stahl & Nagy, 2006). On the other hand, suffixes have relatively less clear meanings. The top seven suffixes accounted for 82% of suffixed words including -s/-es, -ed, -ing, -ly, -er/-or (agent), -ion/-tion/-ation/-ition, -able/-ible. It is clear that inflectional suffixes are more frequently used than derivational suffixes in textbooks. Even though derivational suffixes appear fewer than a quarter of all suffixed words, Stahl and Nagy (2006) still suggest that we teach them because knowing these suffixes assist with learning low-frequency Tier Three words often encountered across content areas in upper grades. For example, the ability to break down "transportation" into its components (e.g., trans [across, through]-port [move]-ation [a noun]) helps children understand other morphologically related words such as import, export, portable, deportation derived from the root word "port." Additionally, transgender, transform, transparent, translate, and so forth, can be understood by combining the of prefix "trans-" and base form (e.g., gender, form). The suffix "ation" helps children identify the word as a noun and its function in the sentence.

However, there are always exceptions to the rules that make utilizing the word learning strategies less straightforward. Carlisle (2007) mentioned two types of morphological transparency that may impede the analysis of the morphological structure. First, the connection between the derived word and root word may be less phonologically transparent when the phonological representation of the root word changes during derivation. For example, "courage" to "courageous," "decide" to "decision" or "decisive," "tragic" to "tragedy." The other issue may arise from semantic transparency, which means the meaning may be very different between the derived word and the root word. Carlisle (2007) used "apply" and "appliance" as an example of a less transparent connection between a root word and its derived form. Besides, Stahl and Nagy (2006) emphasized not to over-generalize the meaning of word parts without referring back to the context and not to assume that affixes have fixed meanings. For example, "re-" in "report" has nothing to do with "again," and "un-" in "unload" and "unhappy" also have different meanings. Incorporating the discussion of common Greek roots (e.g., auto, bio, hypo, micro, mono, hyper, tele), common Latin roots (e.g., port, struct, aqua, ject, multi, rupt, fort), common prefixes (e.g., anti-, de-, dis-, en/em, in-/im-/il-/ir, inter-, non, mis-, pre-, re-) and common suffixes (e.g., -able/ -ible, -al/-ial, -ed, -en, -er, -ful, -ion/-tion/-ation/-ition, -ity/-ty, -less) as suggested in McEwan's book titled "The Reading Puzzle: Word Analysis" (2008) is strongly recommended.

Clinical Implications

Despite the fact that the benefit of teaching word parts is well documented in the literature, morphological analysis is not routinely and explicitly used in the classroom (Kirby & Bowers, 2012; Nunes & Bryant, 2006). Researchers remind us that referring back to a child's curriculum and considering developmental sequences for target selection is the best practice for school-based SLPs. Therefore, compound words should be used with kindergarteners with language deficits since children as young as three may start combining free morphemes to refer to objects with similar functions, such as toothbrush, hairbrush and create new words to label new things, such as finger-brush, cat-brush (Apel & Diem, 2013; Carlisle, 2007). When children move to lower grades, SLPs should emphasize inflectional and early developing derivational morphemes (e.g., -er, -y,-est). Derivational morphemes (e.g., -ness, -tion, -less) and common Latin and Greek word roots (e.g., cent, aud, port, rupt) should be the focus in upper grades (Apel & Diem, 2013; Harris et al., 2011; Helman et al. , 2015). Common Latin and Greek roots can be easily found on the internet (e.g., *Reading Rockets*) and textbooks. Graves, Schneider, and Ringstaff (2017) also suggest a similar sequence to increase the complexity of morphological analysis by starting with inflections, and then followed by prefixes, derivational suffixes, and finally, Latin and Greek roots. It is important to keep in mind that young children with language deficits continue to struggle with inflectional morphemes as they move to elementary school. Therefore, they may experience greater difficulty when learning derivational morphemes (Wolter & Green, 2013).

A common word parts lesson may include the following steps: (1) Look for the root word. Decide if the word can be broken into smaller word parts. See if you know the meaning of the root word. (2) Think about the meaning of each part, including the part before the root word (prefix) and the part after the root word (suffix). (3) Combine the meanings of the parts to build the meaning of the unknown word. (4) Try out your inference to see if the meaning makes sense (Baumann, Edwards, Boland, Olejnik, & Kame'enui, 2003; Graves et al., 2017, p. 536). There are many fun activities to teach morphological analysis, such as word sort and word building, discussed in the literature (Gibson & Wolter, 2015; Kirby & Bowers, 2012). Incorporating visuals such as a matrix, tables, and color-coded cards will help children understand the use of word parts to create new words and derive word meaning. It is always important to keep in mind that using existing words and common affixes reviewed earlier as a starting point can gradually up the ante. Once the child understands the procedure of using morphological analysis and has knowledge of some common affixes, ask the child to look for words used in the curriculum and books and practice using the strategy to infer meanings of new words. As usual, multiple exposures, discussions, and maximal practice are needed for all kinds of learning.

The importance of vocabulary learning has been explicitly stated or implicitly implied in Common Core State Standards across content areas (Fisher & Frey, 2014). In addition, using both context clues and common and grade-appropriate Greek and Latin affixes and roots as clues to access the word meaning are stated in Common Core State Standards of the ELA standards. For example, a second-grader is expected: to determine the meaning of the new word formed when a known prefix is added to a known word (e.g., *happy/unhappy, tell/retell*) (CCSS.ELA-

LITERACY.L.2.4.B); to use a known root word as a clue to the meaning of an unknown word with the same root (e.g., *addition, additional*) (CCSS.ELA-LITERACY.L.2.4.C); and to use knowledge of the meaning of individual words to predict the meaning of compound words (e.g., *birdhouse, lighthouse, housefly; bookshelf, notebook, bookmark*) (CCSS.ELA-LITERACY.L.2.4.D). Based on CCSS ELA standards, third graders are expected to determine the meaning of a new word formed when a known affix is added to a known word (e.g., *agreeable/disagreeable, comfortable/uncomfortable, care/careless, heat/preheat*) (CCSS.ELA-LITERACY.L.3.4.B), and use a known root word as a clue to the meaning of an unknown word with the same root (e.g., *company, companion*) (CCSS.ELA-LITERACY.L.3.4.C). When moving to fifth grade, students are expected to use common, grade-appropriate Greek and Latin affixes and roots as clues to the meaning of a word (e.g., *photograph, photosynthesis*) (CCSS.ELA-LITERACY.L.5.4.B). An example of a CCSS-oriented goal may be "the student will use prefixes and root words to obtain the meaning of the unknown words." Again, consistent with the use of context clues, SLPs need to consider a child's strengths and areas for improvement when identifying the targets.

However, according to Scott, Jamieson-Noel, and Asselin (2003), only 1.4% of instruction time was devoted to teaching vocabulary in social studies, math, science, and 39% of the vocabulary instruction focus on definition and worksheet use (cited in Fisher & Frey, 2014). As per the research highlighted in this chapter, effective and evidence-based vocabulary instructions used by teachers can be modified for children who struggle with language and literacy development.

Chapter Summary

We discussed how typically developing school-age children can expand their vocabulary repertoire through social interaction, environment input, reading books, and instructional strategies. Children with language deficits also benefit from these same inputs and strategies; however, they may need more practice, assistance from an adult, and modifications based on their needs. Knowing what works for their peers can help us plan for the next step; therefore, Common Core State Standards serve as guidance for what children need to develop in language and communication skills. For example, third-grade students are expected to use glossaries or beginning dictionaries, both print and digital, to determine or clarify the precise meaning of key words and phrases (CCSS.ELA-LITERACY.L.3.4.D). However, looking up a word in a dictionary to find the precise meaning is difficult for children with language deficits. Imagine finding the correct meaning of a word in a dictionary when you travel to a foreign country. It feels like you are lost in a sea of words because the definitions may contain other words you do not know, you may get confused by different definitions, and sometimes the examples are hard to understand. That is why children need to have a box of tools (e.g., word part analysis, context clues, using a dictionary) to use in different contexts because some strategies may or may not work in a particular situation.

Besides the difficulty in acquiring new words, children with language deficits also struggle from "learning to read" to "reading to learn." When these children have an early unstable oral language foundation it is more difficult to acquire essential skills for reading such as phonological awareness, word recognition (reading fluency), and reading comprehension. Therefore, SLPs should start with the texts that their clients are familiar with in order to reduce the cognitive load for learning, what may become, too much new information at once. Repetitive reading can also gradually direct the child's attention to new information (new targets) in every read while keeping the cognitive load appropriate for the child. As discussed in Chapter 3, due to limitations in cognitive functions in children with language deficits, it is important to carefully control the number of new targets introduced in every session. Making the connection between newly learned information and existing knowledge explicit, would benefit their learning. No matter if SLPs are working with preschoolers or school-age children with language deficits, we need to constantly evaluate what a child knows, what else the child needs to know, how we can support the child, and how often the child can use the strategies/tools independently.

Discussion Questions

1. Explain how shared book reading is beneficial to lexical development in young children. Find a book appropriate for 3 or 4-year-olds and identify 5 new words you would like to introduce. Develop a lesson plan on how you would introduce new words and facilitate the retention of new words.
2. Discuss different exemplars for semantic mapping for both pre-readers and readers. How does the word class (different nouns, different verbs) influence the use of semantic mapping? What modifications can be implemented to increase the independent use of semantic mapping?
3. Evaluate different types of context, syntactic, and semantic clues along with examples. Find a paragraph from textbooks across different grades (Grade 2, 4, 6, 8, 10) and different subjects (science, math, language arts). Identify 3 to 5 words that may be unknown to children with language deficits. Discuss how effective these clues work on deriving the meaning of unknown words.
4. Search for different activities online to teach word part analysis. Try to make your own materials for the root word "port," prefix "un," and suffix "ness." How would you teach children with language deficits to use word part analysis? What root words, prefixes, and suffixes would you begin with? Why?

References

Anglin, J. M. (1993). Vocabulary development: A morphological analysis. *Monographs of the Society for Research in Child Development, 58*(10) [238], v–165. https://doi.org/10.2307/1166112

Apel, K., & Diem, E. (2013). Morphological awareness intervention with kindergarteners and first and second grade students from low SES homes: A small efficacy study. *Journal of Learning Disabilities, 47*(1), 65–75. https://doi.org/10.1177/0022219413509964

Ard, L., & Beverly, B. (2004). Preschool word learning during joint book reading: Effect of adult questions and comments. *Communication Disorders Quarterly, 26*(1), 17–28. https://doi.org/10.1177/152574010 40260010101

Baleghizadeh, S., & Naeim, M. (2011). Enhancing vocabulary retention through semantic mapping: A single subject study. *The International Journal of Language, Society and Culture,* (32), 11–16. https://www .researchgate.net/publication/266315898

Bang, J., Burns, J., & Nadig, A. (2013). Brief report: Conveying subjective experience in conversation: Production of mental state terms and personal narratives in individuals with high functioning autism. *Journal of Autism and Developmental Disorders, 43*(7), 1732–1740. https://doi.org/10.1007/s10803-012-1716-4

Baumann, J. F., Edwards, E. C., Boland, E., & Font, G. (2012). Teaching word-learning strategies. In E. J. Kame'enui & J. F. Baumann (Eds.), *Vocabulary instruction: Research to practice* (2nd ed., pp. 139–166). Guilford.

Baumann, J. F., Edwards, E. C., Boland, E. M., Olejnik, S., & Kame'enui, E. J. (2003). Vocabulary tricks: Effects of instruction in morphology and context on fifth-grade students' ability to derive and infer word meanings. *American Educational Research Journal, 40*(2), 447–494. https://doi.org/10.3102/00028312040002447

Baumann, J., Font, G., Edwards, E., & Boland, E. (2005). Strategies for teaching middle-grade students to use word-part and context clues to expand reading vocabulary. In E.H. Hiebert & M.L. Kamil (Eds.), *Teaching and learning vocabulary: Bringing research to practice* (pp. 179–205). Erlbaum.

Beck, I., McKeown, M., & Kucan, L. (2002). *Bringing words to life: Robust vocabulary instruction* (2nd ed.). Guilford Press.

Beck, I., McKeown, M., & McCaslin, E. (1983). Vocabulary development: All contexts are not created equal. *The Elementary School Journal, 83*(3), 177–181. https://doi.org/10.1086/461307

Beckage, N., Smith, L., & Hills, T. (2010). Semantic network connectivity is related to vocabulary growth rate in children. *Proceedings of the Annual Meeting of the Cognitive Science Society, 32,* 2769–2774. https://escholarship.org/uc/item/9xm7v9nq

Bloom, P. (2004). Myths of word learning. In D. G. Hall & S. R. Waxman (Eds.), *Weaving a lexicon* (pp. 205–224). MIT Press.

Borovsky, A., Ellis, E., Evans, J., & Elman, J. (2016). Semantic structure in vocabulary knowledge interacts with lexical and sentence processing in infancy. *Child Development, 87*(6), 1893–1908. https://doi .org/10.1111/cdev.12554

Brysbaert, M., Stevens, M., Mandera, P., & Keuleers, E. (2016). The impact of word prevalence on lexical decision times: Evidence from the Dutch Lexicon Project 2. *Journal of Experimental Psychology*, *42*(3), 441–458. https://doi.org/10.1037/xhp0000159

Cain, K. (2007). Deriving word meanings from context: Does explanation facilitate contextual analysis? *Journal of Research in Reading*, *30*(4), 347–359. https://doi.org/10.1111/j.1467-9817.2007.00336.x

Cain, K., & Oakhill, J. (2011). Matthew effects in young readers: Reading comprehension and reading experience aid vocabulary development. *Journal of Learning Disabilities*, *44*(5), 431–433. https://doi.org/10.1177/0022219411410042

Carlisle, J. (2007). Fostering morphological processing, vocabulary development, and reading comprehension. In R. K. Wagner, A. E. Muse, & K. R. Tannenbaum (Eds.), *Vocabulary acquisition: Implications for reading comprehension* (pp. 78–103). Guilford Press.

Dilek, Y., & Yuruk, N. (2012). Using semantic mapping technique in vocabulary teaching at pre-intermediate level. *Procedia- Social and Behavioral Sciences*, *70*, 1531–1544. https://doi.org/10.1016/j.sbspro.2013.01.221

Farrant, B., & Zubrick, S. (2013). Parent-child book reading across early childhood and child vocabulary in the early school years: Findings from the longitudinal study of Australian children. *First Language*, *33*, 280–293. https://doi.org/10.1177/0142723713487617

Fielding-Barnsley, R., & Purdie, N. (2003). Early intervention in the home for children at risk of reading failure. *Support for Learning*, *18*(2), 77–82. https://doi.org/10.1111/1467-9604.00284

Fisher, D., & Frey, N. (2014). Student and teacher perspectives on a close reading protocol. *Literacy Research and Instruction*, *53*(1), 25–49. https://doi.org/10.1080/19388071.2013.818175

Fukkink, R. G. (2005). Deriving word meaning from written context: A process analysis. *Learning Instruction*, *15*(1), 23–43. https://doi.org/10.1016/j.learninstruc.2004.12.002

Fukkink, R. G., & de Glopper, K. (1998). Effects of instruction in deriving word meaning from context: A meta-analysis. *Review of Educational Research*, *68*(4), 450–469. https://doi.org/10.2307/1170735

Gambrell, L. B., Wilson, R. M., & Gantt, W. N. (1981). Classroom observations of task-attending behaviors of good and poor readers. *The Journal of Educational Research*, *74*(6), 400–404. https://doi.org/10.1080/00220671.1981.10885339

Gathercole, S., Service, E., Hitch, G., Adams, A., & Martin, A. (1999). Phonological short-term memory and vocabulary development. *Applied Cognitive Psychology*, *13*(1), 65–77. https://doi.org/10.1002/(SICI)1099-0720(199902)13:1<65::AID-ACP548>3.0.CO;2-O

Gibson, F., & Wolter, J. (2015). Morphological awareness intervention to improve vocabulary and reading success. *Perspectives on Language Learning and Education, 22*(4), 147–155. https://doi.org/10.1044/lle22.4.147

Gombert, J. (1992) Metalinguistic development. *Applied Psycholinguistics, 14*(4), 553–561. https://doi.org/10.1017/S0142716400010742

Graves, M. (1986). Vocabulary learning and instruction. *Review of Research in Education, 13*(1), 49–89. https://doi.org/10.3102/0091732X013001049

Graves, M., Schneider, S., & Ringstaff, C. (2017). Empowering students with word learning strategies: Teach a child to fish. *The Reading Teacher, 71*(5), 533–543. https://doi.org/10.1002/trtr.1644

Hadley, E., Dickinson, D., Hirsh-Pasek, K., & Golinkoff, R. (2018). Building semantic networks: The impact of a vocabulary intervention on preschoolers' depth of word knowledge. *Reading Research Quarterly, 54*(1), 41–61. https://doi.org/10.1002/rrq.225

Harris, M. L., Schumaker, J. B., & Deshler, D. D. (2011). The effects of strategic morphological analysis instruction on the vocabulary performance of secondary students with and without disabilities. *Learning Disability Quarterly, 34*(1), 17–33. https://doi.org/10.1177/0731948711103400102

Helman, A. L., Calhoon, M. B., & Kern, L. (2015). Improving science vocabulary of high school English language learners with reading disabilities. *Learning Disability Quarterly, 38*(1), 40–52. https://doi.org/10.1177/0731948714539769

Hill, T., Maouene, M., Maouene, J., Sheya, A., & Smith, L. (2009). Longitudinal analysis of early semantic networks: Preferential attachment or preferential acquisition. *Psychological Science, 20*(6), 729–739. https://doi.org/10.1111/j.1467-9280.2009.02365.x

Johnson, D., Pittelman, S., & Heimlich, J. (1986). Semantic mapping. *The Reading Teacher, 39,* 778–782. https://www.researchgate.net/publication/234113540

Johnson, D. D., & Pearson, D. P. (1984). *Teaching reading vocabulary* (2nd ed.). Holt, Rinehart & Winston.

Justice, L., Invernizzi, M., & Meier, J. (2002). Designing and implementing an early literacy screening protocol: Suggestions for the speech-language pathologist. *Language, Speech, and Hearing Services in Schools, 33*(2), 84–101. https://doi.org/10.1044/0161-1461(2002/007)

Kirby, J. R., & Bowers, P. N. (2012). Morphology works. *What Works? Research into Practice.* https://collections.ola.org/mon/26007/318854.pdf

Korkmaz, B. (2011). Theory of mind and neurodevelopmental disorders. *Pediatric Research, 69*(5, Pt. 2), 101–108. https://doi.org/10.1203/PDR.0b013e318212c177

Kuhn, M., & Stahl, S. (1998). Teaching children to learn word meanings from context: A synthesis and some questions. *Journal of Literacy Research, 30*(1), 119–138. https://doi.org/10.1080/10862969809547983

Lonigan, C. J. (2007). Vocabulary development and the development of phonological awareness skills in preschool children. In R. K. Wagner, A. E. Muse, & K. R. Tannenbaum (Eds.), *Vocabulary acquisition: Implications for reading comprehension* (p. 15–31). Guilford Press.

McBride-Chang, C., Cho, J., Liu, H., Wagner, R., Shu, H., Zhou, . . . Muse, A. (2005). Changing models across cultures: Associations of phonological awareness and morphological structure awareness with vocabulary and word recognition in second graders from Beijing, Hong Kong, Korea, and the United States. *Journal of Experimental Child Psychology, 92*(2), 140–160. https://doi.org/10.1016/j.jecp.2005.03.009.

McBride-Chang, C., Wagner, R. K., Muse, A., Chow, B. W. -Y., & Shu, H. (2005). The role of morphological awareness in children's vocabulary acquisition in English. *Applied Psycholinguistics, 26*(3), 415–435. https://doi.org/10.1017/S014271640505023X

McEwan, E. K. (2008). *The reading puzzle: Word analysis.* Corwin Press.

Metsala, J. L. (1999). Young children's phonological awareness and nonword repetition as a function of vocabulary development. *Journal of Educational Psychology, 91*, 3–19. https://doi.org/10.1037/0022-0663.91.1.3

Miller, G. (1996). *The Science of words.* Scientific American Library.

Miller, S. A. (2009). Children's understanding of second-order mental states. *Psychological Bulletin, 135*(5), 749–773. https://doi.org/10.1037/a0016854

Mol, S., Bus, A., de Jong, M., & Smeets, D. (2008). Added value of dialogic parent-child book readings: A meta-analysis. *Early Education and Development, 19*(1), 7–26. https://doi.org/10.1080/10409280701838603

Nagy, W. E. (2007). Metalinguistic awareness and the vocabulary-comprehension connection. In R. Wagner, A. Muse, & K. Tannenbaum (Eds.). *Vocabulary acquisition: Implications for reading comprehension* (pp. 53–77). Guilford Press.

Nagy, W. E., & Anderson, R. (1984). How many words are there in printed school English? *Reading Research Quarterly, 19*(3), 304–330. https://doi.org/10.2307/747823

Nagy, W. E., Diakidoy, I.-A. N., & Anderson, R. C. (1993). The acquisition of morphology: Learning the contribution of suffixes to the meanings of derivatives. *Journal of Reading Behavior, 25*(2), 155–170.

Nagy, W. E., & Herman, P. A. (1987). Breadth and depth of vocabulary knowledge: Implications for acquisition and instruction. In M. G. McKeown & M. E. Curtis (Eds.), *The nature of vocabulary acquisition* (p. 19–35). Lawrence Erlbaum Associates.

Nagy, W. E., & Scott, J. A. (2000). *Vocabulary processes.* In M. L. Kamil, P. B. Mosenthal, P.D. Pearson, & R. Barr (Eds.), *Handbook of reading research* (Vol. 3, pp. 269–284). Lawrence Erlbaum Associates.

Nation, P., & Waring, R. (1997). Vocabulary size, text coverage and word lists. In N. Schmitt & M. McCarthy (Eds.), *Vocabulary: Description, acquisition, and pedagogy* (pp. 6–19). University Press.

Nippold, M. A. (2007). *Later language development: School age children, adolescents and young adults.* Pro-Ed.

Nippold, M. A. (2018). The literate lexicon in adolescents: Monitoring the use and understanding of morphologically complex words. *SIG 1 Language Learning and Education, 3*(1), 211–221. https://doi.org/10.1044/persp3.SIG1.211

Nunes, T., & Bryant, P. (2006). *Improving literacy by teaching morphemes.* Routledge. https://doi.org/10.4324/9780203969557

Olson, D. R., & Astington, J. W. (1993). Thinking about thinking: Learning how to take statements and hold beliefs. *Educational Psychologist, 28*(1), 7–23. https://doi.org/10.1207/s15326985ep2801_2

Saeidi, M., & Atmani, S. (2010). Teaching vocabulary through semantic mapping as a pre-reading activity across genders. *Journal of English Studies, 1*(1), 51–64.

Scarborough, H. S. (2001). Connecting early language and literacy to later reading (dis)abilities: Evidence, theory, and practice. In S. Neuman & D. Dickinson (Eds.), *Handbook for research in early literacy* (pp. 97–110). Guilford Press.

Schmitt, N., & McCarthy M. (Eds.). (1997). *Vocabulary: Description, acquisition and pedagogy.* Cambridge University Press.

Schuele, C., & Boudreau, D. (2008). Phonological awareness intervention: Beyond the basics. *Language, Speech, and Hearing Services in Schools, 39*(1), 3–20. https://doi.org/10.1044/0161-1461(2008/002)

Scott, J., Jamieson-Noel, D., & Asselin, M. (2003). Vocabulary instruction throughout the day in twenty-three Canadian upper-elementary classrooms. *The Elementary School Journal, 103*(3), 269–286. https://doi.org/10.1086/499726

Sinatra, R., & Dowd, C. (1991). Using syntactic and semantic clues to learn vocabulary. *Journal of Reading, 35*(3), 224–229. https://doi.org/10.2307/40033183

Sokmen, A. (1997). Current trends in teaching second language vocabulary. In N. Schmitt & M. McCarthy (Eds.), *Vocabulary: Description, acquisition and pedagogy* (pp. 237–257). Cambridge University Press.

Spencer, B., & Guillaume, A. (2006). Integrating curriculum through the learning cycle: Content-based reading and vocabulary instruction. *Reading Teacher, 60*(3), 206–219. https://doi.org/10.1598/RT.60.3.1

Stahl, K., & Stahl, S. A. (2012). Young word wizards! Fostering vocabulary development in preschool and primary education. In J. Baumann, & E. Kame'enui (Eds.), *Vocabulary instruction: Research to practice* (2nd ed., pp. 72–92). Guilford Press.

Stahl, S. A. (1999). *Vocabulary development*. Brookline.

Stahl, S., & Nagy, W. (2006). *Teaching word meanings*. Lawrence Erlbaum Associates

Stahl, S., & Vancil, S. (1986). Discussion is what makes semantic maps works in vocabulary instruction. *Reading Teacher, 40*(1), 62–67.

Stanovich, K. (1986). Matthew effects in reading: Some consequences of individual differences in the acquisition of literacy. *Reading Research Quarterly, 21*(4), 360–407. https://doi.org/10.1598/RRQ.21.4.1

Stroller, F. L., & Grabe, W. (1993). Implementations for L2 vocabulary acquisition and instruction from L1 Vocabulary Research. In T. Huckin, M. Haynes & J. Body (Eds.), *Second language reading and vocabulary learning*. (pp. 24–45). Ablex Publishing.

Verhoeven, L., van Leeuwe, J., & Vermeer, A. (2011). Vocabulary growth and reading development across the elementary school years. *Scientific Studies of Reading, 15*(1), 8–25. https://doi.org/10.1080/10888 438.2011.536125

Wagovich, S., Hill, M., & Petroski, G. (2015). Semantic-syntactic partial word knowledge growth through reading. *American Journal of Speech-Language Pathology, 24*(1), 60–71. https://doi.org/10.1044/ 2014_AJSLP-14-0046

Wasik, B. A., Hindman, A. H., & Snell, E. K. (2016). Book reading and vocabulary development: A systematic review. *Early Childhood Research Quarterly, 37*, 39–57. https://doi.org/10.1016/j.ecresq.2016 .04.003

Westby, C. (2012). Evaluating theory of mind development. *Word of Mouth, 24*(3), 12–16. https://doi.org/10.1177/1048395012465600d

Westby, C., & Robinson, L. (2014). A developmental perspective for promoting theory of mind. *Topics in Language Disorders, 34*(4), 362–382. https://doi.org/10.1097/TLD.0000000000000035

White, T., Sowell, J. & Yanagihara, Y. (1989). Teaching elementary students to use word-part clues. *The Reading Teacher, 42*(4), 302–308. https://www.jstor.org/stable/20200115

Wolter, J. A., & Green, L. (2013). Morphological awareness intervention in school age children with language and literacy deficits: A case study. *Topics in Language Disorders, 33*(1), 27–41. https://doi.org/10.1097/TLD.0b013e318280f5aa

5

VARIABLES THAT AFFECT WORD RETRIEVAL IN ADULTS WITH ACQUIRED LANGUAGE DISORDERS

Kris L. Brock

Chapter Objectives

1. Explain and apply word retrieval variables to clinical practice.
2. Learn how to locate and navigate various lexical databases to select word stimuli based on the knowledge acquired within the chapter.
3. Critically analyze target word lists you have created for PWA and apply word retrieval variables to enhance those lists for more targeted interventions.
4. Discuss the advantages and caveats of single word interventions.

Introduction

While words are the building blocks of language, they are of no use if we cannot store and access them efficiently. This chapter discusses variables that affect word retrieval which contributes to one of the most pervasive symptoms of language breakdown in people with aphasia (PWA): anomia. Of importance to this chapter is the content from Chapter 2 which discusses several models that have been developed and tested in PWA and non-brain-injured participants to understand everything from the intention to communicate through spoken language (Levelt, 1989; Dell et al., 1999). Moreover, these models, notably the Spreading Activation Model (Dell, 1986) and the Speech Production Model (Levelt, 1989), can assist clinicians with a more fine grained analysis of speech and language for PWA. That is, these models provide the ability to determine the locus of deficit in PWA: (a) semantic factors (Hillis et al., 1990), (b) phonological factor (Kay & Ellis, 1987), (c) grammatical factors (Bastiaanse et al., 2016), or (d) a combination of these factors (Howard & Gatehouse, 2006; Kay & Ellis, 1987).

Lexical Production Model

Before discussing the linguistic and non-linguistic variables impacting word storage and retrieval, we must frame these variables in the context of lexical access models. Levelt's (1989) speech production model is used because it is sufficiently complex and provides information that explains everything from concept formation through phonological encoding. Additionally, as Bastiaanse et al. (2016) discussed, Levelt's model also accounts for "grammatical operations on verb production (p. 1222)" as well as verb retrieval.

Levelt (1989) described that the process starts when a concept is triggered, a lemma will also be activated. This lemma contains information about the semantic functions, word class, argument structure, and other features such as gender. Next, the grammatical encoder takes information from the lemma to create a sentence frame or appropriate syntactic pattern. Bastiaanse et al. (2016) noted that grammatical encoding is present for single words such as nouns because those words are seen as a minimal sentence frame. In the case of verbs, the grammatical encoder uses the verb-argument structure found within the lemma to generate this sentence frame. After lemma retrieval, a lexeme is activated, which includes the phonological word form.

Therefore, the lexeme is embedded with the sentence frame, and the phonological encoding process transforms the lemma and sentence frame into speech sounds that follow phonological rules and are now ready for the articulation process and subsequent self-perception of speech.

Unfortunately, the intended word does not always reflect the word produced by a speaker. To account for and predict these errors, researchers created the aphasia model of spoken language for PWA and non-brain injured speakers (Dell et al., 1997). Expanding upon Levelt (1989), Dell et al., (1997) proposed that lexical access is achieved through bidirectional spreading activation where semantic units are activated to retrieve specific words that fit those units. For example, the intended word "Wookie" would activate semantic units and subsequently words that are semantic neighbors ("bear"), phonemically related ("cookie"), or words that are neighbors and also share phonemes ("monkey"). Readers are encouraged to review Chapter 2, Models of Word Production, for a more thorough description.

Variables Impacting Word Retrieval

Previous research has demonstrated that a variety of linguistic and non-linguistic factors affect how words are stored and retrieved in PWA and non-brain-damaged speakers (e.g., Adelman et al., 2006; Bastiaanse et al., 2016; Brown & Thiessen, 2018; Thompson et al., 2013). Word frequency and verb argument structure are examples of linguistic factors while imageability (i.e., mental representation of a word) is an example of a non-linguistic factor. Much to the chagrin of many practicing clinicians, there is no one resource that neatly organizes these factors which would allow for easy selection of target word stimuli for PWA. Moreover, researchers disagree as to which factors are the most important to apply or take into account for intervention purposes. This is because there are too many variables, likely interacting with one another when it comes to language production. For example, Bastiaanse et al. (2016) found that the retrieval of nouns and verbs was influenced by age of acquisition and imageability for PWA. Additionally, the effect of word frequency was only found for noun retrieval and not verb retrieval. Variables such as imageability, frequency, and word class, have significant impacts for both word storage and retrieval as well as spoken language. Therefore, it is important to discuss the impact of each variable to inform clinical decisions being made for over 2 million PWA in the United States alone.

Overview of Word Frequency

If you have ever completed a crossword puzzle, you likely feel excited, King or Queen of "Linguistica." But what about those times you have failed miserably? You know, those days where you cannot think of the word "cat" even if one sat on your face. Good news! It is likely not your fault, but rather the fault of the intern creating the daily crossword puzzle in your newspaper or the programmer of the software that generated the puzzle. This is because these individuals are taking advantage of several variables that we will discuss, but the first variable on the list is the word frequency effect.

Word frequency is calculated many different ways (see Heuven et al., 2014), but most researchers agree that word frequency per million words is the preferable metric for use in experimental publications because it is a standard measure of frequency that is independent of the corpus size (i.e., the number of all words analyzed). There are several corpora that have logged word frequency over the years; however, they are not all created equal. Brysbaert and New (2009) demonstrated that corpora from Kucera and Francis (1967) was outdated and small in terms of the number of words within the corpus as well as how word frequencies were measured. That is, Kucera and Francis (1967) created the corpus using only written sources. Brysbeart and New (2009) pointed out that using only written sources is limiting because the written word tends to be more formal and possibly skewed toward the lower frequency end. Therefore, a more contemporary corpus, such as the free SUB-TLEXus corpus (27 million words), is based on television and movie subtitles because it reflects spoken language use rather than writing. Additionally, the Corpus of Contemporary American English (600 million words; for purchase) includes words from spoken language, fiction, magazines, newspapers, and academic texts. Now find Activity Box 5–1 to utilize the free SUB-TLEXus corpus.

Activity Box 5–1

Have you ever used a word corpus to select words to target for intervention with PWA? Maybe you have, or maybe the thought of 27 million words in single Excel spreadsheet is a bit much. Well, good news! Ctrl+F is your friend. Now go to SUBTLEXus and download the free zip files that include the word corpus. Unzip those files and open the SUBTLEX usExcel2007 file. There are various columns with different word frequency metrics, but the one you will focus on is the SUBTLWF column. If you are interested in learning about the other metrics, the SUBTLEXus site has an explanation of each.

Now think of an individual with non-fluent aphasia who is on your caseload, someone with either anomia or a more sinister spoken language impairment. Think about the words you have been targeting in your treatment sessions: nouns, verbs, prepositions, adjectives, or adverbs. Hit Ctrl+F on the keyboard and search for those words in the corpus. Write down the SUBTLWF number (i.e., the number of times a word was used per million words). Do this for several of your words. What is the average SUBTLWF for all of your words? Do you have any outliers, notably on the lower frequency end? How do you justify the inclusion of those outliers in your therapy?

Clinical Implications

Word frequency is one of the most influential variables when lexical decision time is being investigated, easily accounting for over 40% of the variance in the results (Brysbaert et al., 2011). Duncan (1973) investigated the storage and retrieval of high (100 per million) and low (1 per million) frequency words in non-brain damaged adults using 6-letter words that began with "b." Duncan found that as the word frequency decreased, participants were less likely to recognize a word, recall the word, or produce the word. Participants recognized less than 40% of words with a frequency less than 1 per million while higher frequency words (words at or above 30 per million) were significantly more accurate. Similar results were also found for the recall and production tasks. These results suggest that low frequency words are not stored in the lexicon or have not been used, resulting in poor retrieval. Clinicians who note a lack of progress in word retrieval and production may question whether some of the target words have a low frequency rating. While word frequency is an important variable, it is very rarely the only factor impacting word retrieval.

Imageability, Word Frequency, and Age of Acquisition

Now that you have hopefully seen the utility of a corpus tool to help you make evidence-based decisions regarding words, let us look at some of the literature associated with word frequency because clinical decisions cannot be made on one variable alone. Variables such as imagebility and age of acquisition (AoA) contribute to word familiarity and are almost always controlled in well-designed research and intervention studies with word frequency metrics. This is because the more easily a word can be depicted mentally through graphic representation (i.e., imageable), combined with an early AoA and high word frequency rating, then the easier it will be to store and retrieve (Barry et al., 2006; Garlock et al., 2001). The argument in support of this facilitative effect is grounded in how these variables are closely related to the concepts, lemmas, and lexemes which are frequently accessed together, accessed more often, and at an earlier age (Brysbaert & Ellis, 2016; Sosa & Stoel-Gammon, 2012). This also suggests that motor learning is a variable that interacts with frequency and AoA because of its ties to the lexeme, phonological encoder, and articulatory planning. However, we must be aware that not all words learned early in development are considered high frequency in adulthood. A wonderful example of this can be found in the Disney movie "Inside Out" where the characters are seen dumping low frequency animal words (e.g., leopard) that were acquired at an early age to make room for newly learned material. The newly learned words, including the lemmas, lexemes, and encoders, would be updated along with the new motor plans for speech.

Imageability

Imageability is the how well a word can generate a mental image (Paivio et al., 1968). Words that are highly imageable are easier to retrieve. It is commonly known that nouns, being more concrete, generally lend themselves better to graphic and mental representations because they represent an object (Koul & Harding, 1998). However, the clinical utility of targeting highly imageable nouns in isolation has been called into question because of a lack of generalization to non-trained noun targets (Quique et al., 2019). In contrast, verbs and prepositions can be concrete (e.g., *jump*) and abstract (e.g., *think*). Concrete verbs are generally more imageable than abstract verbs, but verbs are not as imageable as nouns. This is because verbs and some prepositions are inherently dynamic and require movement for correct interpretation. Therefore, instead of a static mental image, one would have a mental video depicting that movement which is arguably more complex to complete cognitively (den Ouden et al., 2009; Höffler & Leutner, 2007).

To reduce the complexity of such a process, researchers in augmentative and alternative communication (AAC) have demonstrated that digital visuographic supports, including videos, are an important aspect of communication within our environments. Notably, regardless of disability, people prefer complex images and videos because of their utility in communicating without words in real time and in digital formats such as Instagram® (Brock et al., 2017; Brown & Thiessen, 2018). Moreover, PWA prefer personalized content when compared to the images found through Google® search (McKelvey et al., 2010). These highly imageable digital tools have been shown to compensate for and restore language function in PWA (Brock et al., 2017; Dietz et al., 2018).

Age of Acquisition and Word Frequency

AoA ratings are interesting databases from a research perspective because we cannot objectively determine when a word is acquired into the lexicon; we have a general idea regarding most words and even some data on a select number of verbs being acquired before the age of three (Huttenlocher et al., 1983). However, with the hundreds of thousands of words in question, researchers obtain subjective ratings from thousands of participants to make more objective decisions about AoA for a word. Before 2012, researchers had only accumulated enough data for a small number of words secondary to the difficulty of amassing such large samples and the time-consuming nature of collecting and analyzing subjective ratings. However, Kuperman et al. (2012) used Amazon Mechanical Turk, a crowdsourcing data collection technology, to collect AoA data for over 30,000 English words with 1,960 participants. The results indicated that AoA was significantly correlated with word frequency, word length, ease of production, ease of defining a word, and imagebility among several other constructs. For the interested reader, see Activity Box 5–2 for Kuperman et al.'s AoA database.

Activity Box 5–2

Do you want to browse another database? Or one that could potentially help you select words for storage and retrieval? Head over to http://crr.ugent.be/archives/806 and download the Kuperman et al. (2012) AoA ratings here. Then find your list of words that you selected for a client from Activity Box 5–1. How do the AoA ratings differ from the word frequency ratings? Would you make any changes to your word list for this client based on what you have found?

In a study of PWA, word frequency was associated with phonological and semantic errors while AoA was associated with phonological errors only (Kittredge et al., 2008). In contrast to Jescheniak and Levelt (1994), Kittredge and colleagues argued that word frequency impacts the lemma (semantic) and lexeme (phonologic) levels of spoken language production while AoA influences the lexeme level. While Kittredge and colleagues make this claim, previous research in this area suggests that frequency impacts only the lemma (semantic) stage (Vitkovitch & Humphreys, 1991; Wheeldon & Monsell, 1992), the lexeme (phonologic) stage (La Heij et al., 1999), or both stages (Knobel et al., 2008). Overall, no conclusions can be made at this time with respect to the spoken language model.

Word frequency effects have also been found when PWA and non-brain injured adults were asked to comprehend sentence level material. Specifically, DeDe (2012) investigated the effects of sentence pairs containing high and low frequency words within a listening task and a reading task. The dependent variables included response time and comprehension question accuracy. The results indicated low frequency words negatively influenced performance of PWA. Additionally, PWA performed poorly in the reading task when low frequency words were present when compared to the high frequency words. In a follow-up study, DeDe (2017) also found that PWA spend more time reading low frequency words when compared to high frequency words.

Overall, it is a combination of AoA and word frequency that predicts word naming accuracy and lexical decision times. The variables are also highly correlated with other word storage and retrieval variables such as imagebility because they are easily depicted in the mind (Kuperman et al., 2012). Therefore, while these are important variables to consider when selecting word targets, they cannot be the only variables taken into consideration. Moreover, as the next section discusses, selecting target words for treatment that have high frequency and AoA ratings are likely *not* going to provide the desired treatment gains in spoken language production. In fact, selecting only high frequency and early AoA words may contribute to an illusion of progress. Moreover, selecting easy target words will not generalize into more difficult words (e.g., low frequency and increased AoA).

Clinical Implications. There is a lot to learn with respect to imageability, AoA, and word frequency, including their interactions. However, there are some concrete takeaways for clinical purposes. First, high imageability facilitates word retrieval; however, those words tend to be nouns that have some clinical utility with respect to communicative functions (e.g., comment or information transfer). Verbs, which have lower imageability ratings, are more clinically useful because other word classes are activated with the target verb (see the section on Word Class and Argument Structure). Second, using digital technologies can make verbs more imageable by providing a cue to facilitate word retrieval. Finally, AoA and word frequency predict word naming and lexical decision times; however, we should not take this as evidence to only include high frequency words learned early in development. On the contrary, we should be incorporating a mixture of words that have high and low frequency and varying AoA ratings secondary to creating varying levels of difficulty in clinic. That is, simple words such as nouns do not generalize to more complex words such as verbs, and the same is true for high word frequency stimuli likely not generalizing to low frequency words. Overall, it is important to have a diverse mixture of word stimuli to challenge PWA and maintain their motivation to continue therapy.

Word Class and Argument Structure

Traditional intervention approaches to word retrieval have primarily focused on nouns (Boyle & Coelho, 1995), but within the last two decades, we have seen increasing interest in verb storage and retrieval (e.g., Edmonds et al., 2009, 2014; Kim & Thompson, 2000; Thompson et al., 2013). With respect to nouns, semantic feature analysis (SFA) is a popular intervention technique that focuses on activating words related to a target (Boyle & Coelho, 1995). Massaro and Tompkins (1994) suggested that retrieval of conceptual information is possible by accessing the semantic network surrounding the target. SFA improves confrontational naming outcomes and those outcomes generalize to untrained words. However, generalization to conversational speech has not been consistently found (Boyle & Coelho, 1995; Coelho et al., 2000), with a recent meta-analysis indicating that generalization did not occur (Quique et al., 2019).

Interestingly, most object naming (i.e., nouns) research in PWA has found a word frequency effect, but that effect is nonexistent in verb naming tasks or sentence production tasks (Bastiaanse et al., 2016; Kemmerer & Tranel, 2000; Luzzatti et al., 2002). There are likely several reasons for this. First, the more complex a lemma is, the more difficulty PWA will have producing the word in isolation or within a sentence. Researchers agree that verbs are more complex than nouns because verbs include additional syntactic and semantic information within the lemma (e.g., Bastiaanse et al., 2016; Bastiaanse & Van Zonneveld, 2004; Kim & Thompson, 2000 McRae et al., 2005; Thompson et al., 2003). Thematic roles and argument structure are activated simultaneously based on the intended message and the processing demands increase when the verb comes with complex argument structures. More specifically, the root cause of the verb naming or sentence production deficits in PWA is not likely due to lemma retrieval because verb comprehension is relatively preserved in people with nonfluent aphasia (Jonkers & Bastiaanse, 2006). The real problem is that the grammatical encoder must encode all of the lemma information (e.g., semantic features, arguments structure, and thematic roles), and this more complex encoding results in spoken language difficulty.

Second, if you read *oven, hot, chef, pastry, pie, cherry, red,* then you likely activated the verb *bake.* As probably noted, *bake* is easily retrieved because it includes several semantic features and is considered a "heavy" verb. In contrast, verbs with very few semantic features (e.g., do) are referred to as "light verbs" (Breedin et al., 1998). Whereas light verbs are the most frequently occurring (e.g., go, have, and do), the majority of verbs are considered heavy, which also contain the light verb or its semantic components within the lemma (Pinker, 2013). For example, the heavy verb *run* is also a derivative of the light verb *go,* which are conceptually related (i.e., state of movement). Previous research indicated that PWA and non-brain damaged controls tend to accurately produce more light verbs than light nouns during sentence generation tasks (Berndt et al., 1997; Kohn et al., 1989). However, Breedin et al. (1998) found that PWA retrieved and produced a greater number of heavy verbs than light verbs during several communicative tasks. They suggested that the additional verb complexity has a facilitative effect in that the greater number of semantic relationships a verb has with nouns, the easier they are to activate than a verb with very few relationships (Breedin et al., 1998; Gentner, 1981; Kintsch, 1974). Extending these complexity results to nouns, Kiran and Thompson (2003) found that training more complex, atypical exemplars for birds and vegetables resulted in enhanced naming of typical items; however, training typical items to name did not generalize to atypical items.

With respect to verb and syntactic complexity, previous research has investigated the effects of verb type and argument structure on verb naming and spoken language production with clinically relevant results (den Ouden et al., 2009; Thompson et al., 2013; Thompson et al., 2003). First, there are several types of verbs: transitive, intransitive, ditransitive, and ambitransitive. Transitive verbs take a direct object ("Mom kissed the baby") whereas ditransitive verbs take on a direct and indirect object ("The mailman delivered the package to the girl."). Transitive and ditransitive verbs are syntactically more complex than intransitive verbs (e.g., "I laugh."), which do not take on a direct object. Ambitransitive verbs can be classified as either transitive or intransitive depending on the context. For example, *broke* can be transitive (e.g., "Ron broke his wand"), or intransitive (e.g., "The Hogwarts oven broke"). PWA typically struggle with transitive and ditransitive verbs because they are more syntactically complex with a greater number of semantic features and thematic roles, as well as a more complex argument structures.

This leads to another useful point; researchers agree that PWA tend to produce one- and two-argument verbs that have fewer thematic roles and arguably fewer semantic relationships with nouns (Thompson et al., 1997, 2003, 2013). Specifically, verbs take on different argument structures (i.e., one-, two-, or three-arguments), increasing the syntactic complexity of natural speech (Thompson et al., 2003). For example, a verb with three arguments (e.g., "the mom [agent] feeds lunch [patient] to her baby [goal]") is more difficult to produce at the sentence level than a verb with two arguments (e.g., "the boy [agent] hugs dad [patient]"). The Argument Structure Complexity Principle indicates that PWA exhibit more difficulty producing verbs with two or more argument structures as compared to verbs with less complex structures (Thompson et al., 2003).

Clinical Implications

Translating this evidence to treatment has been of vital importance to aphasiology. Thompson and colleagues (2003) coined the term "complexity account of treatment efficacy" (CATE), which dictates that simpler, untrained stimuli are found within the lemma of more complex, trained stimuli. CATE not only applies to word class, argument structure, and thematic roles, it also applies to spoken language production levels (e.g., word level and sentence level). Webster and Whitworth's (2012) systematic review of verb treatment in aphasia suggested verbs should be treated in a sentence context and not in isolation because sentence context activates thematic roles, relevant morphological information, and syntactical information. One such intervention, called the Verb Network Strengthening Treatment (VNeST), is a treatment approach that promotes retrieval of verbs and their thematic roles (Edmonds et al., 2014). PWA are required to generate related thematic roles from a given verb in response to Wh- questioning, which simultaneously activates relevant word and world knowledge (Edmonds et al., 2009, 2014; McRae et al., 2005). It is assumed that thematic roles (e.g., book) co-activate with associated verbs (e.g., read). Additionally, the "bidirectional" activation between verbs (e.g., clean) and instruments (e.g., soap) and the priming effect from location to verbs (e.g., swimming pool) are also retrieved (McRae et al., 2005).

Activity Box 5–3

Head over to TactusTherapy.com and search for Verb Network Strengthening Treatment (VNeST). Follow the prompts to select a set of verbs for one of your clients with aphasia. Apply the principles that you learned from the Word Class and Argument Structure section (e.g., verb types) when selecting verbs for this client. Then either review or role-play the Tactus Therapy steps to implement VNeST. Better yet, get access to the publication for first-hand information and then begin (Edmonds, Nadeau, & Kiran, 2009).

Overall, simply treating retrieval at the word level may not reflect the everyday communicative challenges that PWA experience or generalize to spoken sentence production. Best practice for word storage and retrieval starts at the sentence level. Specifically, if we target more syntactically complex structures, complex verbs and nouns, and complex argument structures, then we are more likely to promote generalization to simpler untrained items (Edmonds et al., 2009; Kiran & Thompson, 2003; Thompson et al., 2013; Thompson et al., 2003). Additionally, most sentence level or discourse level treatments such as VNeST or discourse-based AAC interventions maintain their treatment effects and generalize well to different spoken language tasks (Brock et al., 2017; Dietz et al., 2018; Edmonds et al., 2014).

Contextual Distinctiveness, Contextual Diversity, and Semantic Diversity

Contextual Distinctiveness

McDonald and Shillcock (2001) define contextual distinctiveness as the relationship a word (run) has with other words (fast), and that relationship being defined as co-occurrence. Co-occurrence is defined simply as words that are found within a sentence or a limited window of a target word. The word *run* is broad and not tied to a specific linguistic or situational context and, therefore, its contextual distinctiveness is rather high because it is used in a variety of contexts. However, if we have the word *amok*, which almost always follows the word *run*, then *amok* is considered contextually distinctive with a lower rating. They argue that the contextual distinctiveness of a word may facilitate retrieval; however, clinicians must account for the life participation relevance of such words, regardless of how facilitative they are for PWA.

Contextual distinctiveness and word frequency, while similar in concept, are quite different. Researchers of contextual distinctiveness, as defined above, are interested in co-occurring words that surround the target word. Thus, contextual distinctiveness is derived from a distribution of words, while word frequency is independent of any distribution or effects from the surrounding words. In a more practical example, contextual distinctiveness can be used in word prediction algorithms to predict the most likely subsequent word you text secondary to the presence of other words and contextual information surrounding the target word. This is a rather simplified example because word prediction not only takes into account contextual distinctiveness, but also word frequency and syntactic rules among several other variables.

Researchers are able to calculate contextual distinctiveness using large corpora of words using various parameters that are not within the scope of this chapter (McDonald & Shillcock, 2001). Regardless of the computational methodology, contextual distinctiveness and word frequency do have a strong relationship. Specifically, high frequency words have low contextual distinctiveness ratings whereas low frequency words have high contextual distinctiveness ratings; however, there are always exceptions to this principle (Adelman et al., 2006; McDonald & Shillcock, 2001). So what does this mean in terms of therapy?

McDonald and Shillock (2001) found that contextual distinctiveness and response time were significantly related; however, distinctiveness and word frequency were also highly correlated with one another. This indicates that words with high distinctiveness scores (e.g., *amok*) have longer response latencies while words with low distinctiveness scores (indistinctive; *run*) have shorter response latencies. Moreover, these authors analyzed response latency and AoA and found that the two were significantly correlated. When AoA was held constant, distinctiveness and response latency was significant. Overall, the authors concluded that distinctiveness is a better predictor than word frequency, but the analysis of AoA may be a more insightful variable when it comes to lexical decision times.

Contextual Diversity

Adelman et al. (2006) investigated the effect of contextual diversity and word frequency on word naming response latency and lexical decision (judging whether or not the stimulus is a word). Contextual diversity in this study was defined as the number of different contexts (i.e., films and books) in which a word appeared, suggesting that the repeated exposure to words in a variety of contexts should facilitate word retrieval. The results indicated that contextual diversity was more predictive of response latency than word frequency. Moreover, high contextual diversity ratings led to faster responses whereas high word frequency ratings had slower response times. The authors also confirmed that their results were not explained by the high degree of correlation between contextual distinctiveness and word frequency that was found by McDonald and Shillcock (2001). Several additional analyses were run, too many to discuss here, and the results confirmed that contextual diversity was the better predictor of fast responses. In fact, no word frequency effects were found within their subsequent analyses. These results from the early 2000s were rather concerning because word frequency had dominated the lexical landscape for decades. Therefore, researchers began replicating previous work and developing new studies using behavioral as well as more objective electrophysiological methodologies to confirm the contextual diversity effect. The amassed results indicate that the contextual diversity effect was more pronounced than the word frequency effect in the majority of studies (Brysbaert & New, 2009; Johns et al., 2012; Vergara-Martínez et al., 2017). Thus, contextual diversity is an important variable to consider.

Perhaps you noticed that Adelman's definition of contextual diversity was rather constrained (i.e., diversity included the number of times a word appeared in films and books) and may not be applicable to the communicative challenges faced by PWA. Perhaps more applicable to PWA is a definition of contextual diversity as the number of distinctive contexts in which a word appears in several tasks (Rosa et al., 2017). Rosa and colleagues required their third grade participants to read three different items (i.e., a fable, expository text, and math text). Each text included 4 of the 12 experimental words resulting in participants reading each word 3 times corresponding to their experimental condition (high and low contextual diversity). The results indicated that participants in the high contextual diversity condition had better scores on free recall, recognition, multiple choice, and picture matching tasks than their low contextual diversity counterparts. Therefore, contextual diversity, as defined by multiple contextual exposures to words, resulted in greater learning of the new words. Rosa et al.'s (2007) definition of contextual diversity is indeed an interesting concept, but one that needs empirical testing in PWA.

Semantic Diversity

Current evidence in PWA discusses a concept related to contextual diversity called semantic diversity. Hoffman and colleagues (2011), using latent semantic analysis, developed this new measure of semantic diversity defined as "the degree to which a given word is associated with a variety of different senses, meaning, or linguistic contexts" (p. 2434; Hoffman et al., 2011). Similar to contextual diversity, semantic diversity was calculated using a large text-based corpus, with the purpose of creating a variable that was independent of word frequency and captured the different contexts that words were used and had similar meanings. Hoffman et al. (2011) investigated the effects of imageability (i.e., high, medium, or low imageability) and word frequency (high vs. low) in participants with semantic aphasia and semantic dementia (briefly discussed here) using a synonym judgment task (i.e., verbal comprehension by matching synonyms). The result indicated a significant imageability effect with differences between all three levels. That is, highly imageable words were better matched than medium imageable words, and medium words were better matched than low imageable words. Similar to previous studies (e.g., Bastiaanse et al., 2016), results indicated no significant frequency effects were found for the participants with aphasia; however, frequency was significant for participants with dementia (high frequency words were more accurate than low frequency words). The authors suggest that high frequency words have a relatively high degree of semantic diversity, with words being used in so many linguistic contexts that PWA have difficulty accurately retrieving the correct meaning. With respect to low frequency words, PWA continue to have deficits simply because of a lack of exposure to those words on a daily basis, hence the lack of a word frequency effect. To explore this lack of a frequency effect further, a multiple regression analysis was conducted with word frequency, imageability, and semantic diversity. First, the correlation matrix indicated that imageability and semantic diversity were significantly correlated, but frequency was not correlated with any measure. Second, the regression model that included semantic diversity was significant and predicted synonym comprehension scores. In sum, semantic diversity was the greatest predictor of the difficulty PWA experience when judging words. The semantic diversity effect, and PWA's inability to access the multiple meanings of high frequency words, may be the reason previous studies have not found a word frequency effect.

Clinical Implications. Although these studies are important, we need to know how to apply this information. And you, dear reader, are in luck because there is a contextual diversity database for you to browse. Luckily, you have already downloaded the SUBTLEXus database from Activity Box 5–1. This database not only includes word frequency, but also contextual diversity ratings. Therefore, open up your SUBTLEXus database and look for the SUBTLcd column. This column will have a contextual diversity rating, with higher ratings indicating more contextual diversity as defined by Adelman et al. (2006).

However, the use of a corpus including thousands or millions of words may not have clinical utility, especially if you are running from one session to the next. Therefore, you can apply the concepts of contextual distinctiveness, contextual diversity, and semantic diversity in your practice. That is, select words with your clients that are challenging and fall into these three categories. Specifically, contextually distinct words facilitate retrieval, even at very low word frequency ratings and, therefore, may be recalled easily in an attempt to enhance or maintain psychosocial factors, such as motivation. Contextually diverse words, as described by Adelman et al. (2006) and Rosa et al. (2017), can each be manipulated for intervention purposes. Using Rosa's example, therapy can include a subset of words in which PWA are exposed to through various activities (i.e., contextually diverse word exposure). Although this requires some additional preparation, the repeated exposure to words in different situations may facilitate word retrieval and break up the monotony of single, drill-based activities. The astute clinician would then develop generalization word lists and other pre-and post-intervention activities to determine if this contextual diversity approach is facilitating client progress.

Considering semantic diversity, it is important to recall PWA's impaired ability to access the multiple meanings of high frequency words. Thus, clinicians should ask if their target words include a variety of different senses, meaning, or linguistic contexts because this could be one of the issues in which PWA are not making word retrieval progress: too many closely related words (e.g., twist, shake, turn, spin) or multiple meaning words (e.g., bark). Clinicians may therefore adjust their word lists, activities, or treatment intensity levels (e.g., number of trials) to meet the needs of their clients. Regardless, it is important to recall the CATE principle in that easy word targets will not generalize to more complex targets. Thus, clinicians should be selecting challenging words for their generalization benefits.

Neighborhoods and Distance

Based on Levelt et al.'s (1999) model of spoken language, several candidate words are activated simultaneously during word processing. These candidate words within a neighborhood can be similar to the target word with respect to orthography, semantics, phonology, or morphology. An example specific to semantics includes candidate words (tiger, mountain lion, fur, and predator) that are co-activated with the intended target (lion), and these candidate words are called neighbors. As you noted, each of these target words are also similar or have very little semantic distance between them (especially lion [female] vs. mountain lion). The co-activated words compete to be selected, and the intended target word must overcome interference from its neighbors. To investigate word retrieval, the neighborhood density or neighborhood size of these co-activated words plays an important role for all people, regardless of disability. Previous research suggested that high-density semantic neighborhoods (i.e., several co-activated or related words) were facilitative (e.g., faster to identify or name) in nature (McClelland & Rumelhart, 1981), whereas others proposed an inhibitory effect of word production secondary to the competition between competing words (Luce & Pisoni, 1998). Contemporary evidence suggests a more complex interaction between the facilitative and inhibitory effects of semantic neighborhood size/density (Mirman et al., 2008; Mirman & Magnuson, 2009). Therefore, it is important to understand the concept of neighborhoods when targeting specific words for clients with word finding difficulties.

Semantic Neighborhoods

There are two types of semantic neighborhood density: feature-based (taxonomic) and associative-based. Feature-based density refers to the number of features that words share (McRae, Cree, et al., 2005). McRae, Cree, and colleagues asked participants to list features of hundreds of nouns to establish normative data on living and nonliving concepts. For example, respondents read the word *cat,* and were provided with several lines to fill in features, such as *has a tail.* As you may have noted, that approach is labor- and time-intensive for any professional. The supplementary semantic features material from McRae, Cree, et al. (2005) is available behind a paywall from Springer's *Behavior Research Methods* (https://doi.org/10.3758/BF03192726) and may be useful. However, although feature-based approaches work well for more concrete nouns, there are several words and word classes that are considered abstract. In turn, these abstract concepts are harder to describe based on semantic features (e.g., jump and think; Reilly & Desai, 2017). In contrast, associative-based methods (e.g., latent semantic analysis) use large corpora to measure the similarity between concepts. Associative-based semantic density emphasizes thematic relationships between concepts rather than features. An example of the difference between the two includes *cow, milk,* and *bull,* where *cow* and *milk* are considered similar (.60; along a continuum of −1 to 1) using an associative approach because they often co-occur in text, movies, and other media. However, *cow* and *bull,* although taxonomically related and share similar features, have a similarity rating of .21 (Reilly & Desai, 2017). Associative-based approaches, even though useful in the research realm, require extensive knowledge to ensure the modeling analysis yields accurate results. Research has begun to create a hybrid approach that highlights both taxonomic (categorical neighbors; *cow* and *bull*) and associative approaches (*cow* and *milk*) because each approach has an effect on word retrieval.

Reilly and Desai (2017) compared semantic neighborhood densities in a large set of 3,500 abstract and concrete words using a hybrid associative- and feature-based approach. They found that abstract words had sparse neighborhoods when compared to concrete words, meaning that abstract words have very few close neighbors. However, sparse neighborhoods facilitated lexical decisions for concrete words, but not for abstract words. With respect to concrete words, the sparse neighborhood effect occurred because the competition between words was limited and, therefore, easier to select the target word. In contrast, high-density neighborhoods for concrete words introduce "noise" into the system, meaning that these words have large taxonomic and possibly associative overlap. This overlap leads to activation of additional taxonomic units when, for example, the concept for *lion* is activated (e.g., predator units). The additional units slow lexical processing time and subsequently speech and language errors become more prevalent. Additionally, Reilly and Desai (2017) also found that emotionally charged concrete words have dense semantic neighborhoods (e.g., *bully* is related to several other words such as *brat*) compared to concrete words without emotion. Emotionally charged abstract words, in general, have sparse neighborhoods, and no effect was found during lexical decisions tasks.

Mirman and Magnuson (2009) investigated the effects of near and distant semantic neighbors using a visual word recognition paradigm. Near neighbors were classified as words with many related concepts whereas distant neighbors had a few to no related concepts. Their results indicated that non-brain damaged participants recognized words with few or distant neighbors more quickly than words with several near neighbors. Therefore, words with near neighbors inhibited word recognition, whereas words with fewer neighbors facilitated recognition. The effects found by Mirman and Magnuson (2009) also reveal that the combination of neighbor distance and density are not a singular facilitative or inhibitory effect; rather, the effects occur simultaneously. Table 5–1 includes Mirman and Magnuson's (2009) experimental stimuli of target words, near neighbors, distant neighbors, and non-neighbors.

Recent research has also found a similar effect on PWA (Fieder et al., 2016; Mirman, 2011). Specifically, Mirman (2011) and Fieder et al. (2016) investigated the effects of semantic neighborhood density on naming and error types in PWA and primary progressive aphasia. Mirman found that less accurate naming, greater response latencies, and greater semantic error was influenced by target words within dense semantic neighborhoods with semantically similar words (near distance). In contrast, distant semantic neighbors had a facilitative effect on picture naming. Fieder et al., (2016) also found that words with greater semantic neighborhood density and similarity resulted in poor naming accuracy and more semantic errors. However,

Table 5–1. Mirman and Magnuson (2009) Experimental Stimuli of Semantically Similar Concepts

Target	Near Neighbor	Distant Neighbor	Non-neighbor
bayonet	machete	tomahawk	colander
beans	peas	pear	jar
blueberry	raspberry	pineapple	microscope
broccoli	celery	banana	envelope
buffalo	caribou	elephant	clarinet
bus	van	bike	ball
cake	pie	pear	stone
cat	dog	stool (furniture)	doll
cheetah	zebra	bison	tripod
crab	clam	cod	clamp
crow	goose	wasp	snail
dagger	hatchet	shotgun	cello
deer	fox	bear	skis
dove	swan	bat (animal)	hoe
eagle	blackbird	tiger	trumpet
elk	hare	chimp	urn
falcon	partridge	ostrich	sardine
grape	peach	pear	rope
lion	tiger	beaver	crowbar
moose	hare	chimp	sword
owl	hawk	swan	crane (machine)
panther	leopard	zebra	baton
pants	shirt	socks	fork
peacock	blackbird	giraffe	rifle
pelican	flamingo	crocodile	revolver
penguin	starling	otter	missile
pheasant	starling	catfish	cannon
pistol	shotgun	crossbow	banjo
sheep	goat	rat	yacht
sparrow	blackbird	beetle	anchor
spear	bow (weapon)	shield	crown
stork	finch	seal	tank (army)
tomato	strawberry	potato	magazine
trombone	tuba	bagpipe	scooter
truck	van	couch	cheese

Source: From Mirman, D., & Magnuson, J. S. (2009). Dynamics of activation of semantically similar concepts during spoken word recognition. *Memory & Cognition, 37*(7), 1026–1039, p. 1038, Appendix A.

response latency was not influenced by semantic neighborhood density secondary to the requirements of a timed naming task (i.e., generating responses quickly results in incomplete lexical processing). Additionally, Fieder and colleagues found that semantic errors were associated with other variables, such as word frequency and AoA.

Orthographic and Phonological Neighbors

Word production and recognition theories suggest that multiple word candidates are activated simultaneously based not only on their semantic similarity (as discussed above), but also their orthographic and phonological similarity. Orthographic similarity is typically measured using Coltheart's N (Coltheart et al., 1977). This is derived by counting the number of words that can be created from a single word by simply changing one letter. For example, "Sith" can be changed to *myth, sit, sip,* etc. This letter-based similarity demonstrates the facilitative effects found in many orthographic neighborhood studies (Andrews, 1997). However, there are inhibitory effects as well. Specifically, target word recognition is slower when orthographic neighbors are more frequent than the target word. Inhibitory effects are also found for words with a transposed letter during word recognition tasks (e.g., *prefect* vs. *perfect;* Acha & Perea, 2008).

Phonological neighbors, measured by the number of words created by changing a single phoneme of the target word, also exert facilitative effects on visual word recognition (Yates, 2005; Yates et al., 2008). However, during spoken word recognition tasks, inhibitory effects are present (Magnuson et al., 2007). To convolute matters more, PWA have shown the facilitative effects of phonological neighbors during spoken word production tasks (Goldrick et al., 2010). Dell and Gordon (2003) suggest that the reason for these contrasting inhibitory effects for word recognition and facilitative effects for word production is because the tasks are tapping into two separate constructs. Word recognition is a phonological task while word production is a semantic task. To explain this phenomenon, Chen and Mirman (2012) state, " . . . the strongest lexical competitors during word production are semantic neighbors, not phonological neighbors, and therefore the (weak) activation of some phonological neighbors should not substantially increase ambiguity" (p. 4). Moreover, target words overcome semantic neighbor competition through the facilitative effects of phonological neighbors. Kittredge et al. (2008) found evidence for this assumption when they found fewer semantic and omission errors for words within phonologically dense neighborhoods.

Clinical Implications. Calculating neighborhood density using a feature-based (taxonomic) and associative-based method may be a time-consuming endeavor for clinicians; however, the principles can be efficiently applied. We know that sparse neighborhoods facilitate lexical decisions for concrete words (not for abstract words), while dense neighborhoods introduce noise into the retrieval system as evidenced by slower processing and response latencies. However, dense neighborhoods include high frequency words that many PWA are required to use in daily communicative activities. Thus, from a life participation perspective, it is important to include words from semantically dense neighborhoods. Additionally, these dense neighborhoods are challenging, and we must recall the complexity approach to treatment efficacy stating that more difficult stimuli generalizes to stimuli with lower difficulty (Thompson et al., 2003). It is recommended that clinicians include words found in dense and sparse neighborhoods as well as words that are concrete and abstract (see Table 5–1 for an example word list). Clinicians can then track if the more difficult words are generalizing to non-targeted words in sparse neighborhoods or words that are more concrete and imageable. It is ultimately up to the clinician to interpret the effects of these and other variables discussed in this chapter on PWA's word retrieval progress.

The clinical implications of orthographic and phonological neighbors are more straightforward. Clinicians can quickly determine how many words can be created from the target word by changing a single letter (orthographic) or phoneme (phonology). If a clinician can create multiple words by changing one letter, it is likely that one of those words may be higher in frequency than the target word, leading to slower recognition of the target. Moreover, transposing letters to create new words can also be inhibitory and should be closely watched by the clinician.

Morphological Complexity

Morphological errors, although not as common in PWA compared to phonological errors, do occur and can change the meaning of a message. Morphological errors are classified as substitution (*blasted* becomes *blasts*), omissions (*forcefully* becomes *force*), and additions (*seek* becomes *seeker*; Badecker & Caramazza, 2017). Although no reports have been published about PWA with a pure morphological impairment, persons with nonfluent Broca's aphasia have morphosyntactic impairments. However, as the morphological complexity of a word increases so does the word's phonological complexity. Yet phonological complexity does not account for the over-regularizations that PWA use (*sang* becomes *singed*), which are considered phonologically more complex to produce (Bird et al., 2003). Another view posits an impairment in the rules to affix morphemes to base words is the problem (Ullman et al., 1997); however, this theory does not explain the differences between noun and verb morphology or syntactic function (Faroqi-Shah & Thompson, 2007; Kohn & Melvold, 2000). Therefore, it appears that multiple impairments could be responsible for morphological errors (Faroqi-Shah & Thompson, 2007).

To test this argument, the effects of morphological complexity (verb stems, irregular past tense, regular past tense, and progressive "–ing") on verb production accuracy and speed were investigated in PWA and unimpaired adults (Faroqi-Shah & Thompson, 2007). The authors controlled phonological and lexical complexity in the study. The results indicate that there was no morphological complexity effect on accuracy or latency. Specifically, affixed verbs (-ed and -ing) did not differ from the morphologically simpler verbs (stem and irregular verbs). This study's results do not support the impaired affixation account of morphological errors in PWA (Ullman et al., 1997), but rather support the phonological complexity view if PWA have a phonological deficit. More specifically, if phonological complexity is controlled and PWA do not have a phonological deficit, then there will not likely be a morphological complexity effect.

Complex words include multiple morphemes (*agree+able*), which include the base word (*agree*) and the affix (*+able*). The word's frequency will determine how quickly the word can be accessed in a variety of spoken tasks. However, when accounting for morphologically complex words, the surface form's word frequency (i.e., the entire word, base + affix) and the base morpheme frequency (i.e., aggregate frequency of all words containing the base morpheme *agree, agreement, agreeable*, and so on) influence processing in different ways. Of importance to morphological complexity is base frequency in which previous studies have found a facilitative effect (Vannest et al., 2002; Vannest & Boland, 1999). That is, high frequency base words result in faster response latency times.

In another morphological study (Vannest et al., 2011), investigators compared morphological complexity or word type (decomposable, whole-word, and simple) and frequency (high vs. low) with unimpaired adults. Decomposable words were those words that included a base word and the affixes *-able, -ness,* and *-less*. Whole words included a base word and *-ity* and *-ation*. Finally, simple words included monomorphemic words. Each category included 40 high base frequency words and 40 low base frequency words. The results indicated significant main effects for word type and frequency, with a significant interaction between the two. Decomposable words and simple words had a base frequency effect with faster response times in the high frequency condition, whereas no such effect was found for whole-words.

Clinical Implications

Clinically, these results have some utility in the selection of different morphological word types (e.g., monomorphemic). Specifically, whole words (base word and *-ity* and *-ation*) and low base frequency decomposable words appeared to be the most difficult for unimpaired populations. We can argue, using the complexity account of treatment efficacy proposed by Thompson et al. (2003), that by selecting these more difficult word conditions, PWA may generalize treatment to simpler word conditions. However, this claim must be empirically tested. Moreover, the use of low base frequency words for PWA may not be in line with their communicative needs. Therefore, a balance must be struck between life participation and word retrieval variables such as morphological complexity.

Augmentative and Alternative Commination Digital Stimuli

Aphasiologists have long sought for more efficient and effective rehabilitative interventions with the purpose of restoring the natural spoken language of PWA to prestroke levels (Coelho, Sinotte, & Duffy, 2008). For many PWA, a restorative approach is ineffective, and compensatory strategies must be implemented to circumvent communication breakdown secondary to the chronic nature or severity of aphasia (Brock et al., 2017; Dietz et al., 2018). These compensatory interventions, notably augmentative and alternative communication (AAC), rely on static (i.e., nonmoving) and, to a lesser extent, dynamic (i.e., moving) graphic symbols, photographs, and movies to positively supplement natural speech and multimodal message production in PWA (Brock et al., 2017; Brock & Hung, 2021; Dietz et al., 2014, 2018).

Research in the last three decades has primarily explored nouns depicted as static symbols because nouns are easily depicted graphically (Allen et al., 2017). The ease with which nouns are depicted graphically can be explained by several principles such as word frequency (Bastiaanse et al., 2016), AoA (Gentner, 1978), and iconicity (Fuller, Lloyd, & Schlosser, 1992). Given that we have discussed AoA and frequency, let us move to the iconicity principle. The principle states that transparent graphic symbols, which readily depict their referents, are not only easier to teach, but are also acquired for communication purposes much sooner than translucent or opaque symbols (Fuller et al., 1992). In contrast, translucent symbols (i.e., the symbol and the referent are paired by the clinician) and opaque symbols (i.e., no visual relationship with the referent) require additional therapy time to teach the symbol-referent relationship. Most nouns tend to be transparent or translucent. Verbs are not as easily depicted graphically secondary to their inherent movement, but verbs do have the added benefit of activating a lemma (i.e., information associated with a concept), which includes semantic information, thematic roles, and argument structure (Levelt, 1989). For example, the verb feed takes additional arguments in the sentence, "The mom [agent] feeds lunch [patient] to her baby [goal]." Therefore, dynamic verb symbols are more transparent than static verb symbols which enhance verb naming in adults with and without aphasia.

There is a growing research body investigating the effects of symbol format (i.e., graphic line drawings and digitally recorded videos) and verb argument structure (i.e., intransitive and transitive) on verb naming accuracy, identification, and sentence generation (Blankestijn-Wilmsen et al., 2017; Brock & Hung, in press; den Ouden et al., 2009). With respect to symbol format, den Ouden and colleagues (2009) found that participants without aphasia named actions with greater accuracy in the video condition compared to the line drawing condition. They suggested that naming actions from line drawings was less natural and more cognitively demanding than naming verbs from videos. However, it should be noted that their static condition included black and white cartoon drawings, whereas the video condition included a human actor. This difference, though subtle, may have created a threat to internal validity because the two conditions should have been the same with the only exception being movement.

Blankestijn-Wilmsen et al. (2017) studied the effect of static and dynamic symbol format on verb naming and sentence production in PWA using matched stimuli (i.e., each condition was the same with the exception of movement). The verbs grouped into face (e.g., eat), arm (e.g., applaud), and leg (e.g., kick) verbs and matched for frequency, transitivity, and instrumentality. Their results indicated that PWA in the dynamic video condition correctly named more action verbs and produced more sentences than in the static photograph condition. However, the differences were minimal, and it was unclear if the sentence production task was sufficiently difficult to reveal more pronounced differences between the static and dynamic conditions. Specifically, over half of the verbs were intransitive and did not require a direct object to form a sentence (e.g., "to play").

Brock and Hung (2021) investigated the effect symbol format (photograph condition vs. video condition) and verb argument structure (two- and three-argument verbs) on verb naming, verb identification, and spoken sentence production in PWA. The results supported previous research from Thompson and colleagues (1997, 2003, 2013) indicating that the two-argument verbs were easier to name, identify, and use in a sentence when compared to three-argument verbs. While not significant, there was a medium to large effect size where the participants with aphasia accurately named more verbs in the video condition when compared to the photograph condition. Additionally, symbol format did not impact sentence generation scores; however, it should be noted that this study was a processing study, and subsequent investigations need to determine if symbol format effects exist postintervention.

Clinical Implications

Clinically, AAC intervention for many PWA results in spoken language recovery (Dietz et al., 2018), enhanced discourse (Brock et al., 2017; Dietz et al., 2014), and enhanced communicative competence, as rated by participant respondents (Brock et al., 2019). Moreover, PWA can cue themselves using AAC symbols, such as photographs and videos, to enhance their word retrieval and even natural spoken language. The iconic symbol formats lend themselves well to a variety of word classes to treat deficits in word production and sentence generation. AAC is no longer a last resort intervention for PWA.

Chapter Summary

Overall, several variables are likely to impact the ability of PWA to retrieve words. Initially, researchers believed that word frequency was the most important word retrieval variable (Kucera & Francis, 1967); however, more contemporary research found several short-comings related to word frequency calculations from a dataset that included only written work (Brysbeart & New, 2009). Specifically, the written word is more formal and skewed toward lower frequency word inclusion compared to spoken language. Additionally, AoA, imageability, syntax, phonology, morphology, orthographic text, semantic neighborhoods, density, word class, and several others discussed in this chapter were found to be reliable variables affecting word retrieval (Adelman et al., 2006; Andrews, 1997; Barry et al., 2006; Garlock et al., 2001; Hoffman et al., 2011; Kim & Thompson, 2000; McRae, Cree, et al., 2005; Thompson et al., 2003; Vannest et al., 2011; Yates, 2005). There is no agreed upon "recipe" indicating which retrieval variables are the most impactful. Rather, the clinician is encouraged to have an understanding of each to engage in critical thinking with regard to word selection and interpretation of their clients' data.

Discussion Questions

1. Discuss the caveats of using a single word retrieval variable, such as AoA, to make evidence-based decisions.
2. Now combine two or more word retrieval variables and discuss the caveats and benefits these have on your clinical decisions.
3. What are the most important word retrieval variables that you have encountered in clinical practice and why?
4. Discuss the caveats and benefits associated with word level and sentence level treatment approaches. At what level do you begin therapy?

References

Acha, J., & Perea, M. (2008). The effect of neighborhood frequency in reading: Evidence with transposed-letter neighbors. *Cognition*, *108*(1), 290–300. https://doi.org/10.1016/j.cognition.2008.02.006

Adelman, J. S., Brown, G. D. A., & Quesada, J. F. (2006). Contextual diversity, not word frequency, determines word-maming and lexical decision times. *Psychological Science*, *17*(9), 814–823. https://doi.org/10.1111/j.1467-9280.2006.01787.x

Allen, A. A., Schlosser, R. W., Brock, K. L., & Shane, H. C. (2017). The effectiveness of aided augmented input techniques for persons with developmental disabilities: A systematic review. *Augmentative and*

Alternative Communication, 33(3), 149–159. https://doi.org/10.10 80/07434618.2017.1338752

Andrews, S. (1997). The effect of orthographic similarity on lexical retrieval: Resolving neighborhood conflicts. *Psychonomic Bulletin & Review, 4*(4), 439–461. https://doi.org/10.3758/BF03214334

Badecker, W., & Caramazza A., (2017). Morphology and aphasia. In A. Spencer & A.M. Zwicky (Eds.), *The handbook of morphology* (pp. 390–405). John Wiley & Sons. https://doi.org 10.1002/9781405166348

Barry, C., Johnston, R. A., & Wood, R. F. (2006). Effects of age of acquisition, age, and repetition priming on object naming. *Visual Cognition, 13*(7–8), 911–927.

Bastiaanse, R., Wieling, M., & Wolthuis, N. (2016). The role of frequency in the retrieval of nouns and verbs in aphasia. *Aphasiology, 30*(11), 1221–1239. https://doi.org/10.1080/02687038.2015.1100709

Bird, H., Ralph, M. A. L., Seidenberg, M. S., McClelland, J. L., & Patterson, K. (2003). Deficits in phonology and past-tense morphology: What's the connection? *Journal of Memory and Language, 48*(3), 502–526.

Blankestijn-Wilmsen, J., Damen, I., Voorbraak-Timmerman, V., Hurkmans, J., Brouwer de Koning, J., Pross, A., & Jonkers, R. (2017). The effect of static versus dynamic depictions of actions in verb and sentence production in aphasia. *Aphasiology, 31*(10), 1166–1182.

Boyle, M., & Coelho, C. A. (1995). Application of semantic feature analysis as a treatment for aphasic dysnomia. *American Journal of Speech-Language Pathology, 4*(4), 94–98.

Breedin, S. D., Saffran, E. M., & Schwartz, M. F. (1998). Semantic factors in verb retrieval: An effect of complexity. *Brain and Language, 63*(1), 1–31.

Brock, K. L., & Hung, P. F. (2020). The effects of digital symbol format on the naming, identification, and sentence production incorporating verbs for individuals with aphasia. *Aphasiology.* https://doi.org/ 10.1080/02687038.2020.1734528

Brock, K., Koul, R., Corwin, M., & Schlosser, R. (2017). A comparison of visual scene and grid displays for people with chronic aphasia: A pilot study to improve communication using AAC. *Aphasiology, 31*(11), 1282–1306. https://doi.org/10.1080/02687038.2016.1274874

Brock, K. L., Koul, R., Corwin, M., & Schlosser, R. W. (2019). The psychometric properties of the communicative competence scale for individuals with aphasia using speech-generating devices. *Aphasiology, 33*(5), 520–543.

Brown, J., & Thiessen, A. (2018). Using images with individuals with aphasia: Current research and clinical trends. *American Journal of*

Speech-Language Pathology, 27(1S), 504–515. https://doi.org/10.10 44/2017_AJSLP-16-0190

Brysbaert, M., Buchmeier, M., Conrad, M., Jacobs, A. M., Bölte, J., & Böhl, A. (2011). The word frequency effect. *Experimental Psychology, 58*(5), 412–424. https://doi.org/10.1027/1618-3169/a000123

Brysbaert, M., & Ellis, A. W. (2016). Aphasia and age of acquisition: Are early-learned words more resilient? *Aphasiology, 30*(11), 1240–1263. https://doi.org/10.1080/02687038.2015.1106439

Brysbaert, M., & New, B. (2009). Moving beyond Kučera and Francis: A critical evaluation of current word frequency norms and the introduction of a new and improved word frequency measure for American English. *Behavior Research Methods, 41*(4), 977–990. https://doi.org/10.3758/BRM.41.4.977

Chen, Q., & Mirman, D. (2012). Competition and cooperation among similar representations: Toward a unified account of facilitative and inhibitory effects of lexical neighbors. *Psychological Review, 119*(2), 417–430. https://doi.org/10.1037/a0027175

Coelho, C. A., McHugh, R. E., & Boyle, M. (2000). Semantic feature analysis as a treatment for aphasic dysnomia: A replication. *Aphasiology, 14*(2), 133–142.

Coelho, C. A., Sinotte, M., & Duffy, J.R. (2008). Schuell's stimulation approach to rehabilitation. In R. Chapey (Ed.), *Language intervention strategies in aphasia and related neurogenic communication disorders* (pp. 403–449). Wolters Kluwer-Lippincott Williams & Wilkins.

Coltheart, M., Davelaar, E., Jonasson, J. T., & Besner, D. (1977). Access to the internal lexicon. In S. Dornick (Ed.), *Attention and performance* (Vol. 6, pp. 535–556). Erlbaum.

DeDe, G. (2012). Effects of word frequency and modality on sentence comprehension impairments in people with aphasia. *American Journal of Speech-Language Pathology (Online); Rockville, 21*(2), S103–S114A. https://doi.org/10.1044/1058-0360(2012/11-0082)

DeDe, G. (2017). Effects of lexical variables on silent reading comprehension in individuals with aphasia: Evidence from eye tracking. *Journal of Speech, Language, and Hearing Research, 60*(9), 2589–2602. https://doi.org/10.1044/2017_JSLHR-L-16-0045

Dell, G. S. (1986). A spreading-activation theory of retrieval in sentence production. *Psychological Review, 93*(3), 283–321. https://doi.org/10.1037/0033-295X.93.3.283

Dell, G. S., Chang, F., & Griffin, Z. M. (1999). Connectionist models of language production: Lexical access and grammatical encoding. *Cognitive Science, 23*(4), 517–542. https://doi.org/10.1207/s15516709cog2304_6

Dell, G. S., & Gordon, J. K. (2003). Neighbors in the lexicon: Friends or foes. *Phonetics and Phonology in Language Comprehension and Production: Differences and Similarities, 6*, 9–37.

Dell, G. S., Schwartz, M. F., Martin, N., Saffran, E. M., & Gagnon, D. A. (1997). Lexical access in aphasic and nonaphasic speakers. *Psychological Review, 104*(4), 801–838. https://doi.org/10.1037/0033-295X.104.4.801

den Ouden, D.-B., Fix, S., Parrish, T. B., & Thompson, C. K. (2009). Argument structure effects in action verb naming in static and dynamic conditions. *Journal of Neurolinguistics, 22*(2), 196–215. https://doi.org/10.1016/j.jneuroling.2008.10.004

Dietz, A., Vannest, J., Maloney, T., Altaye, M., Holland, S., & Szaflarski, J. P. (2018). The feasibility of improving discourse in people with aphasia through AAC: Clinical and functional MRI correlates. *Aphasiology, 32*(6), 693–719. https://doi.org/10.1080/02687038.2018.1447641

Dietz, A., Weissling, K., Griffith, J., McKelvey, M., & Macke, D. (2014). The impact of interface design during an initial high-technology AAC experience: A collective case study of people with aphasia. *Augmentative and Alternative Communication, 30*(4), 314–328.

Duncan, C. P. (1973). Storage and retrieval of low-frequency words. *Memory & Cognition, 1*(2), 129–132. https://doi.org/10.3758/BF03198081

Edmonds, L. A., Mammino, K., & Ojeda, J. (2014). Effect of Verb Network Strengthening Treatment (VNeST) in persons with aphasia: Extension and replication of previous findings. *American Journal of Speech-Language Pathology, 23*(2), S312–S329.

Edmonds, L. A., Nadeau, S. E., & Kiran, S. (2009). Effect of Verb Network Strengthening Treatment (VNeST) on lexical retrieval of content words in sentences in persons with aphasia. *Aphasiology, 23*(3), 402–424.

Faroqi-Shah, Y., & Thompson, C. K. (2007). Verb inflections in agrammatic aphasia: Encoding of tense features. *Journal of Memory and Language, 56*(1), 129–151.

Fieder, N., Krajenbrink, T., Foxe, D., Hodges, J., Piguet, O., & Nickels, L. (2016). Less is more—Effects of semantic neighbourhood on naming in semantic dementia (svPPA). *Stem-, Spraak-En Taalpathologie, 21*, 65–68.

Fuller, D., Lloyd, L., & Schlosser, R. (1992). Further development of an augmentative and alternative communication symbol taxonomy. *Augmentative and Alternative Communication, 8*(1), 67–74. https://doi.org/10.1080/07434619212331276053

Garlock, V. M., Walley, A. C., & Metsala, J. L. (2001). Age-of-acquisition, word frequency, and neighborhood density effects on spoken word recognition by children and adults. *Journal of Memory and Language*, *45*(3), 468–492.

Gentner, D. (1978). On relational meaning: The acquisition of verb meaning. *Child Development*, 988–998.

Gentner, D. (1981). Verb semantic structures in memory for sentences: Evidence for componential representation. *Cognitive Psychology*, *13*(1), 56–83.

Goldrick, M., Folk, J. R., & Rapp, B. (2010). Mrs. Malaprop's neighborhood: Using word errors to reveal neighborhood structure. *Journal of Memory and Language*, *62*(2), 113–134. https://doi.org/10.1016/j.jml.2009.11.008

Heuven, W. J. B. van, Mandera, P., Keuleers, E., & Brysbaert, M. (2014). SUBTLEX-UK: A new and improved word frequency database for British English. *The Quarterly Journal of Experimental Psychology*, *67*(6), 1176–1190. https://doi.org/10.1080/17470218.2013.850521

Hillis, A. E., Rapp, B., Romani, C., & Caramazza, A. (1990). Selective impairment of semantics in lexical processing. *Cognitive Neuropsychology*, *7*(3), 191–243. https://doi.org/10.1080/02643299008253442

Höffler, T. N., & Leutner, D. (2007). Instructional animation versus static pictures: A meta-analysis. *Learning and Instruction*, *17*(6), 722–738.

Hoffman, P., Rogers, T. T., & Lambon Ralph, M. A. (2011). Semantic diversity accounts for the "missing" word frequency effect in stroke aphasia: Insights using a novel method to quantify contextual variability in meaning. *Journal of Cognitive Neuroscience*, *23*(9), 2432–2446. https://doi.org/10.1162/jocn.2011.21614

Howard, D., & Gatehouse, C. (2006). Distinguishing semantic and lexical word retrieval deficits in people with aphasia. *Aphasiology*, *20*(9), 921–950. https://doi.org/10.1080/02687030600782679

Huttenlocher, J., Smiley, P., & Charney, R. (1983). Emergence of action categories in the child: Evidence from verb meanings. *Psychological Review*, *90*(1), 72. https://doi.org/10.1037/0033-295X.90.1.72

Johns, B. T., Gruenenfelder, T. M., Pisoni, D. B., & Jones, M. N. (2012). Effects of word frequency, contextual diversity, and semantic distinctiveness on spoken word recognition. *The Journal of the Acoustical Society of America*, *132*(2), EL74–EL80.

Jonkers, R., & Bastiaanse, R. (2006). The influence of instrumentality and name-relation to a noun on verb comprehension in Dutch aphasic speakers. *Aphasiology*, *20*(1), 3–16.

Kay, J., & Ellis, A. (1987). A cognitive neuropsychological case study of anomia implications for psychological models of word retrieval. *Brain*, *110*(3), 613–629. https://doi.org/10.1093/brain/110.3.613

Kemmerer, D., & Tranel, D. (2000). Verb retrieval in brain-damaged subjects: 1. Analysis of stimulus, lexical, and conceptual factors. *Brain and Language, 73*(3), 347–392. https://doi.org/10.1006/brln.2000 .2311

Kim, M., & Thompson, C. K. (2000). Patterns of comprehension and production of nouns and verbs in agrammatism: Implications for lexical organization. *Brain and Language, 74*(1), 1–25.

Kintsch, W. (1974). *The representation of meaning in memory.* Lawrence Erlbaum.

Kiran, Swathi, & Thompson, Cynthia K. (2003). The role of semantic complexity in treatment of naming deficits. *Journal of Speech, Language, and Hearing Research, 46*(3), 608–622. https://doi.org/ 10.1044/1092-4388(2003/048)

Kittredge, A. K., Dell, G. S., Verkuilen, J., & Schwartz, M. F. (2008). Where is the effect of frequency in word production? Insights from aphasic picture-naming errors. *Cognitive Neuropsychology, 25*(4), 463–492.

Knobel, M., Finkbeiner, M., & Caramazza, A. (2008). The many places of frequency: Evidence for a novel locus of the lexical frequency effect in word production. *Cognitive Neuropsychology, 25*(2), 256–286.

Kohn, S. E., & Melvold, J. (2000). Effects of morphological complexity on phonological output deficits in fluent and nonfluent aphasia. *Brain and Language, 73*(3), 323–346.

Koul, R., & Harding, R. (1998). Identification and production of graphic symbols by individuals with aphasia: Efficacy of a software application. *Augmentative and Alternative Communication, 14*(1), 11–24.

Kučera, H., & Francis, W. (1967). *Computational analysis of present-day American English.* Brown University Press.

Kuperman, V., Stadthagen-Gonzalez, H., & Brysbaert, M. (2012). Age-of-acquisition ratings for 30,000 English words. *Behavior Research Methods, 44*(4), 978–990.

La Heij, W., Puerta-Melguizo, M. C., van Oostrum, M., & Starreveld, P. A. (1999). Picture naming: Identical priming and word frequency interact. *Acta Psychologica, 102*(1), 77–95.

Levelt, W. J. (1989). *Speaking: From intention to articulation* (Vol. 1). MIT press.

Levelt, Willem J. M., Roelofs, A., & Meyer, A. S. (1999). A theory of lexical access in speech production. *Behavioral and Brain Sciences, 22*(1), 1–38.

Luce, P. A., & Pisoni, D. B. (1998). Recognizing spoken words: The neighborhood activation model. *Ear and Hearing, 19*(1), 1–36.

Luzzatti, C., Raggi, R., Zonca, G., Pistarini, C., Contardi, A., & Pinna, G.-D. (2002). Verb–noun double dissociation in aphasic lexical impairments: The role of word frequency and imageability. *Brain and Language, 81*(1–3), 432–444. https://doi.org/10.1006/brln.2001.2536

Magnuson, J. S., Dixon, J. A., Tanenhaus, M. K., & Aslin, R. N. (2007). The dynamics of lexical competition during spoken word recognition. *Cognitive Science*, *31*(1), 133–156. https://doi.org/10.1080/03640210709336987

Massaro, M., & Tompkins, C. A. (1994). Feature analysis for treatment of communication disorders in traumatically brain-injured patients: An efficacy study. *Clinical Aphasiology*, *22*, 245–256.

McClelland, J. L., & Rumelhart, D. E. (1981). An interactive activation model of context effects in letter perception: I. An account of basic findings. *Psychological Review*, *88*(5), 375.

McDonald, S. A., & Shillcock, R. C. (2001). Rethinking the word frequency effect: The neglected role of distributional information in lexical processing. *Language and Speech*, *44*(3), 295–322. https://doi.org/10.1177/00238309010440030101

McKelvey, M. L., Hux, K., Dietz, A., & Beukelman, D. R. (2010). Impact of personal relevance and contextualization on word-picture matching by people with aphasia. *American Journal of Speech-Language Pathology*, *19*(1), 22–33. https://doi.org/10.1044/1058-0360(2009/08-0021)

McRae, K., Cree, G. S., Seidenberg, M. S., & McNorgan, C. (2005). Semantic feature production norms for a large set of living and nonliving things. *Behavior Research Methods*, *37*(4), 547–559.

McRae, K., Hare, M., Elman, J. L., & Ferretti, T. (2005). A basis for generating expectancies for verbs from nouns. *Memory & Cognition*, *33*(7), 1174–1184.

Mirman, D. (2011). Effects of near and distant semantic neighbors on word production. *Cognitive, Affective, & Behavioral Neuroscience*, *11*(1), 32–43.

Mirman, D., Dixon, J. A., & Magnuson, J. S. (2008). Statistical and computational models of the visual world paradigm: Growth curves and individual differences. *Journal of Memory and Language*, *59*(4), 475–494.

Mirman, D., & Magnuson, J. S. (2009). Dynamics of activation of semantically similar concepts during spoken word recognition. *Memory & Cognition*, *37*(7), 1026–1039

Paivio, A., Yuille, J. C., & Madigan, S. A. (1968). Concreteness, imagery, and meaningfulness values for 925 nouns. *Journal of Experimental Psychology*, *76*(1, Pt.2), 1–25. https://doi.org/10.1037/h0025327

Pinker, S. (2013). *Learnability and cognition: The acquisition of argument structure*. MIT press.

Quique, Y. M., Evans, W. S., & Dickey, M. W. (2019). Acquisition and generalization responses in aphasia naming treatment: A meta-analysis of semantic feature analysis outcomes. *American Journal*

of Speech-Language Pathology, 28(1S), 230–246. https://doi.org/10
.1044/2018_AJSLP-17-0155

Reilly, M., & Desai, R. H. (2017). Effects of semantic neighborhood density in abstract and concrete words. *Cognition, 169,* 46–53. https://doi.org/10.1016/j.cognition.2017.08.004

Rosa, E., Tapia, J. L., & Perea, M. (2017). Contextual diversity facilitates learning new words in the classroom. *PLoS ONE, 12*(6). https://doi .org/10.1371/journal.pone.0179004

Sosa, A. V., & Stoel-Gammon, C. (2012). Lexical and phonological effects in early word production. *Journal of Speech, Language, and Hearing Research, 55*(2), 596–608. https://doi.org/10.1044/1092-43 88(2011/10-0113)

Thompson, C. K., Lange, K. L., Schneider, S. L., & Shapiro, L. P. (1997). Agrammatic and non-brain-damaged subjects' verb and verb argument structure production. *Aphasiology, 11*(4–5), 473–490.

Thompson, C. K., Riley, E. A., den Ouden, D.-B., Meltzer-Asscher, A., & Lukic, S. (2013). Training verb argument structure production in agrammatic aphasia: Behavioral and neural recovery patterns. *Cortex, 49*(9), 2358–2376. https://doi.org/10.1016/j.cortex.2013.02.003

Thompson C. K., Shapiro L. P., Kiran S., & Sobecks J. (2003). The role of syntactic complexity in treatment of sentence deficits in agrammatic aphasia. *Journal of Speech, Language, and Hearing Research, 46*(3), 591–607. https://doi.org/10.1044/1092-4388(2003/047)

Ullman, M. T., Corkin, S., Coppola, M., Hickok, G., Growdon, J. H., Koroshetz, W. J., & Pinker, S. (1997). A neural dissociation within language: Evidence that the mental dictionary is part of declarative memory, and that grammatical rules are processed by the procedural system. *Journal of Cognitive Neuroscience, 9*(2), 266–276.

Vannest, J., Bertram, R., Järvikivi, J., & Niemi, J. (2002). Counterintuitive cross-linguistic differences: More morphological computation in English than in Finnish. *Journal of Psycholinguistic Research, 31*(2), 83–106.

Vannest, J., & Boland, J. E. (1999). Lexical morphology and lexical access. *Brain and Language, 68*(1–2), 324–332.

Vannest, J., Newport, E. L., Newman, A. J., & Bavelier, D. (2011). Interplay between morphology and frequency in lexical access: The case of the base frequency effect. *Brain Research, 1373,* 144–159. https:// doi.org/10.1016/j.brainres.2010.12.022

Vergara-Martínez, M., Comesaña, M., & Perea, M. (2017). The ERP signature of the contextual diversity effect in visual word recognition. *Cognitive, Affective & Behavioral Neuroscience, 17*(3), 461–474. https://doi.org/10.3758/s13416-016-0491-7

Vitkovitch, M., & Humphreys, G. W. (1991). Perseverant responding in speeded naming of pictures: It's in the links. *Journal of Experimental Psychology: Learning, Memory, and Cognition, 17*(4), 664.

Wheeldon, L. R., & Monsell, S. (1992). The locus of repetition priming of spoken word production. *The Quarterly Journal of Experimental Psychology Section A, 44*(4), 723–761.

Yates, M. (2005). Phonological neighbors speed visual word processing: Evidence from multiple tasks. *Journal of Experimental Psychology: Learning, Memory, and Cognition, 31*(6), 1385–1397. https://doi.org/10.1037/0278-7393.31.6.1385

Yates, M., Friend, J., & Ploetz, D. M. (2008). Phonological neighbors influence word naming through the least supported phoneme. *Journal of Experimental Psychology: Human Perception and Performance, 34*(6), 1599–1608. https://doi.org/10.1037/a0011633

6

WORD ACCESS AND RETRIEVAL DIFFICULTY IN DIFFERENT POPULATIONS

Lei Sun and Pei-Fang Hung

Chapter Objectives

1. Explain word retrieval breakdowns using lexical access models.
2. Define word-finding difficulty in children and discuss the underlying lexical access problems in children with developmental language disorders, autism spectrum disorders, and language learning disabilities.
3. Discuss word retrieval difficulty associated with neurogenic language and communication disorders.
4. Identify different error types and clinical characteristics in different neurogenic word retrieval difficulty.

Introduction

This chapter provides an overview of word-finding difficulties (WFD) from the perspectives of developmental and neurogenic language disorders, and reviews the relevant research evidence. After a brief review of lexical access models, the discussion will focus on clinical characteristics and related factors that affect lexical access and retrieval. We will then discuss the studies investigating WFD in different populations with communication disorders, such as developmental language disorders, autism spectrum disorders, learning disabilities, aphasia, cognitive-communication disorders, mild cognitive impairment, and dementia.

A Quick Review of Lexical Access Models and Word Retrieval Breakdowns

As discussed in Chapter 2, Levelt's Speech Production Model (1989) proposes that the word retrieval process starts from a formed conceptual message. Then, in the *grammatical encoding phase*, corresponding words (i.e., lemmas) along with syntactic properties (e.g., word class, gender) will be activated based on the semantic features. In the subsequent phase, *morpho-phonological encoding phase*, the corresponding morphological and phonological properties (lexemes) will be accessed after the target lemma is selected. In other words, lemmas represent semantic and syntactic properties, and lexemes specify morphological and phonological forms (McGregor, 1997). Once the correct phonological form is activated, the word continues to phonetic encoding and articulation, and then the correct words can be uttered accurately (Levelt, 1999, p. 88).

This word retrieval process seems seamless with the activation cascades from the top-level (conceptual level) to the bottom-level (articulation) in a linear fashion. However, competition exists at each level of the process. For example, after the concept is formed, all semantically related features may be activated. Let's use the word "dog" as an example. After seeing a picture of [dog], all semantically related features, such as *animals, four legs, fur*, and so forth, are activated. Each activated feature will further prompt the activation of the corresponding lemmas (words). The word with most activation will be selected for the next stage. Then, it spreads the activation to morpho-phonological encoding where the correct phonemes will be selected from a pool of phonemes, including the onset, nucleus, and coda (e.g., /d/-/ɔ/-/g/) for articulation (Hartsuiker & Vigliocco, 2009; Levelt, 1999).

Slow retrieval and errors can happen at the levels of lemma (word) selection, lexeme (phoneme) selection, or both. A lemma selection error may occur when another competing word is highly activated because of semantic relatedness (e.g., the word "*cat*" (another type of animal pet) for the target word "dog"). Errors may also arise at the lexeme level when selecting the corresponding phonemes. If a competing phoneme has a higher activation level than the intended phoneme, a speech error will occur (Hartsuiker & Vigliocco, 2009, p. 512). For example, if the competing phoneme /f/ is highly activated during the production of "dog", the phonological error /fog/ may occur. A semantic-phonological mixed error may be a result of disruption at both levels. For example, saying "bee" for the target word "flea."

A breakdown at any level or between the levels will result in an error (Nickels, 2001). The scope of this book, and this chapter, is on the semantic representation (i.e., conceptual-semantic and semantic-lexical levels) and phonological representation. Hence, we will not focus on breakdowns that happen after the intended word form is selected and motor processing.

Lexical Access Difficulty in Children

In Chapter 3, we briefly reviewed the underlying cognitive processes for word learning and discussed the process of storing newly learned words in long-term memory. Storage strength means *how well* a person learns the word, and retrieval strength refers to *how easily* the word can be accessed (Nippold, 2007). Storage and retrieval of words are interdependent (Nippold, 2007). This means that the better the words are stored in long-term memory, the easier these words can be retrieved when needed. Also, the more frequently words are used in diverse contexts, the stronger these words can be stored in long-term memory. Thus, lexical storage and retrieval are mutually beneficial and are both important for vocabulary development and lexical access.

Strong word storage requires successful, initial fast mapping and multiple exposures in meaningful contexts, and feedback from using words in diverse contexts to store words in long-term memory, specifically in declarative memory (a.k.a. explicit memory) that contains factual information, past experiences, and concepts. On the other hand, using words requires successful retrieval of the target words when needed. The process for retrieving a target word can be impacted by how frequently the word is accessed, the competition of related words, the presence of cues, and how recently the word was learned (Nippold, 2007).

Define Word Access Difficulty From a Developmental Perspective

Word finding is the ability to retrieve the desired word in an appropriate context (German, 2009). Word finding difficulty in children refers to those children who have naming or lexical access problems (Messer & Dockrell, 2006, p 310), and have difficulty generating specific words when needed (Faust et al., 1997). Characteristics in children with lexical access difficulty can include frequent pauses, circumlocutions, repetitions, reformations, substitutions, excessive use of fillers, and the use of nonspecific words in spontaneous speech (Faust et al., 1997; German & Simon, 1991; Marshall, 2014; Nippold, 2007).

Children develop specific and distinguished forms to store words in long-term memory over time. As they continue to expand their vocabulary, they also develop the sensitivity to the segments of words which is a foundation of metalinguistic skills. Difficulty in accessing words can be found in children with developmental language disorders. Children's naming errors can help clinicians identify the locus of breakdown and the subsequent consequence of the breakdown. For example, inaccessible semantic features can consequently lead to inaccessible phonological forms because of disruption during the activation spreading. According to Messer and Dockrell (2006), lexical access difficulty may originate from different locations throughout the lexical access process and having a sole impairment either in the retrieval of lemma or lexeme is unlikely because both levels may be affected. Nevertheless, it is important to keep in mind that word access difficulties can continue to affect children's language functioning and development as they grow (Messer & Dockrell, 2013).

Word Finding Behaviors and Characteristics

Word finding characteristics in children were defined and reported in several studies (German & Simon, 1991, pp. 311–312; Marks & Strokes, 2010, p. 590; Stiegler & Hoffman, 2001, p.284). German (2009) identified three error patterns of lexical access difficulty in children. The first type is called "*slip of the tongue*" error; this is a type of semantic errors that occurs when there is a failure to access semantic or syntactic information. In other words, after the target concept is selected, the activation somehow does not spread to the corresponding words, or the competing semantically related words receive a higher activation level than the intended word. For example, the child said, "*It is a rabbit . . . no rat . . . oh . . . it is a guinea pig* (target word)."

The second error pattern is called "*tip of the tongue*" error. It shows that there may be a disconnection between the semantic representation and phonological representation. According to Faust et al. (1997), tip-of-the-tongue indicates incomplete activation or access blockage. It prevents children with WFDs from accessing correct phonological forms. Children may start describing "*guinea pig*" without correctly naming it. It indicates that the child knows the word meaning and the correct syntactic information. However, the proper phonological form is not selected because there is a blockage during the activation from lemma to the lexeme level. The error reflects a weak relation between lexical and phonological representations. The third error is called "*twist of the tongue*" error. At the lexeme level where phonological encoding takes place, phonemes in different pools (onset, nucleus, coda) compete with each other. German (2009) referred to this error as a segment-related phonological error that results from incomplete access to correct phoneme sequence or representation.

Table 6–1 summarizes the definitions and examples discussed above, and Table 6–2 lists the different types of word-finding errors and examples adapted from McGregor and Windsor's study in 1996 (p. 1058).

Table 6–1. Word Finding Characteristics, Definition, and Examples

Word-Finding Characteristics	Definition	Example
Repetition	Words within a T-unit has been unnecessarily repeated.	Katy, (Katy) went home.
Reformulation	Words within a T-unit has been changed or replaced. Speaker stops and rewords the message.	She found a (cat), a rat in the room.
Empty words/ Interjection	Words within a T-unit do not add content or specificity to the T-unit.	She found a, (you know), rat in the room.
Insertions/ Explanation	Words or phrases within a T-unit used to comment on the language process.	I want to order...(I forgot what it is called).
Substitutions	Words are replaced by semantically or phonologically similar words.	She is riding a (donkey) (target: horse). The (cats) carry diseases (target: rats).
Indefinite reference	A nonspecific word is used instead of the target word	She found (that thing) in the room.
Delays-unfilled	Pauses of 6 or more seconds without verbalization within a T-unit.	
Time fillers-filled delay	Sounds or syllables inserted to fill in during the retrieval process (e.g., um, uh, er).	

Source: Adapted from German and Simon (1991, pp. 311–312), Marks and Strokes (2010, p. 590), Stiegler and Hoffman (2001, p. 284).

Lexical Access Difficulty in Children With Developmental Language Disorders

Although the term "specific language impairment (SLI)" was commonly used in literature, "developmental language disorders (DLD)" is now a preferred term for referring to the same group

Table 6-2. Word Finding Error Examples

Types of Word-Finding Errors	Target Word (Noun)	Example Error	Target Word (Verb)	Example Error
Semantic errors				
Superordinate	Cat	*"animal"*	Run	*"exercise"*
Coordinate (intrinsic relationship)	Cat	*dog*	Run	*"walk"*
Subordinate	Cat	*American Shorthair*	Run	*"sprint"*
Semantic circumlocution	Cat	*"It says meow."*	Run	*"Like walking, but faster"*
Thematic-related (attributes)	Cat	*"whiskers, jump, paw, scratch"*	Run	*"Sprint, stroll, walk, jog"*
Thematic-association (co-occur)	Cat	*"pet"*	Run	*"move"*
Phonological errors				
Sound substitution	Cat	*"hat"*	Run	*"fun"*
Phonemic circumlocution	Cat	*It sounds like "hat"*	Run	*It sounds like "fun"*
Initial sound	Cat	*"k . . ."*	Run	*"Urrr . . . "*
Mixed semantic and phonological errors				
	Cat	*"rat"*	Hike	*"bike"*
Other types of errors				
No response/ I don't know	Cat	*"I don't know"*	Run	*No response*
Irrelevant	Cat	*"box"*	Run	*"eat"*
Perseveration	Cat	*Repeat previous response/cat*	Run	*Repeat previous response/run*
Neologism	Cat	*"jat"*	Run	*"mun"*

Source: Adapted from McGregor and Windsor (1996, p.1058), McGregor (1997, p.1235).

of children. In this section, we use the term "DLD" to maintain consistency and avoid confusion. Children with DLD have difficulty developing language in general, so it is not uncommon to observe that children with DLD may have difficulty with lexical retrieval due to a smaller vocabulary repertoire, as well as difficulty with semantic mapping, lexical storage, and information organization.

Children with DLD also have core deficits in grammar, so they show significant difficulty in understanding the meaning of a new verb through the use of morphosyntactic information (Kan & Windsor, 2010; McGregor, 2009; Shulman & Guberman, 2007). When compared to typically developing peers, children with DLD show significant difficulty in learning new verbs than novel nouns. Similar to learning new nouns, children with DLD also need significantly more exposures to learn new action verbs (Windfuhr et al., 2002). Children with DLD often have a hard time learning mental state verbs because of abstractness in conceptualization, as well as the sentence complement required for mental state verbs (Ingram, 2002).

Sheng and McGregor (2010) indicated that children with DLD have weak long-term lexical storage and semantic connections between words, which results in naming and word access difficulty. For example, when naming the word [*wasp*], they may select semantically related words instead, such as *fly*, *ladybug*, or *bee* (words in the same semantic category) or *nest*, *sting*, or *pest* (words in the semantically related categories). The more that words overlap (e.g., wasp and bee), the stronger these words coactivate. While developing a dense and rich semantic network, children face the pressure to fine-grain their lexical representations by using more distinct features to differentiate between words. Therefore, the more words a child has acquired, the more sophisticated lexical knowledge the child develops. Children with DLD have insufficient semantic information in lexical storage, thus they do not have sophisticated lexical representations to differentiate among semantic neighbors (Bragard & Schelstraete, 2007; McGregor & Waxman, 1998) which results in lexical access difficulty.

Capone and McGregor (2005) highlighted the importance of semantic representations on naming performance and lexical access in toddlers. They reported that the depth of semantic representations is significantly correlated with word retrieval; rich semantic representations can facilitate the performance of word retrieval. It is important to note that failure in naming/lexical access only indicates weak representations, rather than absent representations. McGregor, Oleson, Bahnsen, and Duff (2013) also reported that both underdeveloped depth and breadth of lexical knowledge was found in school-age children with DLD.

Seiger-Gardner and Schwartz (2008) proposed that lexical access difficulty in children with DLD may be due to an inefficient mechanism that inhibits the activation of competing words because their semantic representations and lexical organization are weak and insufficient. With weak semantic representations, more words in the same semantic category can increase the possibility of competition during the word selection processes. Children with DLD often have underspecified semantic representations, thus they have difficulty differentiating semantically related words (Bragard & Schelstraete, 2007). This may explain the semantic errors made by children with DLD, such as saying "*bee*" for "*wasp*."

On the contrary, Faust and colleagues' study (1997) reported that children with DLD made significantly more phonological errors than typically developing peers. Children with DLD could retrieve semantic information (e.g., identify semantic features) but not the target phonological form, which indicated a phonological cause of naming errors. Hence, Faust et al. (1997) claimed that word access difficulty in children with DLD is due to difficulty in both storage of and access to phonological representations instead of inability to retrieve semantic information. They further recommended that using phonological cues to strengthen lexical-phonological connections may aid the effectiveness of word access/retrieval and minimize the possibility of coactivating competing words.

However, some researchers believe naming and lexical access difficulty in children with DLD is due to lack of both semantic and phonological representations. For example, McGregor and Appel (2002) examined the naming and drawing results from a five-year-old boy with DLD. The child's drawing results (which assessed mental representation) were correlated with his naming performance. They concluded that this child's naming difficulty can stem from both insufficient lexical and phonological representations.

Lexical access and retrieval difficulty in DLD can also be the result of insufficient encoding. For example, adults with a history of DLD continue to struggle with deficiencies in lexical knowledge in both depth and breadth, as well as ongoing lexical learning. They are less able to connect forms to meanings (McGregor et al., 2013). McGregor and colleagues (2017) indicated that once the information is successfully encoded, adults with DLD are better able to retain and retrieve the new words. The deficit in working memory in individuals with DLD hinders information encoding, which in turn adversely affects retention and retrieval of words (McGregor et al., 2017).

In sum, difficulty in lexical encoding, storage, and retrieval may all be related to word access difficulty in children with DLD. This is also related to the deficiency in their cognitive functions (e.g., working memory and language abilities [or, syntax]). Therefore, children with DLD have difficulty using the required semantic and syntactic information to access lexicon and aid the mapping between meanings and forms (Kan & Windsor, 2010).

Lexical Access Difficulty in Children With Language-Based Learning Disability

In this section, our discussion focuses on lexical access difficulty in the group of children who have difficulty learning academically due to chronic and undiagnosed language disorders or weak language skills. There are many terms used to describe this population. For example, the term *"specific learning disability (SLD)"* is one of the categories listed in the Individuals with Disabilities Education Act (IDEA, 2004). SLD means

> *a disorder in one or more of the basic psychological processes involved in understanding or in using language, spoken or written, that may manifest itself in the imperfect ability to listen, think, speak, read, write, spell, or to do mathematical calculations . . .* (34 D.F.R.§ 300.8 (c)(10.ii))

According to IDEA (2004), SLD does not include "learning problems that are primarily the result of visual, hearing, or mental retardation, of emotional disturbance, or of environmental, cultural, or economic disadvantage" (34 D.F.R.§ 300.8 (c)(10. ii)). Another example is the term *"learning disabilities (LD)."* The National Joint Committee on Learning Disabilities (NJCLD) defines LD as "a heterogeneous group of disorders of presumed neurological origin" that covers different groups of children who struggle academically due to problems in both spoken and written language (NJCLD, 2001). In this section, we will not use either SLD or LD. Instead, we will use the term "language-based learning disability (LLD)." According to Sun and Wallach (2014), the term LLD captures the concept that "language disorders change over time."

Language-based learning disability (LLD) is a term used to highlight academic learning difficulties as a result of limitations in the development of oral and written languages (Butler & Wallach, 1980). Because of their chronic language disorders in oral language, children's difficulties manifest and significantly affect their ability to learn to read and write. Reading is a critical resource to lexical development (Nagy, Herman, & Anderson, 1985). Reading comprehension is a complex process that requires word recognition, decoding of written words, and strong oral language skills. Scarborough's (2001) Reading Rope specifies all the necessary skills required to become a skilled reader. It is crucial to keep in mind that deficits in word recognition and decoding may negatively affect reading comprehension. For example, when reading an article in biology with more than 50% of unknown words, reader's understanding and comprehension could be comprised. However, poor reading comprehension can also happen in children with intact word recognition and phonological processing skills (Catts, Adlof, & Weismer, 2006). These children may have relatively mild language impairments, which negatively impact their comprehension.

Similar to learning new words orally, children can pick up the partial meaning of an unknown word incidentally during reading (Fukkink, Blok, & de Glopper, 2001). How typically developing children expand vocabulary is discussed in depth in Chapter 4. The differences in lexical learning through reading between children with LLD and their typically developing peers lay in the quality and quantity of word learning during reading.

"Matthew Effect" reminds us that children who start with sparse lexical knowledge may have difficulty retaining and expanding their lexical knowledge, which in turn increases the gap between children with LLD and their peers. Scarborough and Dobrich's (1990) illusory recovery provides a great explanation of why the gap between children with LLD and their peers becomes wider. When the amount of unknown words increase during reading, children with LLD are less interested in reading; this makes expanding the breadth and depth of their lexical knowledge even more challenging (Nagy, Herman, & Anderson, 1985). It is not surprising that children with LLD are slower in picking up the meaning of new words incidentally and struggle more with reading fluency and comprehension than their peers (Steele & Watkins, 2010). Steele (2015) suggested that lexical learning difficulty exists in both spoken and written language and may be related to cognitive limitations, immature language skills across phonology, semantics and syntax, insufficient reading level, and cumulative vocabulary deficit. Interestingly, children with LLD can infer word meanings like their typically developing peers when the reading materials match their current reading level. The deficit in fast mapping continues in adults with LLD, thus it suggests that people with LLD "do not outgrow their vocabulary deficit over time" (McGregor, Eden, Arbisi-Kelm, & Oleson, 2020, p. 3126). Therefore, increasing the number of repetition and exposure of the new words, explicit instruction on the use of semantic, phonological, and contextual cues may be needed for children with LLD to learn words through reading (Steele, 2015; Steele & Watkins, 2010; Steele, Willoughby, & Mills, 2013).

Children With Stand-Alone Lexical Access/Word Finding Difficulty

Children can have stand-alone word finding difficulty without having developmental language disorders or language-based learning disabilities. Clinically, children with stand-alone WFD have adequate receptive vocabulary knowledge, but only struggle with naming and retrieving certain words. Researchers have different viewpoints on stand-alone WFD in children. Some researchers state there is no stand-alone WFD because they believe it is part of developmental language delay/disorders. For example, Kail and Leonard (1986) indicated that word finding/word access difficulty is a byproduct of delayed language development. However, some researchers believe that there is stand-alone WFD, and it can be the result of difficulty in accessing the learned lexical items (Faust et al., 1997; Wolf & Segal, 1992). Lastly, some researchers think WFD in children can be a more pronounced characteristic of a developmental language delay (Dockrell et al., 1998).

Regardless of the perspectives on stand-alone WFD, many researchers support that the root problem of pronounced WFD in children may lie in the level of semantic representations. McGregor (1997) reported that children with noticeable WFD consistently made more semantic errors than other types of errors (e.g., phonological or mixed semantic-phonological errors). She explained that these children may have incomplete or limited knowledge of certain words, so they use semantically related words to fill the lexical gaps. In other words, the evident WFD can be the result of immaturity in developing the semantic specifications of words and retrieval mechanisms (McGregor, 1997). Messer and Dockrell (2013) also specifically pointed out that children with pronounced WFD had a greater deficit in semantics than phonological abilities because their study participants showed strengths in phonological skills demonstrated by their performance in spelling, single-word reading, and phonological awareness tasks. Thus, they concluded that deficits in semantic representations are likely to be the source of word retrieval difficulty. Dockrell and Messer (2007) also supported that deficits in semantic representations are the underlying problems of pronounced WFD. The children that participated in their study showed within average receptive language abilities, which makes them different from children with developmental language disorders who typically have below average receptive language abilities.

A way to identify children with stand-alone WFD is to discover a significant discrepancy between receptive and expressive vocabulary (Messer & Dockrell, 2006). It is because children with DLD or LLD often show "similar delays" in developing or acquiring both receptive and expressive vocabulary. In Messer and Dockrell's review (2006), they concluded that semantic errors were the most frequent naming error found in children with stand-alone WFD. Children with WFDs often use semantic substitutions (e.g., "*cat*" for [rat]) or phonological substitutions (e.g., "*bat*" for [rat]). German (2009) indicated that a word may not be accessible due to the competition with other semantically related words or closely related phonemes during the selection process. However, it should be noted that identifying children with stand-alone WFD is clinically challenging because children with mild DLD or LLD can also show similar clinical characteristics, such as more semantic errors than phonological or mixed errors.

Messer and Dockrell (2006) remind clinicians to view word retrieval difficulty in children in a big picture as it involves a range of cognitive and linguistic processes, such as disruption at the semantic level, a weak connection between lexical and phonological representations, and limitation in information processing speed. Although word access difficulty is commonly associated with developmental language disorders, there may be a group of children who only have difficulty in word access and retrieval without having other language disorders. Hence, these children may require different intervention strategies to support development of lexical knowledge and to promote retrieval of target words when needed.

Lexical Access Difficulty in Children With Autism Spectrum Disorders

According to the *Diagnostic and Statistical Manual of Mental Disorders 5th edition* (DSM–5; American Psychiatric Association, 2013), autism spectrum disorders (ASD) is defined as a complex neurodevelopmental disorder characterized by repetitive behaviors and impairments in social communication. Children with ASD demonstrate different levels of language functioning depending on the presence of concomitant language impairments. Study results show that only children with both ASD and language disorders presented immature word associations and insufficient word knowledge similar to those with DLD (McGregor et al., 2012). Children with both ASD and language disorders also experience comparable language difficulties as children with DLD, such as early language delays and limited lexical knowledge in breadth and depth (Haebig et al., 2015). Children with DLD tend to struggle more with syntax than children with ASD, whereas children with ASD have more, significant difficulty in pragmatics than children with DLD (Conti-Ramsden et al., 2006). Generally speaking, children with ASD have difficulty using social information or cues to aid word learning due to delays and deficits in mutual engagement and theory of mind, which is critical for inferring and mapping meaning to the referent (McGregor, 2009). As discussed in Chapter 3, mutual engagement directs a child's focus to the referent and further facilitates the word-referent mapping (Tomasello, 1995). Mutual engagement also brings a child's attention to the adult's communicative cues, such as gestures and eye gaze, which assist in inferring the meaning of the word (Shneidman et al., 2009).

Norbury (2005) found that children with DLD and children with both ASD and language disorders were less familiar with subordinate items (e.g., hawk, robin, sparrow for bird) suggesting that they had limited knowledge on less frequent and alternative meaning of words. McGregor et al. (2012) also reported that children with both ASD and language disorders showed limited depth of lexical knowledge similar to children with DLD. However, children with DLD showed a larger knowledge gap between abstract and concrete nouns and verbs across high and low-frequency words whereas children with ASD did not. Because language abilities in children with ASD can be on a spectrum, it is important not to make clinical decisions about a child's lexical knowledge and processing skills solely based on the results of standardized tests. Speirs, Yelland, Rinehart, and Tonge (2011) recommended that ongoing intervention is still needed for children with ASD due to underlying deficits in lexical processing despite their relatively better language skills.

Children with ASD show strengths and limitations in learning words. Studies have shown that children with ASD may learn words from context like their typically developing peers (Brock et al., 2008; Lucas et al., 2017). However, children with ASD may have a greater difficulty learning new words from a more extended and less explicit context due to their deficits in inferencing (Lucas et al., 2017). In addition, children with both ASD and language impairments show deficiency in utilizing context to resolve lexical ambiguities (Norbury, 2005).

Children with ASD show adequate syntactic bootstrapping abilities to learn verbs due to their relative strength in syntactic skills (Shulman & Guberman, 2007). Horvath and colleagues (2018) also support that children with ASD are able to use syntactic bootstrapping to identify the thematic role and assign the possible meaning of the novel verbs without the presence of any social or visual cues. This means that children with ASD can use syntactic information to learn non-social words. It is important for clinicians to have good understanding on diverse language skills within ASD and the impact of their different strengths on lexical learning. Understanding their strengths and limitations can help speech-language pathologists plan effective interventions.

Summary

It is essential to identify the strengths and challenges in lexical learning. Using children with ASD as an example, a subgroup of children with ASD and language impairments show very similar challenges in lexical learning as children with DLD. However, some children with ASD are able to use adequate syntactic bootstrapping abilities and contextual cues to infer the word meaning. Children with DLD and those with LLD share very similar profiles of deficits in spoken and written language. These children have difficulties in learning both semantic and phonological information of new words. Also, children with DLD or LLD show more difficulty in learning new words incidentally through listening and reading. In sum, children with language impairments either as a primary or secondary disorder struggle with lexical learning due to limitations in phonological lexical memory, impaired fast mapping abilities, sparse exiting lexical knowledge to expand on, and less effective in using syntactic bootstrapping abilities and contextual cues (Nash & Donaldson, 2005).

Children with language disorders are less able to learn, retain, and retrieve words both in quality and quantity compared to typically developing peers. They need significantly more repetition and exposure to new words than their peers, and they benefit from explicit teaching. In addition, careful control of the learning context to reduce competing resources when introducing new words may facilitate word learning. It is important to consider limitations in working memory capacity in children with language disorders as well as their root cause of lexical learning difficulty when developing lexical treatment programs. In order to tackle lexical difficulties, it requires comprehensive understanding of different contributing factors to lexical challenges, such as difficulty in using social cues in children with ASD and difficulty in using syntactic cues in children with DLD. Clinicians also need to be aware of the within-group variations and recognize individual differences in lexical learning and retrieval. Speech-language pathologists should carefully analyze a child's lexical errors and responses to cues during their lexical learning and retrieval process and closely monitor each child's response to the intervention. The breakdowns can help clinicians pinpoint the underlying linguistic problem and develop effective treatment programs accordingly. More information about lexical assessment and intervention can be found in the following chapters.

Word Finding Difficulty in Adults

In this section, our discussion focuses on word finding difficulty in adults with neurogenic language disorders, such as aphasia, and other related communication disorders, such as word retrieval difficulty in traumatic brain injury and dementia. It should be highlighted that cognitive functions (e.g., attention, memory, and executive functions) can also significantly influence word retrieval behaviors in adults.

Figure 6–1 is a framework that explains word production, and lays out how the target word [cat] is selected and produced based on Levelt et al.'s speech production model (1989). A word production starts from concept preparation that involves presentations of concepts without the involvement of language. Based on the conceptual representations, features are activated

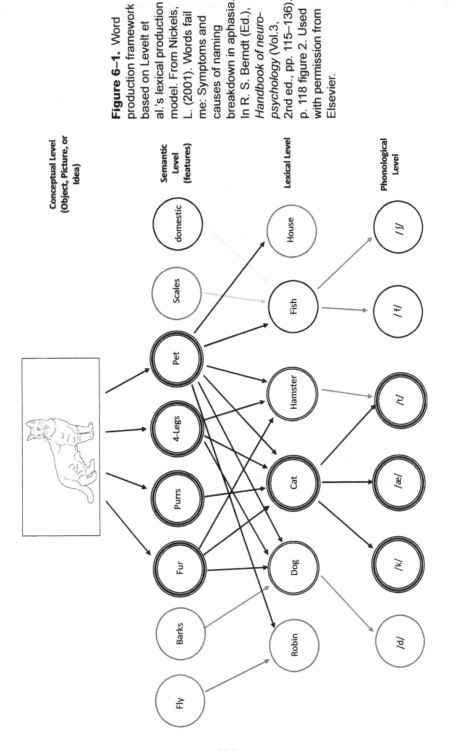

Figure 6–1. Word production framework based on Levelt et al.'s lexical production model. From Nickels, L. (2001). Words fail me: Symptoms and causes of naming breakdown in aphasia. In R. S. Berndt (Ed.), *Handbook of neuropsychology* (Vol. 3, 2nd ed., pp. 115–136). p. 118 figure 2. Used with permission from Elsevier.

at the semantical level. The activated semantic features lead to selecting a corresponding lexicon at the lexical level. Then, the corresponding phonemes are retrieved and further processed by encoding its syllable and stress information at the phonological level. Breakdowns at any level or the combinations of levels may result in word production errors.

Word Finding Difficulty in Aphasia

Aphasia is an acquired language disorder due to damage to the language processing areas in the brain, primarily in the dominant cerebral hemisphere (i.e., left cerebral hemisphere for most individuals). Brain damages can affect both receptive and expressive language across all modalities. The most common cause of aphasia is a stroke, and other causes of aphasia include brain tumors, traumatic brain injury, anoxia, and other encephalopathy. The National Institute on Deafness and Other Communication Disorders (NIDCD; 2015) estimated that 1 in 250 people in the United States live with aphasia, and the estimated new cases of aphasia is about 180,000 per year. According to the National Aphasia Association, about one-third of strokes result in aphasia and at least 2,000,000 people in the United States live with aphasia. Aphasia symptoms and severity vary depending on the lesion location and extent of the damage to the perisylvian cortex of the dominant hemisphere (i.e., language areas). Regardless of the type of aphasia, word finding difficulty, a.k.a. *anomia*, is the most pervasive symptom in aphasia among symptoms across spoken and written language (Laine & Martin, 2006). We first discuss different error types and word production breakdowns in people with aphasia and then review relevant research studies regarding word finding difficulty (WFD) in aphasia.

Word Finding Error Types

As reviewed in Chapter 2, Dell et al.'s two-step interactive model was proposed based on the errors observed in individuals with aphasia. Based on this interactive model, WFD in aphasia can be the results of (a) incomplete or incorrect activation at either lemma (lexical) or lexeme (phonological) levels or (b) failure or disruption of the connection between these two levels. This interactive model is bidirectional which can be used to explain both top-down and bottom-up influences. This means the lower level (e.g., phonological level) can have an impact on the upper level (e.g., semantic level). Based on this two-step interactive model, Dell et al. (1997) identified five types of aphasic naming errors below.

1. Semantic errors
   - Semantic errors are real words that can be strongly associated to the target word (e.g., superordinate or subordinate) or synonyms of the target word.
   - Example: Saying "*dog*" for the target word [cat].
   - This type of errors occurs at the semantic level where conceptual features are activated. A semantically competing word instead of the target word is selected because the competing word receives stronger activation than the target word.
2. Phonological errors (word from errors)
   - Phonological errors are real words that share phonological features with the target words.
   - Example: Saying "*hat*" or "*chat*" for the target word [cat].
   - This type of errors may occur either at the lexical-semantic access or phonological level. Due to the interactive and bidirectional activation between lemma (lexical) and lexeme (phonological) levels, words that share similar phonological features with the target words may compete at the lexical level because of the feedback from the phonological level. These errors result from either (a) failure at word selection due to inaccurate feedback from the phonological level or (b) disruption during phonological retrieval (Middleton & Schwartz, 2010).
     a. If "*hat*" was activated, the error follows both the syntactic constraint (the error is also a *noun*) and also shares phonological features with the target word [cat].
     b. If "chat" was activated, the error only follows phonotactic constraints (i.e., phonological sequence) but not syntactic constraints (the error is a *verb*).

3. Mixed semantic-phonological errors
   - Mixed semantic-phonological errors are real words that have both semantic and phonological similarity.
   - Example: Saying "*rat*" for the target word [cat].
   - According to Schwartz et al. (2006), this type of error is the most common type of errors observed in aphasic anomia. It means both semantic and phonological information simultaneously influenced at the lexical selection level (Dell et al., 1997). Due to the influences from both top-down (i.e., semantic to lexical) and bottom-up (i.e., phonological to lexical), the competing word was selected rather than the target word. The mixed errors result from shared semantic features and feedback from shared phonemes. In this example, the error (*rat*) shares similar semantic features (e.g., *animal, four legs, tail*) and phonological features (e.g., /at/) with the target word [cat].
4. Unrelated word errors
   - Unrelated word errors are real words that do not share semantic or phonological similarities with the target word (Schwartz, 2013).
   - Example: Saying "*fog*" for the target word [cat].
   - This type of errors happens when there is access difficulty at both lexical and phonological levels or when the connection between the lemma and its word form is disrupted. For example, "*fog*" is an unrelated error because it does not share any semantic or phonological features with the target word [cat].
5. Neologistic errors (neologism)
   - Neologistic errors are not real words. These nonword errors are strings of phonemes that do not follow the phonotactic rule in a given language; however, these errors may share some phonological similarity with the target word (Schwartz, 2013).
   - Example: Saying "*caf*" or "*dat*" for the target word [cat].
   - This type of errors may be the result of severe disruption at phonological access or difficulties at both lexical and phonological levels (Dell et al., 1997). For example, "*caf*" or "*dat*" sound similar to the target word [cat] but are not real words.

Although Dell et al.'s (1997) categorization covers a wide range of speech errors, few errors produced by people with aphasia are still not well explained by this model, such as mis-ordering of phonemes (e.g., saying /tæk/ for the word [cat]. Therefore, Nickels (2001) proposed the following error types to describe lexical impairments based on the breakdown in the word production process.

1. Conceptual-semantic impairments
   - Error types: Semantically related words, semantically unrelated words, or no response.
   - Commonly seen in people with semantic dementia.
   - Clinical expression: These clients often have difficulty in both linguistic and non-linguistic tasks, such as sorting pictures. The breakdown is the result of progressive deterioration of semantic information, so only some typical semantic features may be activated which are not salient enough for the target lemma to be selected.
2. Lexical-semantic impairments
   - Error type: Semantically related words.
   - Clinical expression: These clients often have preserved conceptual-semantic representations, so they do well on non-linguistic tests but not linguistic tests. The errors result from disrupted or weakened connections between conceptual-semantic and lexical-semantic levels. Thus, the semantically-related, completing node is more strongly activated than the target node.
3. Post-lexical access impairments
   - Errors: Phonologically related words or unrelated non-words in severe cases.
   - Clinical expression: These clients tend to have preserved conceptual-semantic and lexical-semantic representations. Some phonemes in the word are omitted or replaced by other random phonemes, such as saying "*cad*" for the word [cat]. The incorrect association between the phoneme and syllable position may also cause an error (Nickels, 2001). For example, saying "*tac*" for the word [cat].

Table 6–3 summarizes the explanations of different word finding errors from Dell et al. (1997) and Nickels (2001).

Table 6–3. Two Different Classifications of Word-Finding Error Types in Aphasia

Error Types	Dell et al. (1997)	Nickels (2001)
Semantic Errors	• Disruption occurs at the lemma level. • A similar meaning word is selected instead of the target word. • Potential errors: synonym, superordinate, subordinate.	• Clients may (1) have preserved conceptual-semantic representation but weakened connections between levels or (2) have difficulty accessing salient semantic features. • The errors result from disrupted or weakened connections between conceptual-semantic and lexical-semantic levels.
Phonological Errors	• (1) Similar sounding words that follow the syntactic constraints may compete at the lemma level due to feedback from the lexeme level or (2) competition exclusively at the lexeme level. • A similar-sounding word is selected instead of the target word. • Potential errors: words that rhyme.	• Clients have preserved conceptual-semantic and lexical-semantic representations. Errors caused by interruption at the phonological level (post lexical access). • Some phonemes in the word are omitted or replaced by other random phonemes).
Mixed Errors	• The most common type used by PWA. • Words that share semantic and phonological similarities are activated simultaneously during lemma access. • Potential errors: similar meaning and sounding words that follow the syntactic constraints.	

Table 6–3. *continued*

Error Types	Dell et al. (1997)	Nickels (2001)
Unrelated Errors	• Access difficulty at both lexical and phonological levels. • Real words that do not share semantic nor phonological similarities with the target cat.	• Deterioration of semantic information (semantic unrelated errors). • Quick decay at the phonological level that results in an incorrect association between the phoneme and syllable position (post lexical access).
Neologisms or Nonwords	• Severe disruption at phonological access or difficulties at both lemma and phoneme access. • Words or strings of phonemes that share some phonological similarities with the target words.	• Severe deterioration of semantic information. • Severe decay at the phonological level.

It is always a challenge to identify the underlying cause of a naming error. Naming errors may result from impaired semantic specifications or decreased access to semantic representations. Impaired semantic specifications may activate several semantic related competitors, making activation of the target lemma difficult or even impossible. A naming error may also arise when correct phonological representations are not accessible, resulting in the activation of semantically and phonologically similar nontargets.

Correct word production is a complex process that involves successful activation, selection, and connections in many subprocesses. As reviewed in Chapter 5, several psycholinguistic variables, such as word imageability and frequency, may contribute to the effectiveness of word retrieval. For example, Middleton and Schwartz (2010) reported that naming accuracy in individuals with aphasia may be higher in words from high neighborhood density (i.e., words that share many phonological features) than words from low neighborhood density. Besides the linguistic variables, Howard and Gatehouse (2006) also reminded clinicians not to assume that the client has sufficient semantic knowledge based solely on the results of a receptive language test (e.g., identifying objects or follow simple commands). Also, for clients showing similar naming errors, the underlying nature of the impairment may be different, and different clients require different word retrieval strategies to remediate their word retrieval difficulty.

The Role of Distinct Semantic Features in Word Retrieval

Semantic features are critical to successful word retrieval, because lexical-semantic representations are composed of bundles of semantic features (Wallace & Mason-Baughman, 2012). Distinct semantic features play a more important role than prototypical/ common features in constructing a lexical-semantic representation. For example, distinct features for the word [cat] would be *chasing a mouse* and *saying meow*, which are more facilitative in word retrieval than prototypical features, such as *animal, pet,* and *four legs*. Distinct features are critical for effective and successful word retrieval because these can facilitate differentiating semantically related words from the target. Taking the word [cat] as an example, prototypical features may not effectively distinguish "cat" from "dog".

Impairment at the level of lexical-semantical representations is common in people with aphasia. Wallace and Mason-Baughman (2012) found that people with aphasia who were able to discriminate between semantically related items had better performance in word retrieval. They also stated that lexical treatment in aphasia should include training distinct features. Mason-Baughman and Wallace (2013) reported that the richness of semantic representations was critical to the differentiation of semantically related items and word retrieval ability. Inability to discriminate between semantically related concepts can lead to difficulty in lexical comprehension and word retrieval. Antonucci and MacWilliam (2015) asked 21 people with aphasia to describe living and nonliving objects and found that the clients produced predominantly common features that are insufficient for retrieving the target word. Hence, they suggested that lexical treatment in aphasia should emphasize the salient and distinct features of target words in order to facilitate lexical access.

Words are building blocks and are essential to morphological application, sentence construction, and discourse generation in both spoken and written forms. Most research studies on word retrieval difficulty in aphasia focus on the word level; however, word finding difficulty also happen at other levels. Therefore, it is critical for speech-language pathologists to pay attention to the changes in word retrieval at the sentence and discourse levels and compare the differences among these levels.

Word Finding Difficulty in Traumatic Brain Injury and Right Hemisphere Damage

Both communication (e.g., semantic processing and pragmatic function) and cognitive functions (e.g., attention, memory, executive functions) may get affected after traumatic brain injury or right hemisphere damage. Traumatic brain injury (TBI) is the disruption of normal brain function caused by an external force, usually a blow or a jolt to the head. TBI can be the result of a fall, motor vehicle accident, or severe sports injury (Centers for Disease Control and Prevention, 2019). Forty to fifty percent of TBI requiring hospitalization are due to diffuse axonal injuries (Meythaler, Peduzzi, Eleftheriou, & Novack, 2001); diffuse axonal injuries are the result of shearing forces generated by sudden acceleration and deceleration of the brain to the white matter tracts of the brain (Faul & Coronado, 2015). Right hemisphere damage (RHD), also known as right hemisphere disorder, is usually a type of acquired brain injury caused by stroke, TBI, brain tumor, or other encephalopathy.

Individuals with cognitive communication disorders due to TBI or RHD often experience difficulties in pragmatics and macrostructural language, such as cohesion and coherence of discourse, story grammar, and information organization. These individuals may also show deficits at the microstructural level, such as semantic processing of words and syntax (Coelho, Lê, Mozeiko, Hamilton, Tyler, Krueger, & Grafman, 2013; Lê, Coelho, Mozeiko, Krueger, & Grafman, 2014; Marini, Galetto, Zampieri, Vorano, Zettin, & Carlomagno, 2011). Difficulty in finding words is one of the complaints that people with TBI or RHD commonly report. The characteristics of WFD in TBI or RHD are decreased naming accuracy in timed naming tasks or during fast-paced conversation. They usually present good semantic knowledge and can access the semantic network but have decreased efficiency in retrieving and accessing certain types of semantic information (e.g., specific visual features), or delay in processing information. For example, people with TBI tend to provide poorer word definitions, less specific perceptual features when describing the objects, or fewer superordinate categories than normal controls (Constantinidou & Kreimer, 2004; McWilliams & Schmitter-Edgecombe, 2008).

People with RHD or TBI may show different error patterns and varying degrees of naming accuracy depending on the size and location of the lesion, time post onset, severity of injury, comorbidity (e.g., aphasia, motor speech disorders), the client's age, education level, medical history before and after brain injury, and so forth. The extensive discussion on cognitive-communication disorders due to TBI and RHD is beyond the scope of this book. Readers who are interested in getting more information on this topic can visit the American Speech-Language-Hearing Association's Practice Portal (https://www.asha.org/practice-portal).

When evaluating WFD in people with cognitive communication disorders, it is crucial to consider how cognitive deficits may negatively affect their word retrieval ability. WFD may reflect their deficits in the semantic memory organization and resource allocation (Popescu et al., 2017). In addition, naming errors in TBI or RHD may reflect the reduced information processing speed, memory deficit, and dysexecutive syndrome rather than damage to specific language areas (Barrow et al., 2003). In the study of Crawford, Knight, and Alsop (2007), the participants with post-concussive syndrome retrieved fewer words in verbal fluency tasks than normal controls. The authors suggested that a global reduction in information processing capacity may explain the slowness in verbal fluency tasks.

Clinicians need to keep in mind that WFD in people with TBI or RHD may not show on standardized tests, and simple naming tasks may not be sensitive to identify their WFD, especially mild cases (Riès et al., 2016). King et al. (2006) indicated that timed naming tasks may be more sensitive to identify WFD in TBI because it requires efficient cognitive processing. Barrow et al. (2006) also stated that standardized tests may not accurately capture subtle cognitive deficits or WFD in people with mild TBI because they still have the required cognitive capacity to perform well in standardized tests. However, time-constrained tasks, such as verbal fluency tasks, may be sensitive due to the increased processing demands. It was also found that people with mild TBI had decreased accuracy in naming more advanced words than normal controls (Barrow et al., 2006).

In sum, clinicians must be aware of the root cause and neurological etiologies of WFD. Word retrieval difficulty in TBI or RHD may reflect the reduced processing speed, memory, inhibition efficiency, and executive functions rather than the direct damage to underlying language systems. Therefore, it is essential for clinicians to consider how and to what extent cognitive deficits may affect word retrieval in people who sustained a TBI or with RHD. Clinicians should also keep in mind that cognitively demanding tasks, such as timed tasks or unstructured discourse, may be more sensitive to identify word retrieval difficulty in these clients. Generating a more cognitive-demanding type of discourse (e.g., argumentative and expository discourse) requires more cognitive resources and processing, so it is more sensitive in identifying WFD than a less cognitive-demanding discourse tasks (e.g., simple picture description tasks). Understanding the underlying deficits and contributing factors to WFD can help clinicians select appropriate and sensitive measures to capture word retrieval problems and develop effective and individualized interventions to remediate WFD.

Age-Related Word Finding Difficulty

Studies showed that language performance, both production and comprehension, declined with advancing age due to *decrement in processing speed* (Kwong See & Ryan, 1995; Waters & Caplan, 2005), *working memory* (Carpenter et al., 1994; Gunter et al., 1995; Kwong See & Ryan, 1995; Waters & Caplan, 2005), *verbal working memory* (DeDe et al., 2004), and *inhibitory efficiency* (Burke, 1997; Kwong See & Ryan, 1995). It has been reported that difficulties in naming, reduced syntactic complexity, and decrement in verbal fluency are commonly observed in people who are at age 70 or over (Ardila & Rosselli, 1996). Elders might have difficulty in accessing appropriate lexical items, producing syntactically complex sentences, and organizing a cohesive discourse (Juncos-Rabadan & Iglesias, 1994). Both spoken and written language production consistently shows age-related declines. Common deterioration observed in elders' language production includes word finding difficulty, disfluency in speech, and ambiguous references (Burke & MacKay, 1997). Moreover, older adults tended to produce less complex sentences compared to younger adults to avoid high cognitive demands (Kemper et al., 2001; Kemper, Herman, & Lian, 2003; Kemper, Herman, & Liu, 2004).

Most research supported that older adults experience more difficulty in processing abstract and complex sentences and connected speech because these tasks require high cognitive demands. Although some researchers suggested that language deterioration may be associated with healthy aging (Emery, 1986; Olber & Albert, 1989), it is noted that there are different levels of deterioration in language functions. The results of Juncos-Rabadan and Iglesias's study (1994) showed that aging was associated with linguistic deterioration in syntax, morphology, phonology, and semantics. The deterioration was especially observed in synonyms, antonyms, word definition, repeating complex sentences, and discourse. Kemper and Zelinski (1994) compared the language changes in healthy elders to the individuals with dementia and found that people with healthy aging had mild word-finding difficulties due to decreased lexical retrieval ability. On the other hand, word-finding difficulties were a prominent symptom in people with dementia, which occurred in every sentence.

It should be noted that when evaluating age-related language decline (e.g., word retrieval difficulty), many variables should be taken into consideration, such as verbal ability, prior level of functioning, education level, gender differences, and so forth. Several studies have shown the impact of these variables on older adults' language abilities (Ardila & Rosselli, 1996; Harris et al., 1998; Juncos-Rabadan & Iglesias, 1994; Juncos-Rabadan, 1996; Mackenzie, 2000). Additionally, different types of assessment tasks can play a role in different performance observed in older adults, such as simple naming tasks versus cognitive demanding discourse generating tasks, due to different cognitive demands (Burke & MacKay, 1997; Glosser & Deser, 1992; Radvansky, 1999).

Tip-of-the-Tongue Phenomenon in Normal Aging

The term "tip of the tongue (a.k.a. TOT)" phenomenon describes the experience when someone feels they know the word but are unable to successfully produce the word. The frequency of experiencing TOT increases as people get older; several studies show that naming performance starts to decline at age 70 and beyond (Burke et al.,1991). TOTs do not occur until later in life because adults' extensive and rich vocabulary and advanced cognitive abilities help them compensate for temporary word retrieval problems. TOTs start mostly in proper nouns and then extend to common nouns (Burke, et al., 1991). Proper nouns include specific names for a particular person, place, or entity, such as *Martin Luther King Jr.* (person), *Philadelphia* (place), *Toyota* (entity), and so forth. Ramsay and colleagues (1999) also found an age-related decline in verb naming. They found that verb naming decline becomes observable at the age of 60, but may start as early as the ages of 40 to 50.

The common word retrieval errors in TOT include delay in response (e.g., saying "*um*" while retrieving words), disfluency/repetition (e.g., saying "*we just went, went, went to the park*"), circumlocution (e.g., saying "*using this thing to hit nails*" for the word [hammer]), substitution errors (e.g., saying "*pinwheel*" for the word [windmill] or "*tennis bat*" for [tennis racquet]), word reformulations/revision (e.g., saying "*he can't . . . he won't play baseball*"), and empty/ambiguous responses (e.g., saying "*you know that thing*" or "*that guy*," etc.). Schmitter-Edgecombe et al. (2000) stated that older adults have reduced access to word forms despite the types of errors. Older adults experience more noticeable TOTs than younger adults during discourse production than picture naming tasks (Schmitter-Edgecombe et al., 2000). Therefore, utilizing discourse tasks to evaluate TOT or word-finding difficulty is suggested because of the nature of the task and sensitivity to WFD in older adults.

The occurrence of TOT does not indicate deterioration of semantic, lexical, or phonological knowledge but rather the weak connections between these levels due to increased transmission deficits associated with healthy aging. Burke et al. (1991) claimed that the connections between semantic and lexical representations (i.e., lemma) and lexical and phonological representations (i.e., lexeme) become weaker as people age. Weakening connections associated with aging made the activation of intended lemma or lexeme difficult, and the weakening connections make word retrieval difficult.

The presence of TOT suggests that the partial phonological information (e.g., initial sound) is available, but the complete phonological form is inaccessible at the time. Burke et al. (1991) claimed that TOT indicated adequate activation of semantic and lexical representations but failed or incomplete activation of phonological information of the word (lexeme). In addition, age-related TOT can be the result of insufficient semantic activation, so phonological information becomes even less available during retrieval. This explanation was also supported by the finding that providing phonologically related words can promote successful naming in elders. Burke and colleagues (2004) found that the occurrence of TOT reduces and the naming accuracy increases after providing homophones of the target words (e.g., "*cherry pit*" primed "*Brad Pitt*") in older adults but not younger adults.

The brain imaging studies suggested the involvement of the left anterior insula in TOT. Shafto and colleagues (2007) reported the correlation between left insula atrophy and increasing age-related TOT. Shafto et al. (2010) provided additional neuroimaging evidence to support the role of the left insula in phonological production and claimed that age-related TOT is due to retrieval failure at the phonological level. Besides the involvement of left insula in the word retrieval process, Wierenga and colleagues (2006) reported a more significant activity in the frontal network was found in older adults than younger adults during word retrieval. Besides, more bilateral and robust activations in Brodmann area 45 of the right hemisphere (Broca's area homologue) were found in older adults indicating that compensatory brain response was needed to maintain naming accuracy. They suggested that WFD (or TOT) may arise from compromised higher-order functions involving in selecting and retrieving semantic-lexical information, not the loss of semantic representations.

Age-related cognitive changes have been reported in literature. Baciu et al. (2016) claimed that a general decline in executive functions, delay in processing speed, and deficit in accessing certain phonological information are mainly attributed to age-related WFD. Based on their fMRI study, they stated that decreased efficiency in executive functions contributes to age-related word retrieval difficulty. In addition, executive functions are the first cognitive function to decline, and the decline becomes more noticeable when managing tasks that require high cognitive demands. Baciu et al. (2016) further stated that age-related word finding problems are associated with ineffective access to certain lexical processes due to a decline in executive functions and processing speed. In other words, semantic knowledge does not deteriorate as people age, but the ability to effectively and efficiently search, select, and access words decreases over time due to aging.

In summary, age-related TOT occurs late in life and may be compensated by older adults' rich and well-established semantic knowledge, effective self-correction, and internal and external cueing strategies. Changes in brain structures, as well as cognitive functions, seem to be the possible causes of age-related TOT. In other words, age-related TOT is associated with brain atrophy in specific regions as well as a decline in executive functions and/or other cognitive processes. Specifically, age-related word retrieval difficulty is not the result of the deterioration of semantic knowledge. It is more likely due to reduced effectiveness and efficiency in accessing phonological or semantic information. Therefore, commonly implemented cueing strategies, such as semantic and phonemic cues, are beneficial to improve word retrieval performance in people with age-related word finding difficulty.

Word Finding Difficulty in Dementia

Dementia is a type of neurodegenerative disease that affects many cortical functions and is progressive, so its clinical symptoms gradually worsen over a number of years. Dementia is diagnosed when someone's cognitive and behavioral symptoms significantly interfere with his/her function at work and daily activities. There are several different types of dementia, such as Alzheimer's disease, vascular dementia, Lewy body dementia, frontotemporal dementia, and so forth. Alzheimer's disease is the most common cause of dementia and accounts for 60% to 80% of dementia cases (Alzheimer's Association, 2021). Alzheimer's disease is not a normal part of aging; it is a progressive neurodegenerative disease that affects cognitive and linguistic functions over time. Individuals with dementia typically show impairments in at least two of the following domains, including memory (e.g., difficulty remembering newly learned information), executive functions (e.g., problem solving and handling complex tasks), visuospatial abilities (e.g., recognizing faces or common objects), language functions (e.g., word retrieval, discourse production) and personality changes (e.g., lack of initiation, loss of drive) (McKhann et al., 2011). As Alzheimer's disease is the most common cause of dementia, our discussion in this section will focus only on dementia in Alzheimer disease.

The word retrieval difficulty in Alzheimer's disease is different from the age-related word finding difficulty (or TOT) in healthy aging adults. TOT in normal aging is the result of the change in lexical access due to aging. However, individuals with Alzheimer's disease have difficulty retrieving words because of the impaired semantic network, memory deficits, and loss of semantic information, so WFD in Alzheimer's disease is the result of impairments in conceptual and semantic knowledge. Kraut and colleagues (2006) reported that 70% of participants with Alzheimer's disease in their study showed word finding difficulty, along with semantic memory deficits. Impairment in semantic memory in the early stage of Alzheimer's disease was further supported by their difficulty with all lexical tasks, such as object matching, naming, verbal fluency, and word association (Adlam, Bozeat, Arnold, Watson, & Hodges, 2006).

Balthazar, Cendes, and Damasceno (2008) stated that individuals with Alzheimer's disease have partially preserved semantic knowledge, and the naming difficulties may result from a combination of loss of semantic knowledge, impaired lexical access, and diminished cognitive functions (e.g., inhibitory control). Because semantic deterioration is the major contributing factor to their naming difficulty, phonological cues may be more beneficial than semantic cues in naming (Lin et al., 2013). Salehi, Reisi, and Ghasisin (2017) elaborated that word finding difficulty may lie in the retrieval process at an early stage of Alzheimer's disease, but the degradation of concepts coupled with the increasing difficulty in accessing lemma and lexeme may be the reason for word finding difficulty in late stages of Alzheimer's disease.

Individuals with Alzheimer's disease show difficulties in recognizing common objects, retrieving words for recognized objects, and verbal fluency. This can be the results of the deteriorations in temporal lobes (damage to the semantic network) and frontal lobes (inability to retrieve information from the semantic network) (Melrose et al, 2011). Mickes and colleagues (2007) further emphasized that the functions of temporal lobes (e.g., memory, semantic knowledge) seem to be more impaired than the functions of frontal lobes (e.g., executive functions, initiation) during the very early phase (preclinical phase) of Alzheimer's disease.

Lexical retrieval tasks may serve as a sensitive measure to evaluate cognitive and linguistic impairments in individuals with mild cognitive impairment and suspected Alzheimer's disease (Taler & Jarema, 2006). However, lexical retrieval tasks alone may not be sensitive enough. It is important to examine word retrieval in connected speech (e.g., picture description, storytelling, conversation) because individuals with Alzheimer's disease tend to use more simple, shorter, and frequent words in connected speech than their healthy peers (Kave & Goral, 2016). Pekkala and colleagues (2013) also stated written discourse tasks are more sensitive in revealing word retrieval difficulty in Alzheimer's disease than confrontation naming and verbal fluency tasks. Therefore, clinicians could consider incorporating discourse tasks (spoken and written) in addition to the lexical retrieval tasks when evaluating word finding difficulty in Alzheimer's disease.

When working with individuals with neurogenic word retrieval difficulty, it is essential to take the different neurological etiologies and underlying causes of word finding difficulty into consideration. In other words, word finding difficulty can stem from different etiological causes, such as aphasia, cognitive-communication impairment due to traumatic brain injury or right hemisphere damage, or Alzheimer's disease. Hence, identifying the root cause helps clinicians plan an effective intervention and tailor the intervention plan to address individual needs, such as addressing lexical access difficulty in individuals with aphasia or dealing with the deterioration in semantic knowledge in individuals with Alzheimer's disease.

Chapter Summary

In this chapter, we discuss word-finding difficulty in different types of language and communication disorders. The purpose of this chapter is to help readers understand word access and retrieval difficulty from different perspectives and in a more holistic view from word learning to lexical retrieval. Using the lexical access models, we examine different errors commonly made by individuals with word access or retrieval difficulty from both developmental and neurogenic perspectives. We also highlight the clinical symptoms and different underlying causes of word access and retrieval difficulty across different types of language and communication disorders.

Clinicians should keep in mind that the cause of word access difficulty in developmental language disorders is different from word retrieval difficulty in neurogenic language/communication disorders. It is important to focus on the etiological causes rather than age when determining the best possible treatment options. For example, a 30-year-old individual with Down syndrome requires different treatment approaches than a 30-year-old adult with neurogenic language/communication disorders (e.g., aphasia). Clients with developmental language disorders, regardless of age, often have difficulty in consolidating and storing semantic and lexical information in long-term memory. In addition, because the semantic and lexical information is not well-organized, such as linking words with similar features together, clients with developmental language disorders have difficulty in accessing words effectively. On the other hand, word finding difficulty in neurogenic communication disorders often results from inability to access the semantic or phonological representations during lexical processing. Therefore, it is critical not to reteach vocabulary when working with clients with neurogenic word retrieval difficulty. Instead, treatment should focus on reestablishing a more effective way for effectively accessings lexical information. With this knowledge foundation, we can now move on to discussing clinical assessment and intervention approaches to address word access and retrieval difficulty in the next three chapters.

Discussion Questions

1. How are lexical access difficulties different in children with developmental language disorders, children with language-based learning disabilities, and children with autism spectrum disorders?
2. What are the common lexical errors observed in children with word access difficulty? What may contribute to these lexical errors?
3. What are the different etiological and underlying causes of neurogenic word retrieval difficulty?
4. Describe different types and examples of aphasic naming errors discussed in the chapter.
5. Describe age-related, tip-of-the-tongue phenomenon and discuss how this is different from the word finding difficulty in dementia.

References

Adlam, A., Bozeat, S., Arnold, R., & Watson, P., Hodges, J. (2006). Semantic knowledge in mild cognitive impairment and mild Alzheimer's disease. *Cortex, 42,* 675–684.

Alzheimer's Association. (2021, May 17). *What is dementia?* https://www.alz.org/alzheimers-dementia/what-is-dementia

American Psychiatric Association. (2013). *Diagnostic and statistical manual of mental disorders* (5th ed.). Author.

Antonucci, S. M., & MacWilliam, C. (2015). Verbal description of concrete objects: A method for assessing semantic circumlocution in persons with aphasia. *American Journal of Speech-Language Pathology, 24*(4), 823–837. https://doi.org/10.1044/2015_ajslp-14-0154

Ardila, A., & Rosselli, M. (1996). Spontaneous language production and aging: Sex and educational effects. *International Journal of Neuroscience, 87*(1-2), 71–78. https://doi.org/10.3109/00207459608990754

Baciu, M., Boudiaf, N., Cousin, E., Perrone-Bertolotti, M., Pichat, C., Fournet, N., . . . Krainik, A. (2016). Functional MRI evidence for the decline in word retrieval during normal aging. *AGE, 38*(3), 1–22. https://doi.org/10.1007/s11357-015-9857-y

Balthazar, M., Cendes, F., & Damasceno, B. (2008). Semantic error patterns on the Boston Naming Test in normal aging, amnestic mild cognitive impairment, and mild Alzheimer's disease: Is there semantic disruption? *Neuropsychology, 22*, 703–709.

Barrow, I. M., Hough, M., Rastatter, M. P., Walker, M., Holbert, D., & Rotondo, M. F. (2006). The effects of mild traumatic brain injury on confrontation naming in adults. *Brain Injury, 8*, 845–855.

Barrow, I. M., Hough, M., Rastatter, M.P., Walker, M., Holbert, D., & Rotondo, M. (2003). Can within category naming identify subtle cognitive deficits in mild traumatic brain injured patients? *Journal of TRAUMA, Injury, Infection, and Critical Care, 54*(5), 1–10.

Bragard, A., & Schelstraete, M. (2007). Word-finding difficulties in French-speaking children with SLI. *Clinical Linguistics and Phonetics, 21*(11–12), 927–934. https://doi.org/10.1080/02699200701615211

Brock, J., Norbury, C., Einav, S., & Nation, K. (2008). Do individuals with autism process words in context? Evidence from language-mediated eye-movements. *Cognition, 108*(3), 896–904. https://doi.org/10.1016/j.cognition.2008.06.007

Burke, D. M. (1997). Language, aging, and inhibitory deficits: Evaluation of a theory. *The Journals of Gerontology, 52*(6) 254–264. https://doi.org/10.1093/geronb/52B.6.P254

Burke, D. M., Locantore, J. K., Austin, A. A., & Chae, B. (2004). Cherry pit primes Brad Pitt: Homophone priming effects on young and older adults' production of proper names. *Psychological Science, 15*(3), 164–170. https://doi.org/10.1111/j.0956-7976.2004.01503004.x

Burke, D., & MacKay, D. (1997). Memory, language and ageing. *Philosophical Transactions of the Royal Society B, 352*(1363), 1845–1856. https://doi.org/10.1098/rstb.1997.0170

Burke, D., MacKay, D., Worthley, J., & Wade, E. (1991). On the tip of the tongue: What causes word finding failures in young and older adults. *Journal of Memory and Language, 30*(5), 542–579. https://doi.org/10.1016/0749-596X(91)90026-G

Butler, K., & Wallach, G. (1980). Language disorders and learning disabilities. *Topics in Language Disorders, 1*(1).

Capone, N., & McGregor, K. (2005). The effect of semantic representation on toddlers' word retrieval. *Journal of Speech, Language and Hearing Research, 48*(6), 1468–1480. https://doi.org/10.1044/1092-4388(2005/102)

Carpenter, P., Miyake, A., & Just, M. (1994). A capacity approach to syntactic comprehension disorders: making normal adults perform like aphasic patients. *Cognitive Neuropsychology, 11*(6), 671–717. https://doi.org/10.1080/02643299408251989

Catts, H. W., Adlof, S., & Weismer, S. (2006). Language deficits in poor comprehenders: A case for the simple view of reading. *Journal of Speech, Language, and Hearing Research, 49*, 278–293.

Centers for Disease Control and Prevention. (2019). *Surveillance report of traumatic brain injury-related emergency department visits, hospitalizations, and deaths by age group, sex, and mechanism of injury—United States, 2016/2017.* U.S. Department of Health and Human Services. https://www.cdc.gov/traumaticbraininjury/pdf/TBI-surveillance-report-2016-2017-508.pdf

Coelho, C., Lê, K., Mozeiko, J., Hamilton, M., Tyler, E., Krueger, F., & Grafman, J. (2013). Characterizing discourse deficits following penetrating head injury: A preliminary model. *American Journal of Speech-Language Pathology, 22*, S438–S448.

Constantinidou, F., & Kreimer, L. (2004). Feature description and categorization of common objects after traumatic brain injury: The effects of a multi-trial paradigm. *Brain and Language, 89*, 216–225.

Conti-Ramsden, G., Simkin, Z., & Botting, N. (2006). The prevalence of autistic spectrum disorders in adolescents with a history of specific language impairment. *The Journal of Child Psychology and Psychiatry, 47*(6), 621–628. https://doi.org/10.1111/j.1469-7610.2005.01584.x

Crawford, M. A., Knight, R. G., & Alsop, B. L. (2007). Speed of word retrieval in postconcussion syndrome. *Journal of the International Neuropsychological Society, 13*(1), 178–182. https://doi.org/10.1017/S135561770707021X

DeDe, G., Caplan, D., Kemtes, K., & Waters, G. (2004). The relationship between age, verbal working memory, and language comprehension. *Psychology and Aging, 19*(4), 601–616. https://doi.org/10.1037/0882-7974.19.4.601

Dell, G. S., Schwartz, M. F., Martin, N., Saffran, E. M., & Gagnon, D. A. (1997). Lexical access in aphasic and nonaphasic speakers. *Psychological Review, 104*(4), 801–838. https://doi.org/10.1037/0033-295X.104.4.801

Dockrell, J., & Messer, D. (2007). Language profiles and naming in children with word finding difficulties. *Folia Phoniatrica et Logopaedica, 59*(6), 318–323. https://doi.org/10.1159/000108338

Dockrell, J., Messer, D., George, R., & Wilson, G. (1998). Notes and discussion children with word finding difficulties—prevalence, presentation and naming problems. *International Journal of Language and Communication Disorders, 33*(4), 445–454.

Emery, O. (1986). Linguistic decrement in normal aging. *Language & Communication, 6*(1-2), 47–64. https://doi.org/10.1016/0271-5309 (86)90005-4

Faul, M., & Coronado, V. (2015). Epidemiology of traumatic brain injury. *Handbook of Clinical Neurology, 127*, 3–13. https://doi.org/10.1016/ B978-0-444-52892-6.00001-5

Faust, M., Dimitrovsky, L., & Davidi, S. (1997). Naming difficulties in language disabled children. *Journal of Speech, Language, and Hearing Research, 40*(5), 1026–1036. https://doi.org/10.1044/jslhr.4005.1026

Fukkink, R. G., Blok, H., & de Glopper, K. (2001). Deriving word meaning from context: A multi-componential skill. *Language Learning 51*(3), 477–496.

German, D. J. (1991). *Test of Word Finding in Discourse (TWFD): Administration, scoring, interpretation, and technical manual.* Pro-Ed.

German, D. J. (2009). Child word finding. *The ASHA Leader, 14*(2), 10–13. https://doi.org/10.1044/leader.FTR2.14022009.10

German, D., & Simon, E. (1991). Analysis of children's word finding skills in discourse. *Journal of Speech, Language, and Hearing Research, 34*(2), 309–316. https://doi.org/10.1044/jshr.3402.309

Glosser, G., & Deser, T. (1992). A Comparison of changes in macrolinguistic and microlinguistic aspects of discourse production in normal aging. *Journal of Gerontology, 47*(4), 266–272. https://doi .org/10.1093/geronj/47.4.P266

Gunter, T., Jackson, J., & Mulder, G. (1995). Language, memory, and aging: An electrophysiological exploration of the N400 during reading of memory-demanding sentences. *Psychophysiology, 32*(3), 215–229. https://doi.org/10.1111/j.1469-8986.1995.tb02951.x

Haebig, E., Kaushanskaya, M., & Ellis Weismer, S. (2015). Lexical processing in school-age children with autism spectrum disorder and children with specific language impairment: The role of semantics. *Journal of Autism and Developmental Disorders, 45*, 4109–4123. https://doi.org/10.1007/s10803-015-2534-2

Harris, J., Rogers, W., & Qualls, C. (1998). Written language comprehension in younger and older adults. *Journal of Speech, Language, and Hearing Research, 41*(3), 603–617. https://doi.org/10.1044/jslhr .4103.603

Hartsuiker, R., & Vigliocco, G. (2009). Word production. In L. R. Squire (Ed.), *Encyclopedia of neuroscience* (pp. 509–516). Academic Press.

Horvath, S., McDermott, E., Reilly, K., & Arunachalam, S. (2018). Acquisition of verb meaning from syntactic distribution in preschoolers with autism spectrum disorder. *Language, Speech, and Hearing Services in Schools, 49*(3S), 668–680. https://doi.org/10.1044/2018 _LSHSS-STLT1-17-0126

Howard, D., & Gatehouse, C. (2006). Distinguishing semantic and lexical word retrieval deficits in people with aphasia. *Aphasiology, 20*(9), 921–950. https://doi.org/10.1080/02687030600782679

Individuals With Disabilities Education Act (IDEA), 20 U.S.C. § 1400. (2004).

Ingram, D. (2002). The measurement of whole-word productions. *Journal of Child Language, 29*(4), 713–733. https://doi.org/10.1017/ S0305000902005275

Juncos-Rabadán, O. (1996). Narrative speech in the elderly: Effects of age and education on telling stories. *International Journal of Behavioral Development, 19*(3), 669–685.

Juncos-Rabadán, O., & Iglesias, F. (1994). Decline in the elderly's language: Evidence from cross-linguistic data. *Journal of Neurolinguistics, 8*(3), 183–190. https://doi.org/10.1016/0911-6044(94)90025-6

Kail, R., & Leonard, L. (1986). Word-finding abilities in language-impaired children. *ASHA Monographs, 25.*

Kan, P., & Windsor, J. (2010). Word learning in children with primary language impairment: A meta-analysis. *Journal of Speech, Language, and Hearing Research, 53*(3), 739–756. https://doi.org/10.1044/ 1092-4388(2009/08-0248)

Kavé, G., & Goral, M. (2016). Word retrieval in picture descriptions produced by individuals with Alzheimer's disease. *Journal of Clinical and Experimental Neuropsychology, 38*(9), 958–966. https://doi.org/ 10.1080/13803395.2016.1179266

Kemper, S., Greiner, L. H., Marquis, J. G., Prenovost, K., & Mitzner, T. L. (2001). Language decline across the life span: Findings from the nun study. *Psychology and Aging, 16*(2), 227–239. https://doi.org/ 10.1037/0882-7974.16.2.227

Kemper, S., Herman, R. E., & Lian, C. H. T. (2003). The costs of doing two things at once for young and older adults: Talking while walking, finger tapping, and ignoring speech of noise. *Psychology and Aging, 18*(2), 181–192. https://doi.org/10.1037/0882-7974.18.2.181

Kemper, S., Herman, R., & Liu, C. (2004). Sentence production by young and older adults in controlled contexts. *The Journals of Gerontology: Series B, 59*(5), 220–224. https://doi.org/10.1093/geronb/59.5 .P220

Kemper, D., & Zelinski, E. (1994). Language in dementia and normal aging. In F. A. Huppert, C. Brayne, & D. W. O'Connor (Eds.), *Dementia and normal aging* (pp. 331–364). Cambridge University Press.

King, K., Hough, M. S., Vos, P., Walker, M., & Givens, G. (2006) Word retrieval following mild traumatic brain injury: Implications for categorical deficits. *Aphasiology*, 20, 233–245.

Kraut, M., Cherry, B., Pitcock, J., Vestal, L., Henderson, V., & Hart Jr, J. (2006). The Semantic Object Retrieval Test (SORT) in normal aging and Alzheimer disease. *Cognitive and Behavioral Neurology*, 19(4), 177–184. https://doi.org/10.1097/01.wnn.0000213922.41008.22.

Kwong See, S. T., & Ryan, E. B. (1995). Cognitive mediation of adult age differences in language performance. *Psychology and Aging*, 10(3), 458–468. https://doi.org/10.1037/0882-7974.10.3.458

Laine, M., & Martin, N. (2006). *Brain damage, behaviour and cognition. Anomia: Theoretical and clinical aspects*. Psychology Press.

Lê, K., Coelho, C., Mozeiko, J., Krueger, F., & Grafman, J. (2014). Does brain volume loss predict cognitive and narrative discourse performance following traumatic brain injury? *American Journal of Speech-Language Pathology*, 23(2), S271–S284.

Levelt, W. J. (1989). *Speaking: From intention to articulation* (Vol. 1). MIT press.

Levelt, W. J. (1999). A Blueprint of the speaker. In C. Brown & P. Hagoort (Eds.), *The neurocognition of language* (pp. 83–122). Oxford Press.

Lin, J., O'Connor, E., Rossom, R., Perdue, L., & Eckstrom, E. (2013). Screening for cognitive impairment in older adults: A systematic review for the U.S. preventive services task force. *Annals of Internal Medicine*, 159(9). 601–612.

Lucas, R., Thomas, L., & Norbury, C. (2017). Can children with autism spectrum disorders learn new vocabulary from linguistic context. *Journal of Autism and Developmental Disorders*, 47, 2205–2216. https://doi.org/10.1007/s10803-017-3151-z

Mackenzie, C. (2000). Adult spoken discourse: The influences of age and education. *International Journal of Language and Communication Disorders*, 35(2), 269–285. https://doi.org/10.1080/136828200247188

Marini, A., Galetto, V., Zampieri, E., Vorano, L., Zettin, M., & Carlomagno, S. (2011). Narrative language in traumatic brain injury. *Neuropsychologia*, 49, 2904–2910. https://doi.org/10.1016/j.neuropsychologia.2011.06.017

Marks, I., & Strokes, S. (2010). Narrative-based intervention for word-finding difficulties: A case study. *International Journal of Language and Communication Disorders*, 45(5), 586–599. https://doi.org/10.3109/13682820903277951

Marshall, C. R. (2014). Word production errors in children with developmental language impairments. *Philosophical Transactions of the Royal Society B, 369*(1634), 1–8. https://doi.org/10.1098/rstb.2012.0389

Mason-Baughman, M. B., & Wallace, S. E. (2013). The role of commonality, distinctiveness and importance of semantic features in persons with aphasia. *Brain Injury, 27*(4), 399–407. https://doi.org/10.3109/02699052.2012.750748

Mason-Baughman, M. B., & Wallace, S. E. (2014). Role of importance and distinctiveness of semantic features in people with aphasia: A replication study. *Communication Disorders Quarterly, 35*(3), 158–166. https://doi.org/10.1177/1525740113518342

McGregor, K. K. (1997). The nature of word finding errors of preschoolers with and without word-finding deficits. *Journal of Speech, Language, and Hearing Research, 40*(6), 1232–1244. https://doi.org/10.1044/jslhr.4006.1232

McGregor, K. (2009). Semantics in child language disorders. In R. G. Schwartz (Eds.), *The handbook of child language disorders.* (2nd ed., pp. 365–387). Psychology Press.

McGregor, K., & Appel, A. (2002). On the relation between mental representation and naming in a child with specific language impairment. *Clinical Linguistics and Phonetics, 16*(1), 1–20. https://doi.org/10.1080/02699200110085034

McGregor, K., Berns, A., Owen, A., Michels, S., Duff, D., Bahnsen, A., & Lloyd, M. (2012). Associations between syntax and lexicon among children with or without ASD and language impairment. *Journal of Autism and Developmental Disorders, 42*, 35–47. https://doi.org/10.1007/s10803-011-1210-4

McGregor, K. K., Oleson, J., Bahnsen, A., & Duff, D. (2013). Children with developmental language impairment have vocabulary deficits characterized by limited breadth and depth. *International Journal of Language and Communication Disorders, 48*(3), 307–319. https://doi.org/10.1111/1460-6984.12008

McGregor, K., Gordon, K., Eden, N., Arbisi-Kelm, T., & Oleson, J. (2017). Encoding deficits impede word learning and memory in adults with developmental language disorders. *Journal of Speech, Language, and Hearing Research, 60*(10), 2891–2905. https://doi.org/10.1044/2017_JSLHR-L-17-0031

McGregor, K., Licandro, U., Arenas, R., Eden, N., Stiles, D., Bean, A., & Walker, E. (2013). Why words are hard for adults with developmental language impairments. *Journal of Speech, Language, and Hearing Research, 56*(6), 1845–1856. https://doi.org/10.1044/1092-4388(2013/12-0233)

McGregor, K., Eden, N., Arbisi-Kelm, T., & Oleson, J. (2020). The fast-mapping abilities of adults with developmental language disorder. *Journal of Speech, Language, and Hearing Research, 63*(9), 3117–3129.

McGregor, K., & Waxman, S. (1998). Object naming at multiple hierarchical levels: A comparison of preschoolers with and without word-finding deficits. *Journal of Child Language, 25*(2), 419–430. https://doi.org/10.1017/S030500099800347X

McGregor, K., & Windsor, J. (1996) The effects of priming on the naming accuracy of preschoolers with word finding deficits. *Journal of Speech, Language, and Hearing Research, 39*(5), 1048–1058. https://doi.org/10.1044/jshr.3905.1048

McKhann, G., Knopman, D., Chertkow, H., Hyman, B., Jack Jr. C., Kawas, C., . . . Phelps, C. (2011). The diagnosis of dementia due to Alzheimer's disease: Recommendations from the National Institute on Aging-Alzheimer's Association workgroups on diagnostic guidelines for Alzheimer's disease. *Alzheimers Dement, 7*(3), 263–269

McWilliams, J., & Schmitter-Edgecombe, M. (2008). Semantic memory organization during the early stage of recovery from traumatic brain injury. *Brain Injury, 22*(3), 243–253. https://doi.org/10.1080/02699050801935252

Melrose, R., Ettenhofer, M., Harwood, D., Achamallah, N., Campa, O., Mandelkern, M., & Sultzer, D.(2011). Cerebral metabolism, cognition, and functional abilities in Alzheimer disease. *Journal of Geriatric Psychiatry and Neurology, 24*(3), 127–134. https://doi.org/10.1177/0891988871140533324/3/127

Messer, D., & Dockrell, J. (2006). Children's naming and word-finding difficulties: Descriptions and explanations. *Journal of Speech, Language, and Hearing Research, 49*(2), 309–324. https://doi.org/10.1044/1092-4388(2006/025)

Messer, D., & Dockrell, J. (2013). Children with word finding difficulties: Continuities and profiles of abilities. *First Language, 33*(5), 433–448. https://doi.org/10.1177/0142723713493345

Meythaler, J. M., Peduzzi, J. D., Eleftheriou, E., & Novack, T. A. (2001). Current concepts: Diffuse axonal injury–associated traumatic brain injury. *Archives of Physical Medicine and Rehabilitation, 82*(10), 1461–1471. https://doi.org/10.1053/apmr.2001.25137

Mickes, L., Wixted, J., Fennema-Notestine, C., Galasko, D., Bondi, M., Thal, L., & Salmon, D. (2007). Progressive impairment on neuropsychological tasks in a longitudinal study of preclinical Alzheimer's disease. *Neuropsychology, 21*(6), 696–705. https://doi.org/10.1037/0894-4105.21.6.696

Middleton, E., & Schwartz, M. (2010). Density pervades: An analysis of phonological neighborhood density effects in aphasic speakers with different types of naming impairment. *Cognitive Neuropsychology, 27*(5), 401–427. https://doi.org/10.1080/02643294.2011.57 0325

Nagy, W. E., Herman, P. A., & Anderson, R. C. (1985). Learning words from context. *Reading Research Quarterly, 20*(2), 233–253. https://doi.org/10.2307/747758

National Aphasia Association. (n.d.). *Aphasia fact sheet.* https://www .aphasia.org/aphasia-resources/aphasia-factsheet/

National Institute on Deafness and Other Communication Disorders. (2015). *Aphasia.* https://www.nidcd.nih.gov/health/aphasia

National Joint Committee on Learning Disabilities. (2001). Learning disabilities: Issues on definition. In the National Joint Committee on Learning Disabilities (Ed.), *Collective perspectives on issues affecting learning disabilities: Position papers, statements, and reports* (2nd ed., pp. 27–32). Pro-Ed. http://www.ldonline.org

National Joint Committee on Learning Disabilities. (2001). *What are LD?* https://njcld.org/ld-topics/

Nash, M., & Donaldson, M. (2005). Word learning in children with vocabulary deficits. *Journal of Speech, Language, and Hearing Research, 48,* 439–458.

Nickels, L. (2001). Spoken word production. In B. Rapp (Ed.), *Handbook of cognitive neuropsychology: What deficits reveal about the human mind* (pp. 291–320). Psychology Press.

Nippold, M. A. (2007). *Later language development: School age children, adolescents, and young adults.* Pro-Ed.

Norbury, C. (2005). The relationship between theory of mind and metaphor: Evidence from children with language impairment and autistic spectrum disorder. *Developmental Psychology, 23*(3), 383–399. https://doi.org/10.1348/026151005X26732

Obler, L. K., & Albert, M. (1989). Language decline in aging. *International Journal of Applied Linguistics, 83,* 63–73. https://doi.org/10.1075/itl.83-84.06obl

Pekkala, S., Wiener, D., Himali, J. J., Beiser, A. S., Obler, L. K., Liu, Y., . . . Au, R. (2013). Lexical retrieval in discourse: An early indicator of Alzheimer's dementia. *Clinical linguistics & Phonetics, 27*(12), 905–921. https://doi.org/10.3109/02699206.2013.815278

Popescu, M., Hughes, J., Popescu, E-A., Mikola, J, Merrified, W., DeGraba, M., . . . DeGraba, T. (2017). Activation of dominant hemisphere association cortex during naming as a function of cognitive performance in mild traumatic brain injury: Insights into mechanisms of lexical access. *NeuroImage: Clinical, 15,* 741–752.

Radvansky, G. A. (1999). Memory retrieval and suppression: The inhibition of situation models. *Journal of Experimental Psychology: General, 128*(4), 563–579. https://doi.org/10.1037/0096-3445.128.4.563

Ramsay, C. B., Nicholas, M., Au, R., Obler, L. K., & Albert, M. L. (1999). Verb naming in normal aging. *Applied Neuropsychology, 6*(2), 57–67. https://doi.org/10.1207/s15324826an0602_1

Riès, S. K., Dronkers, N. F., & Knight, R. T. (2016). Choosing words: Left hemisphere, right hemisphere, or both? Perspective on the lateralization of word retrieval. *Annals of the New York Academy of Sciences, 1369*(1), 111–131. https://doi.org/10.1111/nyas.12993

Salehi, M., Reisi, M., & Ghasisin, L. (2017). Lexical retrieval or semantic knowledge? Which one causes naming errors in patients with mild and moderate Alzheimer's disease? *Dementia and Geriatric Cognitive Disorders Extra, 7*(3), 419-429. https://doi.org/10.1159/000484137

Scarborough, H. S. (2001). Connecting early language and literacy to later reading (dis)abilities: Evidence, theory, and practice. In S. Neuman & D. Dickinson (Eds.), *Handbook for research in early literacy* (pp. 97–110). Guilford Press.

Scarborough, H. S., & Dobrich, W. (1990). Development of children with early language delay. *Journal of Speech & Hearing Research, 33*(1), 70–83. https://doi.org/10.1044/jshr.3301.70

Schmitter-Edgecombe, M., Vesneski, M., & Jones, D. (2000). Aging and word-finding: A comparison of spontaneous and constrained naming tests. *Archives of Clinical Neuropsychology, 15*(6), 479–493. https://doi.org/10.1093/arclin/15.6.479

Schwartz, M. (2013). Patterns of speech production deficit within and across aphasia syndromes: Application of a psycholinguistic model. In M. Coltheart, G. Sartori, & R. Job (Eds.). *The cognitive neuropsychology of language* (pp. 163–196). Taylor & Francis Group.

Schwartz, M., Dell, G., Martin, N., Gahl, S., & Sobel, P. (2006). A case-series test of the interactive two-step model of lexical access: Evidence from picture naming. *Journal of Memory and Language, 54*(2), 228–264. https://doi.org/10.1016/j.jml.2005.10.001

Seiger-Gardner, L., & Schwartz, R. G. (2008). Lexical access in children with and without specific language impairment: A cross-modal picture-word interference study. *International Journal of Language & Communication Disorders, 43*(5), 528–551. https://doi.org/10.1080/13682820701768581

Shafto, M., Burke, D., Stamatakis, E., Tam, P., & Tyler, L. (2007). On the tip-of-the-tongue: Neural correlates of increased word finding failures in normal aging. *Journal of Cognitive Neuroscience, 19*(12), 2060–2070. https://doi.org/10.1162/jocn.2007.19.12.2060

Shafto, M., Stamatakis, E., Tam, P., & Tyler, L. (2010). Word retrieval failures in old age: The relationship between structure and function. *Journal of Cognitive Neuroscience, 22*(7), 1530–1540. https://doi .org/10.1162/jocn.2009.21321

Sheng, L., & McGregor, K. (2010). Lexical-semantic organization in children with specific language impairment. *Journal of Speech, Language, and Hearing Research, 53*(1), 146–159. https://doi.org/ 10.1044/1092-4388(2009/08-0160)

Shneidman, L., Buresh, J., Shimpi, P., Knight-Schwarz, J., & Woodward, A. (2009). Social experience, social attention and word learning in an overhearing paradigm. *Language Learning and Development, 5*(4), 266–281. https://doi.org/10.1080/15475440903001115

Shulman, C., & Guberman, A. (2007). Acquisition of verb meaning through syntactic cues: A comparison of children with autism, children with specific language impairment (SLI) and children with typical language development (TLD). *Journal of Child Language, 34*(2), 411–423. https://doi.org/10.1017/S0305000906007963

Speirs, S., Yelland, G., Rinehart, N., & Tonge, B. (2011). Lexical processing in individuals with high-functioning autism and Asperger's disorder. *Autism, 15*(3), 307–325. https://doi.org/10.1177/1362361310386501

Steele, S. C. (2015). Does language learning disability in school aged children affect semantic word learning while reading? *International Journal of Speech-Language Pathology. 17*(2), 172–184. https://doi .org/10.3109/17549507.2014.979872

Steele, S. C. & Watkins, R. W. (2010). Learning word meanings during reading by children with language learning disability and typically-developing peers, *Clinical Linguistics and Phonetics, 24*(7), 520–539.

Steele, S. C., Willoughby, L. M., & Mills, M. T. (2013). Semantic word learning during reading: Effects of phonological and semantic cues on children with language impairment. *International Journal of Speech-Language Pathology, 15*(2), 184–197.

Stiegler, L. N., & Hoffman, P. R. (2001). Discourse-based intervention for word finding in children. *Journal of Communication Disorders, 34*(4), 277–303. https://doi.org/10.1016/S0021-9924(01)00051-X

Sun, L., & Wallach, G. (2014). Language disorders are learning disabilities: Challenges on the divergent and diverse paths to language learning disability, *Topics in Language Disorders, 34*(1), 25–38. https://doi.org/10.1097/TLD.0000000000000005

Taler, V., & Jarema, G. (2006). On-line lexical processing in AD and MCI: An early measure of cognitive impairment? *Journal of Neurolinguistics, 19*(1), 38–55.

Tomasello, M. (1995). Joint attention as social cognition. In C. Moore & P. J. Dunham (Eds.), *Joint attention: Its origins and role in development*. (p. 103–130). Lawrence Erlbaum Associates.

Wallace, S. E., & Mason-Baughman, M. B. (2012). Relationship between distinctive feature knowledge and word retrieval abilities in people with aphasia. *Aphasiology, 26*(10), 1–20. https://doi.org/10.1080/02 687038.2012.702886

Waters, G., & Caplan, D. (2005). The relationship between age, processing speed, working memory capacity, and language comprehension. *Memory, 13*(3-4), 403–413. https://doi.org/10.1080/0965 8210344000459

Wierenga, C., Benjamin, M., Gopinath, K., Perlstein, W., Leonard, C., Rothi, L., . . . Crosson, B. (2006). Age related changes in word retrieval: Role of bilateral frontal and subcortical networks. *Neurobiology of Aging, 29*(3), 436–451. https://doi.org/10.1016/j.neurobiol aging.2006.10.024

Windfuhr, K., Faragher, B., & Conti-Ramsden, G. (2002). Lexical learning skills in young children with specific language impairment (SLI). *International Journal of Language and Communication Disorders, 37*(4), 415–432. https://doi.org/10.1080/1368282021000007758

Wolf, M., & Segal, D. (1992). Word finding and reading in the developmental dyslexias. *Topics in Language Disorders, 13*(1), 51–65. https://doi.org/10.1097/00011363-199211000-00007

7

ASSESSMENT OF LEXICAL KNOWLEDGE AND WORD PRODUCTION

Lei Sun and Pei-Fang Hung

Chapter Objectives

1. Discuss considerations for assessing lexical knowledge and spoken word production.
2. Identify assessment procedures for evaluating lexical knowledge and word production.
3. Discuss the strengths and limitations of formal and informal assessment procedures to assess lexical knowledge and spoken word production.
4. Explain the recommended practices in clinical data analysis and interpretation.

Introduction

Lexical production is a multifaceted concept and has been extensively studied in several disciplines, such as psychology, linguistics, and education. In the previous chapters, we have briefly reviewed theoretical frameworks for lexical access and production from psychological perspectives and theories for lexical development from linguistic and educational perspectives. The two commonly applied lexical theoretical models are Levelt's Speech Production Model and Dell's Two-Step Interactive Model. Based on these models, word access/production breakdowns can happen due to a weak connection between conceptual-semantic or semantic-lexical representations of the intended target word or strong activation of the competing words. A reliable assessment plan is essential to help clinicians understand and identify the breakdowns.

When evaluating lexical knowledge and word production, speech-language pathologists often administer confrontation naming tasks or standardized vocabulary tests as part of language assessment processes. However, clinicians are often uncertain if results of a simple confrontation-naming task can accurately reflect clients' lexical knowledge and word retrieval function. In this chapter, we discuss general assessment considerations, available tools, and approaches for a comprehensive assessment plan to evaluate lexical knowledge and word production, and analysis and interpretations of the collected clinical data.

Pre-Assessment: Considerations for Assessing Lexical Knowledge and Word Production

Evaluating lexical knowledge is a multifaceted and complex process. It starts with a question, "How do we know someone knows a word?" As discussed in the previous chapters, people know a word when they know the meaning, associated morphological and syntactic knowledge, phonological form, spelling, and can use the word accurately in diverse contexts. When developing an assessment plan, clinicians should incorporate the World Health Organization's International Classification of Functioning, Disability and Health (WHO-ICF) model (World Health Organization, 2001). The WHO-ICF framework guides clinicians to not just focus on impairments (e.g., deficits in lexical knowledge and word production) but also to investigate how deficits may impact clients' daily activities and how their social interaction and community participation may be restricted due to the deficits. Clinicians should also consider both personal factors (e.g., motivation, overall language skills, cognitive functions, health condition) and environmental factors (e.g., support system, access to treatment) that may influence assessment results. In this section, we discuss several factors for speech-language pathologists (SLPs) to consider before conducting vocabulary assessment, including the breadth and depth of lexical knowledge, the difference between receptive and expressive word knowledge, assessment across different contexts, lexical organization and automaticity, and word form, meaning, and use.

The Breadth and Depth of Lexical Knowledge

The first consideration is the breadth and depth of lexical (word) knowledge. The breadth (size) of lexical knowledge is defined as *how many* words are known, and the depth (quality) of lexical knowledge is defined as *how well* the words are known (Anderson & Freebody, 1981). The depth of lexical knowledge can range from none, to partial to complete knowledge (Henriksen, 1999). Qian (2002) further added that depth of word knowledge should include the knowledge of all word characteristics, including phonemic, graphemic, morphemic, syntactic, semantic, and collocational properties.

Word size and depth do not necessarily grow in parallel because the child may have learned a small size of words with great knowledge or may know many words but only with shallow word knowledge. Although both breadth and depth of lexical knowledge expand over time, clinicians cannot assume that the vocabulary depth grows equally to the same degree for all words. Schmitt (2014) pointed out that the vocabulary tests evaluating "*size*" usually examine explicit word knowledge, such as meaning and form, whereas the tests evaluating "*depth*" intend to evaluate implicit word knowledge, such as associations and collocations (words usually go together, e.g., *pay attention, take a shower, give a ride*).

Additionally, both word size and depth are important to reading comprehension. Regarding vocabulary size, readers have to know about 98% to 99% of the words in a text in order to understand it well (Hu & Nation, 2000). Without the depth of word knowledge, readers can get confused about the intended meaning of words with multiple meanings (e.g., *cabinet, charge, sentence*), words with multiple derived forms (e.g., *transform, transport, transaction, transparent*), or words that look or sound alike (e.g., *access* vs. *assess, affect* vs. *effect, lie* vs. *lay*). Children learn most Tier One vocabulary (i.e., basic words) through conversation and learn Tier Two (i.e., high frequency/multiple meaning) and Tier Three (subject-related) vocabulary through reading, direct instruction, formal education, and personal interests. Understanding different "shades" of word meanings is strongly correlated to the development of the depth of vocabulary knowledge (Stahl & Bravo, 2010). Both size and depth of vocabulary knowledge are crucial for reading comprehension because large vocabulary size enables the readers to infer the meanings whereas the depth of vocabulary improves the result of the inferencing process (Qian, 2002). Therefore, both the size and depth of word knowledge are essential for efficient word use and should be included in vocabulary assessment (Ishii & Schmitt, 2009).

The Difference Between Receptive and Expressive Language

The difference between receptive lexical knowledge and expressive word production should also be taken into consideration when conducing vocabulary assessments. Word learning is a complex and continuous developmental process that involves multiple linguistic and cognitive processes to form comprehensive understanding of words. The understanding of words evolves through the expansion of world knowledge and demands from different contexts. Melka (1997) stated that receptive and expressive vocabulary knowledge develops on a continuum that is a gradual shift from receptive mastery to productive mastery, and cumulative word knowledge develops gradually over time. Schmitt (2014) further explained that more advanced word knowledge, such as associations and collocations, are crucial for the development of expressive vocabulary; this advanced word knowledge usually takes time to develop.

It is also important to keep in mind that when people do not have a full understanding of words, they can still use inferential strategies and context cues to figure out an approximate meaning (Henriksen, 1999). In other words, children who perform well in receptive vocabulary tests may only have partial word knowledge. It is because receptive vocabulary tests are usually implemented via a multiple-choice format, such as requiring examinees to point to the picture that matches to the target word. Examinees can perform well by applying partial knowledge along with using strategies (e.g., eliminating the outliers). Additionally, it is not uncommon to observe higher receptive vocabulary scores and lower expressive vocabulary scores in children with language disorders (with only partial understating of the target words) because vocabulary comprehension usually precedes expressive vocabulary.

Multiple Assessments Across Different Contexts

Word knowledge functions on a continuum, from no knowledge to partial, then to solid and comprehensive knowledge and from context-bound knowledge, to rich and decontextualized knowledge, including its metaphorical uses (Beck et al., 2002; Beck et al., 1987). A child's word knowledge evolves based on his/her world knowledge development and personal interests. Therefore, until the point someone can use the target word appropriately in various contexts to meet different demands, it is difficult to measure the breadth and depth of word knowledge. For example, the word [company], a multiple-meaning word for students to learn in Grades 6 to 8, can be used in the different contexts, such as *"It is an international company"* and *"I am expecting company."* The child who demonstrates a good understanding of the word meaning should be able to use the word correctly in different contexts based on its meaning.

The ability to define a word, to use the word in an appropriate context, to recognize multiple meanings of the word, and to understand the relationship between words should be taken into consideration when conducing vocabulary assessments (Beck et al., 2002). Comprehensive and solid word knowledge means that an individual understands meanings, associations, and word use in various contexts correctly and independently (Hoffman et al., 2013). Thus, clinicians cannot have a complete picture of a child's word knowledge in a short period of time from a single assessment session and need to be cautious not to form a clinical judgment prematurely just based on the result of a single measure. In other words, assuming that a child has a comprehensive or limited lexical knowledge based on the result of a simple naming task or a picture-pointing task should be avoided. A child's word knowledge should be evaluated at different points in time and different contexts because lexical knowledge is acquired incrementally. Clinicians can also observe the strategies the child uses to figure out the word meaning (e.g., inferencing from the context, syntactic structure), the linguistic context where the incorrect word use occurs (e.g., words with multiple meanings, collocation errors), and the approaches the child uses to retrieve a word when experiencing difficulty. Because word meanings change depending on the linguistic contexts and situations, clinicians may want to assess a child's lexical knowledge in both contextualized and decontextualized formats. With the support of contextual information, clinicians may determine how much and what kind of prompts and support that a child may need to succeed (Pearson et al., 2007).

Lexical Organization and Automaticity

According to Qian (2002), the lexical organization refers to "storage, connection, and representation of words in the mental lexicon" (p. 516). As discussed in previous chapters, how well words are linked, and how well words are organized, are strongly correlated with how effective and efficient the word can be used. The lexical organization is also crucial for the development of receptive and expressive vocabulary knowledge. Strong lexical organization and accurate lexical connections facilitate the development of lexical production, whereas weak and fragile lexical connections can only keep the vocabulary knowledge at the receptive level (Meara, 1997; Schmitt, 2014).

Automaticity or fluency means the adequate speed in word recognition during reading and listening and adequate retrieval speed in speaking and writing (Laufer & Goldstein, 2004;

Schmitt, 2010). The better the lexical knowledge is stored and organized, the easier and faster word retrieval can be. In addition, commonly used words also have stronger storage strength than words that are recently acquired or rarely used.

Word Form, Meaning, and Use

Nation (2001) utilized *"form," "meaning,"* and *"use"* to further organize the aspects involved in word knowledge in both receptive and expressive fashion. *"Form"* includes pronunciation, spelling, and word parts (e.g., root words and affixes). For example, knowing the meaning of the word *"uncomfortable"* means that a person knows how to pronounce the word and the word parts by recognizing the prefix *"un-"* which means "not" and suffix *"-able"* which indicates the word is an adjective and the root word *"comfort."* Because knowing the phonological and morphological structures of the word, this person can pronounce and spell the word "uncomfortable" correctly.

"Meaning" refers to an understanding of word components, concepts and referents, and associations (Nation, 2001). Continuing the word "uncomfortable" as an example, a person understands that the meanings of the affixes and root word, which means "not comfort." The concepts and referents help this person connect the word to the past experience that makes him/her uncomfortable. Associations may also be activated, such as synonyms (e.g., "discomfort", "harsh"), antonyms (e.g., "comfy"), and homonyms.

"Use" refers to how someone uses a word by considering its grammatical functions, collocations, and constraints on use. Let's continue using the word "uncomfortable" again as an example. The suffix indicates the grammatical function (i.e., adjective); therefore, it has to be used to describe a noun (e.g., *an uncomfortable situation*), or a feeling (e.g., *I feel uncomfortable after speaking with my boss*). Regarding constraints on use, when someone doesn't feel good in a situation or about something, he/she can use the word "uncomfortable." Thus, when a speaker is telling unpleasant personal stories, the listener would expect the speaker uses the word "uncomfortable" to describes the situation and his/her feelings.

A solid word knowledge requires all three aspects we discussed (i.e., form, meaning, and use). Table 7–1 lays out the aspects of knowledge involved in knowing a word (adapted from Nation, 2001, p. 27).

Table 7–1. The Aspects of Knowledge Involved in Knowing a Word

Form	Spoken	R	What does the word sound like?
		E	How is the word pronounced?
	Written	R	What does the word look like?
		E	How is the word written and spelled?
	Word parts	R	What parts are recognizable in this word?
		E	What word parts are needed to express this meaning?
Meaning	Form and meaning	R	What meaning does this word form signal?
		E	What word form can be used to express this meaning?
	Concept and referents	R	What is included in the concept?
		E	What items can the concept refer to?
	Associations	R	What other words does this make us think of?
		E	What other words could we use instead of this one?
Use	Grammatical functions	R	In what patterns does this word occur?
		E	In what patterns must we use this word?
	Collocations	R	What words or types of words occur with this one?
		E	What words or types of words must we use with this one?
	Constraints on use (register, frequency . . .)	R	Where, when, and how often would we expect to meet this word?
		E	Where, when, and how often can we use this word?

R = Receptive; E = Expressive.
Source: Adapted from Learning Vocabulary in Another Language by Paul Nation (2001, p. 27). Reproduced with permission of the Licensor through PLSclear.

Additional Considerations for Assessing Neurogenic Word Retrieval Difficulty

Several factors have been identified that can affect the success of word retrieval in individuals with neurogenic communication disorders, including grammatical word class, imageability, word frequency, and word length. Readers are encouraged to review Chapter 5 for extensive discussion on these factors. Moreover, the types of neurological condition(s) (e.g., stroke, traumatic brain injury, dementia), lesion size and site, time post onset, types of neurogenic communication disorders (e.g., aphasia, cognitive-communication disorders due to brain injury), and co-occurring speech disorders can affect the effectiveness of lexical production and word retrieval.

Also, the influence of co-occurring disorders should be ruled out for an accurate diagnosis. For example, acquired, neurogenic speech disorders, such as dysarthria and apraxia of speech, should be evaluated because deficits in motor planning, motor programming or motor execution can affect word production. These difficulties result from the breakdowns in motor phases, not at lexical processing phases. Because the processes beyond phonological encoding is beyond the scope of this book, readers are recommended to review information related to motor processing of word production and motor speech disorders.

Assessment Plan for Evaluating Lexical Knowledge and Word Production

A comprehensive assessment plan for evaluating lexical knowledge and word production should consider a client's present level and takes the aforementioned factors into consideration. Clinically, lexical knowledge and word retrieval can be evaluated through testing comprehension of word meaning, verbal word production, word associations, or multiple parameters simultaneously (Laufer & Goldstein, 2004). Similar to assessments in other language domains, lexical knowledge and word production should be evaluated through the combination of standardized and nonstandardized measures with the focus on lexical production across different linguistic units (i.e., word, sentence, discourse).

Evaluating Lexical Knowledge and Production at Word Level

The most common type of assessment tasks for evaluating lexical knowledge at word level is a picture-pointing task. Examinees are asked to point to the picture or object that matches the target word from an array of choices, for example, four line-drawing pictures. On the other hand, the most commonly conducted word production assessment task is a confrontation naming task. It is also a straightforward task by asking examinees to name line-drawing pictures or photographs. This can also be done by asking the examinee to name common objects.

Several other types of assessment tasks for evaluating word retrieval include verbal fluency, synonym/antonym tasks, cloze tests, and word definitions. Verbal fluency tasks are also known as generative naming tasks. Examinees are required to generate words from a given semantic or phonemic category in a pre-determined time period. For example, an examinee is asked to name as many *animals* as possible in one minute. Any semantically related words are counted as correct responses, such as *dog, giraffe, dolphin*, and so forth. Another example is asking an examinee to name as many words starting with letter 'F' as possible in one minute, such as *fun, flower, fabulous*, and so forth. Another type of tasks for evaluating word retrieval is requiring an examinee to say synonyms and antonyms of a word. Examinees are required to say a word with the same or similar meaning (synonyms) of the stimulus word or to think of a word with the opposite meaning (antonyms). For example, saying "*large*" (synonym) and "*small*" (antonym) for the stimulus word [big]. Word retrieval can also be evaluated via fill-in-the blank questions similar to a cloze test or using one word to answer questions posted by clinicians. For example, examinees are asked to complete the sentence "*It's raining cats and _____.*" (*dogs*) or to answer the question "*What do you slice steak with?*" (*knife* or *steak knife*). Lastly, clinicians can ask examinees to verbally define a stimulus word or describe what a given word means. For example, ask clients to describe the function of "*fork*" or the meaning of the word "*happy.*" This task requires higher spoken language skills, so it is not suitable for clients with limited verbal output. The results of these word production tasks can help clinicians evaluate the accuracy and efficiency of word retrieval and the types of errors, for example, phonologically or semantically linked to target words. However, these tasks are generally decontextualized because limited to no contextual cues may be available to aid naming and word production.

Standardized Measures for Evaluating Lexical Knowledge and Production

For the pediatric population, lexical knowledge and word use can be evaluated through the subtests in comprehensive norm-referenced language batteries, such as Clinical Evaluation of Language Fundamentals (CELF-5; Wiig et al., 2013) and Test of Language Development-Primary (TOLD-P5; Newcomer & Hammill, 2019a). Some subtests, such as Word Classes subtest in CELF-5 and Relational Vocabulary subtest in TOLD-P5, assess a child's understanding of word associations either through spoken words or picture stimuli. The Word Definition subtests in CELF-5 and TOLD-P5 can be used to evaluate a child's ability to define a word verbally. These subtests provide valuable information about a child's lexical knowledge. However, the word definition subtest may not be suitable for children younger than age five because it is metalinguistic in nature and requires the child to reflect on how words are used. Some children with language disorders struggle with semantics and morphosyntax, thus, they may struggle with word definition tests. Therefore, clinicians may consider modifying the test by offering choices (e.g., Do you think [stimulus word] means A or B?) to minimize the demands of the task to obtain additional information about the child's lexical knowledge.

The two norm-referenced tests designed especially for children with suspected word finding difficulties are the Test of Word Finding-3rd edition (TWF-3; German, 2015) and Test of Adolescent/Adult Word Finding-2nd edition (TAWF-2; German, 2016). The TWF-3 is designed for children between ages 4 years, 6 months and 12 years, 11 months, and to identify if the child has word finding difficulty. The child is asked to retrieve nouns and verbs through picture naming and sentence naming tasks. Clinicians identify semantic- or phonological-based word finding difficulty based on analyzing the results of error patterns, including (1) lemma related semantic errors, (2) form related blocked errors, and (3) form and segment related phonological errors. The child's response to cues is also recorded. Additionally, the comprehension task of TWF-3 helps clinician further evaluate if the error is due to word finding difficulty or insufficient lexical knowledge. The TAWF-2 can be used for individuals ages 12 through 80 years who experience WFD. Similar to TWF-3, the examinee is asked to name nouns, verbs, and categories through picture naming and sentence completion tasks, and the comprehension section is used to identify if the error is a result of WFD or poor comprehension. Clinicians can conduct five informal analyses including phonemic curing procedure, imitation procedure, substitution analysis, delayed response procedure and the secondary characteristics analysis (gestures and extra verbalization) to obtain more information. Both TWF-3 and TAWF-2 offer specific information about the client's WFD through well-structured measures and analyses.

For adults with neurogenic word finding difficulties, the commonly administered norm-referenced test is the Boston Naming Test–Second Edition (BNT-2; Kaplan et al., 2001). The BNT-2 is a stand-alone confrontation naming test embedded within the Boston Diagnostic Aphasia Examination, Third Edition (BDAE-3; Goodglass et al., 2001). In addition, the Western Aphasia Battery Revised (WAB-R; Kertesz, 2006), a comprehensive aphasia battery, has several subtests that can be utilized to evaluate a client's naming and word finding ability, including confrontation naming, word fluency, responsive naming, and sentence completion. The Pyramids and Palm Trees Test (PPT; Howard & Patterson, 1992), another standardized test, can be administered to evaluate semantic knowledge in adults. It measures the examinee's ability to access the semantic information through written words and pictures. It tests whether there is a modality-specific difficulty in accessing semantic knowledge and can be used to evaluate semantic memory in adults (Gamboz et al., 2009).

Commonly utilized norm-referenced tests that evaluate lexical knowledge and production across age groups are listed in Appendix 7–1, such as Boston Naming Test, Peabody Picture Vocabulary Test–5th Edition, Expressive Vocabulary Test–3rd Edition, Receptive/Expressive One Word Picture Vocabulary Test–4th Edition, and so forth.

Strengths and Limitations of Standardized Vocabulary and Naming Tests

One of the strengths of these standardized vocabulary and naming tests is that the administration of these tests is straightforward, especially when examinees are able to follow the directions and cooperate. The test protocols and procedures are well established, thus clinicians just need to review the test manual before administering a standardized vocabulary or naming test. It should be noted that when deviating from the administration instructions, the normative data should not be applied. Another strength is that the stimulus words are presented in a hierarchical fashion with increasing difficulty. For example, the test items in BNT-2 start from simple, high-frequency vocabulary (e.g., *bed*) to rare words (e.g., *abacus*). Lastly, using the established scoring system, a standardized test can estimate naming accuracy in a quantitative manner with the availability of standard scores and percentiles, which can be used for comparisons and progress monitoring.

However, standardized vocabulary and naming tests also have several disadvantages and limitations. First, standardized vocabulary/naming tests are decontextualized and static in nature, thus these only give a snapshot of a client's function at the moment of assessment. Secondly, because the format of standardized tests relies on picture pointing or confrontation naming, most test items are nouns, and some picture stimuli consist of ambiguous and outdated illustrations. Lastly, assessments with a multiple-choice format may not truly evaluate a client's lexical knowledge. For pediatric population, it is important to keep in mind that a child may be able to name a picture without having sufficient lexical knowledge. Therefore, clinicians should take these limitations and other factors (e.g., client's cultural and linguistic background) into consideration when interpreting test results.

Hoffman et al. (2013) also raised concerns about using normed referenced vocabulary tests because they do not include curriculum-related words nor do they measure the depth of word knowledge. Even though they recommend definitional measures for preschool children, the child's ability to convey word meaning may compromise the test result. It is important to keep in mind that defining words is a metalinguistic skill. Thus, an alternative measure, such as using follow-up questions, may be appropriate when evaluating preschoolers' word knowledge. Hence, we cannot assume that the child has full knowledge of word meaning based on the results of receptive vocabulary and naming tests.

In summary, speech-language pathologists should be mindful that standardized vocabulary and naming tests give only a snapshot of a client's lexical knowledge and production at the time of assessment and the result cannot be generalized to the client's overall language skills. Clinicians also should keep in mind not to overgeneralize the assessment result beyond the scope of the assessment battery. Therefore, a stand-alone vocabulary/naming test can be viewed as an ad hoc measure in addition to a comprehensive language assessment especially when a client's lexical knowledge/production is an area of concern or requires a more in-depth evaluation.

Clinical Observations

Lexical knowledge and word production can be informally evaluated by administering assessment tasks with different types of lexical stimuli. Firstly, the format of assessment tasks can be confrontation naming, verbal fluency, answering open-ended questions, or a combination of all. Although the test formats are similar to standardized test, informal assessment tests provide clinicians additional flexibility. For example, the BNT-2 is a timed test and gives examinees only 20 seconds to respond to each picture stimulus. For clients with delayed information processing, additional time may improve their naming accuracy or offer clinicians additional information for clinical decision making. Secondly, the informal assessment task can be conducted and structured at a client's present level. Clinicians can select words that are commonly used in the client's daily life across different settings (e.g., *home, school, workplace*), words from different word classes (e.g., *nouns, verbs, adjectives*), and words for different functions (e.g., *greetings, requesting, commenting*). For clients who have better expressive language skills, clinicians may probe word production by asking open-ended questions about the target word or asking the client to describe/explain the target word further. The follow-up questions may be structured based on the semantic features, such as "*what do you do with* ___?" "*where can you find* ___?" "*who uses* ___?" "*how do you feel when you think of* ___?" The purpose of probing is to learn more about the breakdowns during word learning or word retrieval.

For pediatric populations, clinicians can develop a list of words that a child is able to say or understand for clinical observations. This list of words can be used to establish a baseline and also to monitor the child's progress and development over time. For example, clinicians can select words based on a child's present level of expressive language and zone of proximal development. For a 3-year-old boy with only 15 expressive words, a clinician can evaluate his word knowledge of the known words and probe his comprehension of other early developing words (find more details in Chapter 3). For an 8-year-old girl whose language function is at the preschool range, a clinician could evaluate words commonly used by preschoolers and probe for additional responses and productions. These probing activities can be delivered during conversation, shared book reading activities, or play, to keep the probing as natural as possible. Through these activities, clinicians can observe how a child's vocabulary are being used and grouped.

Hart and Risley (1992) claimed that there is a strong correlation between the number and type of words that children use and words used in the children's environment, including family values, cultural and linguistic background, and socio-economic status of the family. In addition, the development of word knowledge is a gradual process. Quick incidental learning (QUIL) tasks, developed based on research, may be suitable to evaluate a child's ability of forming an initial mapping during the beginning of the word learning process or first exposures (Burton & Watkins, 2007). For example, clinicians can select several unknown words before a book reading activity and then incorporate these words during the book reading. The initial word learning ability can be measured by asking the child to name the target word during the follow-up activities. Children with developmental language disorders show slowness at fast mapping and require more exposures than their typically developing peers. Thus, this QUIL task provides clinicians an informal measure of initial word learning process. It helps differentiate between children with developmental language disorders and typically developing children with limited lexical knowledge due to cultural and linguistic differences (Burton & Watkins, 2007).

Self-Evaluation and Caregiver Reports

Speech-language pathologists can generate a list of questions to better understand the impact of word retrieval difficulty on a client's daily communication and how they deal with the difficulty. These questions may help clinicians and clients to work together on planning for treatment. Some sample questions are listed below.

- What do you do when you cannot successfully say a word that you want to say?
- How often does it happen when you cannot successfully say a word that you want to say?
- How do you feel when you cannot successfully say a word that you want to say?
- Does word finding difficulty affect your communication effectiveness? If so, how do you overcome this challenge?
- What words do you have hard time retrieving? Do you notice a pattern, such as certain words that are more difficult for you?
- What strategy works best for you to retrieve a word successfully?

For clients with limited verbal output or younger children, clinicians can have caregivers or parents to answer these questions and share their insights. There are also published questionnaires available for clinicians. For example, ASHA Functional Assessment for Communication Skills for Adults (ASHA FACS; Frattali et al., 1995) can be administered to estimate a client's functional communication skills in everyday life. The questionnaire is based on a 7-point rating scale and the target areas include (i) social communication, (ii) communication of basic needs, (iii) reading, writing, number concepts, and (iv) daily planning. For pediatric population, MacArthur-Bates Communicative Developmental Inventories (MB-CDIs) (Fenson et al., 2007) is an instrument that helps clinicians get a parent report on their young children's developmental abilities, including vocabulary comprehension, production, gestures, and grammar. Parent reports have been found to be valid and reliable in learning about a child's vocabulary development (Watkins & DeThorne, 2000). The inventories are widely used in the evaluation of young children across languages. Administration resources and adaptations in other languages can be found at MacArthur-Bates CDIs website (https://mb-cdi.stan ford.edu).

Clinicians can use self-evaluation checklists to monitor school-age children's vocabulary growth and development of lexical knowledge. SLPs can ask school-age children to create a sentence with the target word and discuss how difficult this type of activity is to them. Self-report and evaluations are more appropriate for older children because they involve metalinguistic skill that requires them to reflect what they know. This piece of information can serve as a baseline for progress monitoring and facilitate intervention planning, which can be built on the child's existing knowledge.

School-age children encounter more Tier Two and Tier Three vocabulary that often have multiple meanings and involve more advanced word knowledge. In addition, word meaning may change depending on the context and content area. For example, the word "*square*" has different meanings in mathematics and language arts and the word "*address*" has different meanings when functioning as a noun verses a verb. Stahl and Bravo (2010) suggested that generating a checklist of words based on the school-age children's word use is beneficial to monitor their vocabulary growth and use. Also, comparing their self-evaluation of word knowledge before and after learning is a useful curriculum-based vocabulary assessment. Even though Stahl and Bravo's suggestions (2010) are offered to teachers, speech-language pathologists can easily adapt this method as an informal measure to monitor school-age children's growth in academic related lexical knowledge. Table 7–2 shows an example for self-assessment of lexical knowledge. In addition, clinicians

Table 7–2. An Example of Self-Assessment of Word Knowledge

Target Word	Heard of the word before but has no knowledge about it.	Can use the word in a specific context with emerging knowledge.	Can correctly explain the word and use it beyond the specific situation.	Knows the word well and can use and understand in various contexts correctly.
Cabinet				
Record				
Coach				

Source: Adapted from Beck, McKeown, and Kucan (2002).

can also ask school-age children to identify their knowledge level of selected words based on the categories suggested by Stahl and Bravo (2010). Table 7–3 shows an example of using self-assessment for evaluating lexical knowledge of mental state verbs.

Evaluate Lexical Knowledge and Word Production in Connected Speech

The understanding of collocations and word relations is key to sentence formation and morphological application. Without using proper words and parts of speech correctly, a sentence cannot be formed. Additionally, *"knowing a word"* means that the individual has all aspects of lexical knowledge across the meaning, form, and use (Nation, 2001). Therefore, it is essential to holistically evaluate lexical knowledge and word use through different types of spoken discourse, such as conversation, narrative discourse (e.g., retelling or generating a story), and expository discourse (e.g., explaining how to play and win a favorite game). Constructing and generating different types of spoken discourse may pose different cognitive and linguistic demands to the examinees. Hence, it provides clinicians valuable information about how word-finding difficulty may manifest because of different processing demands. Clinicians can also evaluate if clients

Table 7–3. Example of Self-Assessment of Mental-State Words for School-Age Children

Word	I don't remember having heard of this word before.	I have heard of this word before, but I don't know what it means.	I have heard of this word before, and I think it means ___.	I know this word. It means ___.	I can use this word in a sentence. My sentence is ___.
Suspicious					
Ashamed					
Disgusted					
Amused					

Word	Give a situation when you may experience this feeling.	Give a word and a situation that you may feel the opposite.	Find a facial expression online to reflect the word meaning.
Suspicious			
Ashamed			
Disgusted			
Amused			

Source: Adapted from Stahl and Bravo (2010).

could use words correctly in diverse contexts to serve different purposes and also observe their communication effectiveness and social communication.

Dynamic Assessment for Children From Culturally and Linguistically Diverse Backgrounds

Dynamic assessment (DA), developed and based on Vygotsky's sociocultural theory (1978), is another non-standardized measure to capture the dynamic process of word learning. Gutierrez-Clellen and Peña (2001) recommended that test-teach-retest is the most suitable approach to differentiate *language differences* from *language disorders* because static assessments do not capture a child's learnability and learning potential and heavily rely on the child's prior knowledge and experiences. Other types of dynamic assessment, such as testing the limits and gradual prompting, may be more appropriate for determining readiness for treatment intervention. When conducting *test-teach-retest* in dynamic assessment, a child's current lexical knowledge is assessed during the first *test* period. Secondly, during the *teaching* phase, mediated learning experience (MLE) is delivered through teaching the child problem-solving strategies and observing the changes in the child's learning and response to teaching. Lastly, during the retest phase, clinicians evaluate the child's learning within his/her zone of proximal development and the response to instruction (Peña et al., 2001). Gutierrez-Clellen and Peña (2001) further discussed four essential ingredients of MLE and the role of mediator, including *intentionality* (i.e., the mediator explains the goal of the activity), *meaning* (i.e., the mediator explains the importance and value of the activity), *transcendence* (i.e., the mediator facilitates the connection between newly learned skills and the individual's experience to encourage independent thinking and learning), and *competence* (i.e., the mediator encourages the individual use newly learned strategies and encourages generalization).

The differences between static assessment (SA) and DA include (1) DA focuses on what a child *can learn* whereas static measure pays attention to what the child *has learned*, (2) DA emphasizes *the process* of learning whereas SA focuses on *the product* of learning, (3) interaction, contextual assessment, and scaffolding are prohibited in SA but allowed in DA (Hessamy & Ghaderi, 2014; Kapantzoglou et al., 2012). The reliability of diagnosing bilingual children with language impairments using DA has been supported by research through different word learning tasks (Kapantzoglou et al., 2012). Children from non-mainstream cultures without language impairments show significant gains after MLE, whereas children with language impairments show no to little changes between test and retest in vocabulary learning (Gutierrez-Clellen & Peña, 2001; Kapantzoglou et al., 2012; Peña et al., 2001; Petersen et al., 2020). It is undoubtable that DA is an excellent tool to assess learning potential for children from non-mainstream cultures. Whereas dynamic assessment can capture partial word learning, the static assessment may provide information from other aspects of word knowledge. Thus, Burton and Watkins (2007) suggested that both measures for the word learning process and word knowledge should be used in the vocabulary assessment.

Two measures for evaluating MLE are Learning Strategies Checklist (Peña, 1993) and Modifiable Scale (Peña, 1993). Learning Strategies Checklist (LSC) evaluates *attention* (e.g., student's sustained attention to task-relevant stimuli), *comparative behavior* (e.g., focus on specific teaching and the student's response to a targeted learning task), *planning* (e.g., student's use of systematic strategy), *self-regulation* (e.g., student's awareness to seek help when needing it, self-correct, and reward self), *motivation* (e.g., student's enthusiasm and persistence in learning), and *transfer* (e.g., student applies strategies within and between tasks). While rating the student's use of learning strategies (LSC) during the session, the examiner also rates on the modifiable scale (MS) based on examiner's effort (the amount of effort required to induce change during teaching), student's responsivity (student's response to instruction), and ability to transfer (student's ability to apply the learned strategies to new tasks). Both LSC and MS have been reported as useful and effective for differentiating language differences from language disorders (Gutierrez-Clellen & Peña, 2001; Peña, 2000).

In sum, evaluating lexical knowledge and word production via just one type of assessment tool can provide only limited information. It is critically important to have a clear picture of word access or word retrieval difficulty based on the result of a comprehensive assessment. A naming error may be related to insufficient lexical knowledge, fragile semantic relations, or weak semantic-lexical connections. For example, a 9-year-old boy with developmental language disorder may successfully point to the correct picture but fail to name the target word because he has only a superficial understanding of the word. Because of the limited language skills, the boy is not able to define the word, discuss attributes of the word, or use the word in a sentence. In summary, understanding the type of information gathered from different types of assessment tasks can help clinicians select appropriate measures and put together the most accurate profile of the client's lexical knowledge and word retrieval ability. Table 7–4 summarizes the commonly used tasks for evaluating lexical knowledge and word production across settings.

Post-Assessment: Analyzing and Interpreting Assessment Results

Naming Accuracy

The formula for calculating naming accuracy consists of taking the number of correctly named responses and then dividing it by the total number of items given. In other words, naming accuracy rates mean the percentage of items correctly named. It can be used to track a client's progress and compare the changes before and after treatment. However, when interpreting naming accuracy, clinicians should take the number of total test items into consideration. For example, three correct responses out of five targets and 80 correct responses out of a total of 100 targets both result in 80% naming accuracy. The more test items that are given, the more reliable the result could be.

Table 7–4. Tasks for Evaluating Lexical Knowledge and Word Production

Target Area	Procedure	Examples	Strengths	Limitations
Lexical knowledge at word level	Point to pictures that go together, or verbally explain how two words are alike.	Pyramids and Palm Tree (PPT), PPVT-5, ROWPVT-relational vocabulary (TOLD-P5), word class (CELF-5)	+ Quick + Semantic knowledge + Semantic network + Lexical organization + Semantic relations	– Superficial word knowledge – A chance of guessing – Mostly nouns due to illustration limitation – Word selection may be culturally insensitive – Do not reflect the word learning process
Word production at word level	• Confrontation naming • Define a word • Synonyms and antonyms • Sentence completion	Boston Naming Test WAB-R naming subtests EVT-4, EOWPVT-5	+ Elicit some information about the depth of word knowledge using definitional measures + Relatively quick	– Naming does not provide too much information about the depth of word knowledge – Besides accuracy, no other qualitative data can be obtained. – Definitional measures are metalinguistic-based. Not suitable for young children. – Do not consider the influence of context on word use.
Verbal fluency (generative naming)	Name items in the same category in 1 minute	Name as many as fruits as possible in 1 minute	+ Lexical organization + Semantic relations	– Involves information processing speed. – Time constrain may create anxiety which in turn affects performance – Similar limitations mentioned in norm-referenced tests (vocabulary use)

Target Area	Procedure	Examples	Strengths	Limitations
Spoken discourse	Analyze errors and responses to cues across different types of discourse.	Number of Different Words (NDW) Type-Token Ration (TTR)	+ Lexical diversity. + Can get normative data using language sample analysis programs (e.g., SALT) + Word use in a natural context.	– Involves language sample analysis. Time-consuming. – The result of TTR may vary due to sample size.
Self-reports or parent/ caregiver reports	Complete checklists	MB-CDIs ASHA -FACS Informal checklist	+ Functional information can be gathered. + Cost-effective and efficient.	– Subjective perception – Word selection may be culturally insensitive.
Dynamic assessment	Identify unknown words and then engage activities to evaluate initial word learning	Quick incidental learning (QUIL) Test-teach-retest	+ Can capture word learning potential. + Focus on the word learning process, not just word knowledge + Differentiate language difference from language disorder + Consider the influence of non-mainstream culture and language	– The procedure is not standardized. Variations exist in the implementation. – The measurement may be subjective. – More preparation from the clinician.

continues

Table 7–4. *continued*

Target Area	Procedure	Examples	Strengths	Limitations
Curriculum-based assessment	Collect student's work and collaborate with teachers	Teacher created exams, word journals, word games, observation, homework	+ Target selection is based on content areas + Functional for school-age children + Increase generalization from therapy to classroom + Can monitor vocabulary knowledge growth + Vocabulary knowledge and use is measured by various methods and multiple points in time.	– Measures may be subjective. – More preparation from the clinician.
Use of other means of communication	Spontaneous vs. promoted drawing or gesturing when experiencing lexical access difficulty	The use of gestures when student cannot think of a word (How frequent? What types of words?) The use of drawing when student cannot think of a word (self-initiated or promoted)?	+ Can reflect the client's semantic knowledge when verbally naming is not an option. + Have the potential to facilitate word retrieval in adults. + Aids communication effectiveness	– Interpretation may be subjective. – Physical disability may limit use.

Source: Adapted from Watkins and DeThorne (2000, p. 241).

Naming Response Time

Naming response time can also be used to identify and evaluate the severity of word finding difficulty. Some standardized naming tests, such as Boston Naming Test (BNT), have a specific time limit for verbal responses, such as 20 seconds. During confrontation naming and verbal fluency tasks, clinicians should record the time it takes for an examinee to name each item and make notes to the words that the examinee needs additional time to respond. During discourse tasks, clinicians can track delayed responses, pauses, or use of fillers (e.g., "um"). A longer response time reflects slower information processing or/and a greater effort needed to produce the target word.

Frequency of Occurrence of Different Error Types

Speech-language pathologists can also calculate the frequency of occurrence for each error type made by a client. The frequency can be calculated by taking the number of specific type of errors and dividing it by the total number of errors. For example, if a clinician wants to get the frequency of occurrence for semantic substitutions in a 3-minute conversation sample, the clinician can take the number of occurrences (e.g., 10 semantic substitutions) and divide it by the total number of all errors made in the language sample (e.g., 20 errors). This means half (50%) of the errors were semantic substations presented in this language sample. The frequency of total error occurrence can be calculated by taking the number of T-units with one or more word-finding characteristics (details listed in Table 6–1) divided by the total number of T-units in the sample (German, 1991). This information is helpful for clinicians to learn the error types commonly made, and it is valuable for clinical decision making and treatment planning.

Error Analysis and Response to Cues

Analyzing errors and client's response to diffident types of cues (e.g., phonological cues, semantic cues, gestural cues, etc.) can provide clinicians with additional information about the challenge in acquiring lexical knowledge or retrieving words. For example, if a client says *"cap"* when naming the picture of a cat, clinicians can probe more on the client's semantic and lexical representations of *"cat"* by asking the client to describe distinct attributes. Clinicians can also discuss with the client about how *"cap"* to *"cat"* sounds different. It is important to keep in mind that this task requires a certain level of auditory comprehension and metalinguistic skills because the client needs to focus on analyzing the language components instead of simply saying the target word correctly. Clinicians can observe if there is a pattern in a client's naming errors. For example, a client tends to replace target words by using words with similar meanings or words in the same semantic category. Clinicians can discuss the similar and different semantic features of the target word and the error to prompt for more responses. Carefully analyzing the error patterns can help clinicians pinpoint the potential treatment goals and objectives, such as strengthening lexical representations or phonological representations.

Clinicians should also document the compensatory strategies used by an examinee when experiencing word-finding difficulty. The compensatory or self-cuing strategies during word retrieval process are a piece of valuable information for treatment planning, such as circumlocutions, using writing/drawing/gestures, phonemic cues, and so on. It is also essential to document (1) the context when word finding difficulty happens (e.g., longer and complex sentences, specific topics, certain word categories), (2) the context when the examinee uses a certain type of coping strategy, and (3) if the compensatory strategy was effective. This piece of information can help clinicians identify the context of word finding difficulty and the examinee's strength in overcoming challenges.

An analysis of error patterns can provide speech-language pathologists with insightful information about the breakdowns in word retrieval process in spoken discourse. In other words, analysis of naming errors and responses to different types of cues across different linguistic units and genres of discourse is beneficial for clinicians in pinpointing the breakdown and in facilitating the treatment planning.

Analyzing Lexical Diversity

For the pediatric population, lexical diversity (i.e., word variety) should also be measured as children with developmental language disorders usually have less diverse vocabulary than their typically developing peers. Lexical diversity can be evaluated via different measures, including number of different words (NDW) and type-token ration (TTR). The NDW is calculated by dividing the number of different words by the total number of words (TNW) spoken in a language sample. When calculating the number of types, words that occur more than once (e.g., [the], [a]) can only be counted once. The normative data for NDW can be found in the Systematic Analysis of Language Transcripts (SALT) database at https://www.saltsoftware.com. The TTR is calculated by dividing NDW by total number of words (TNW) in a spoken or written sample (Miller, 1981). A TTR that is close to 1.0 reflects a great diversity of words that a child is able to express. A TTR below .5 indicates that a child uses the same words repeatedly, which is commonly seen in children with developmental language disorders. An online tool, Text Inspector (https://textinspector.com), can be used to analyze up to 250 words for free, and TTR is included in the basic statistics report generated by Text Inspector. However, TTR should be interpreted with caution because the results may vary depending on the language sample size and other variables, such as the topic of interest. Therefore, analyzing multiple language samples across different contexts is highly recommended to develop a more comprehensive understanding of the child's word use.

Chapter Summary

In this chapter, we have discussed the components of a comprehensive plan for evaluating lexical knowledge and word production based on current research evidence. We also review the considerations for assessing lexical knowledge and word production. It should be noted that different factors need to be considered when assessing developmental lexical learning disorders verses a neurogenic word retrieval deficit. Understanding what is involved in the speech production process and why clients with developmental or acquired language disorders may struggle with word retrieval gives speech-language pathologists a good foundation for evaluating lexical knowledge and word production. It is critical to not rely on a single measure when conducing assessments. Clinicians should not just administer a confrontation naming test at word level but should consider evaluating word production in different contexts and spoken discourse to further assess word retrieval and lexical learning difficulty. Additionally, error analyses and clinical observations can help clinicians make clinical decisions based on the identified strengths and limitations.

Speech-language pathologists should continue evaluating clients' improvement by monitoring their progress over time; therefore, ongoing assessment is essential. It is critical to first identify the treatment targets based on the initial assessment results and then continuously collect ongoing clinical data after implementing treatment plans to track progress. Measuring improvement in lexical knowledge and word learning in children can be accomplished through evaluating vocabulary size and depth of word knowledge. For measuring word retrieval in adults with neurogenic language disorders, progress monitoring may be structured based on the intervention approach implemented. Commonly implemented treatment approaches to address developmental lexical learning and neurogenic word retrieval difficulty are discussed in the next two chapters.

Discussion Questions

1. What are some standardized tasks that can be used to evaluate lexical knowledge and word production?
2. When evaluating lexical knowledge and word production in a client who comes from a non-mainstream culture background and speaks a primary language other than English, what factors do you need to consider during the assessment? Why?

3. What different aspects should clinicians consider when evaluating a preschool child with developmental language disorders versus an adult with aphasic word retrieval difficulty? What aspects of word retrieval ability should be considered when evaluating the adult with anomia but who has good semantic knowledge?

References

Anderson, R. C., & Freebody, P. (1981). Vocabulary knowledge. In J. Guthrie (Ed.), *Comprehension and teaching: Research reviews* (pp. 77–117). International Reading Association.

Beck, I., McKeown, M., & Kucan, L. (2002). *Bringing words to life: Robust vocabulary instruction* (2nd ed.). Guilford Press.

Beck, I. L., McKeown, M. G., & Omanson, R. C. (1987). The effects and uses of diverse vocabulary instructional techniques. In M. G. McKeown & M. E. Curtis (Eds.), *The nature of vocabulary acquisition* (pp. 147–163). Lawrence Erlbaum Associates.

Bowers, L., Huisingh, R., LoGiudice, C., & Orman, J. (1990). *The Word Test 3—Elementary*. LinguiSystems.

Burton, V. J., & Watkins, R. V. (2007). Measuring word learning: Dynamic versus static assessment of kindergarten vocabulary. *Journal of Communication Disorders*, *40*(5), 335–356. https://doi.org/10.1016/j.jcomdis.2006.06.015

Dunn, D. M. (2019). *Peabody Picture Vocabulary Test* (5th ed.). NCS Pearson.

Fenson, L., Marchman, V. A., Thal, D. J., Dale, P. S., Reznick, J. S., & Bates, E. (2007). *MacArthur-Bates Communicative Development Inventories: User's guide and technical manual* (2nd ed.). Brookes.

Frattali, C., Thompson, C., Holland, A., Wohl, C., & Ferketic, M. (1995). *The American Speech-Language-Hearing Association Functional Assessment of Communication Skills for Adults (ASHA FACS)*. ASHA.

Gamboz, N., Coluccia, E., Iavarone, A., & Brandimonte, M. (2009). Normative data for the Pyramids and Palm Trees Test in the elderly italian population. *Neurological Sciences*, *30*, 453. https://doi.org/10.1007/s10072-009-0130-y

German, D. J. (1991). *Test of Word Finding in Discourse (TWFD): Administration, scoring, interpretation, and technical manual*. Pro-Ed.

German, D. J. (2015). *Test of Word Finding* (3rd ed.). Pro-Ed.

German, D. J. (2016). *Test of Adolescent/Adult Word Finding* (2nd ed.). Pro-Ed.

Goodglass, H., Kaplan, E., & Barresi, B. (2001). *The Boston Diagnostic Aphasia Exam* (3rd ed.). Lippincott Williams & Wilkins.

Gutierrez–Clellen, V. F., & Peña, E. (2001). Dynamic assessment of diverse children. *Language, Speech, and Hearing Services in Schools, 32*(4), 212–224. https://doi.org/10.1044/0161-1461(2001/019)

Hamaguchi, P. & Ross-Swain, D. (2015). *Receptive, expressive, and social communication assessment*. Super Duper Publications.

Hart, B., & Risley, T. R. (1992). American parenting of language-learning children: Persisting differences in family-child interactions observed in natural home environments. *Developmental Psychology, 28*(6), 1096–1105. https://doi.org/10.1037/0012-1649.28.6.1096

Henriksen, B. (1999). Three dimensions of vocabulary development. *Studies in Second Language Acquisition, 21*(2), 303–317. https://doi.org/10.1017/S0272263199002089

Hessamy, G., & Ghaderi, E. (2014). The role of dynamic assessment in the vocabulary learning of Iranian EFL learners. *Procedia—Social and Behavioral Sciences, 98*, 645–652. https://doi.org/10.1016/j.sbspro.2014.03.463

Hoffman, J. L., Teale, W. H., & Paciga, K. A. (2013). What do children need to succeed in early literacy—and beyond? In K. G. Goodman, R. C. Calfee, & Y. M. Goodman (Eds.), *Whose knowledge counts in government literacy programs?: Why expertise matters* (pp. 179–186). Routledge.

Howard, D., & Patterson, K. (1992). *The Pyramids and Palm Trees Test*. Thames Valley Company.

Hresko, W. P., Reid, K., & Hammill, D. D. (2018). *Test of Early Language Development* (4th ed.). Pro-Ed.

Hu, H. M., & P. Nation. (2000). What vocabulary size is needed to read unsimplified texts? *Reading in a Foreign Language, 8*, 689–696.

Ishii, T., & Schmitt, N. (2009). Developing an integrated diagnostic test of vocabulary size and depth. *RELC Journal, 40*(1), 5–22. https://doi.org/10.1177/0033688208101452

Kapantzoglou, M., Restrepo, M. A., & Thompson, M. S. (2012). Dynamic assessment of word learning skills: Identifying language impairment in bilingual children. *Language, Speech, and Hearing Services in Schools, 43*(1), 81–96. https://doi.org/10.1044/0161-1461(2011/10-0095)

Kaplan E., Goodglass H., & Weintraub, S. (1983). *Boston Naming Test*. Lea & Febiger.

Kaplan, E., Harold, H., & Weintraub, S. (2001). *Boston Naming Test– Second Edition (BNT-2)*. Pro-Ed.

Kertesz, A. (2006). *Western Aphasia Battery–Revised (WAB-R)*. Pro-Ed.

Laufer, B., & Goldstein, Z. (2004). Testing vocabulary knowledge: Size, strength and computer adaptiveness. *Language Learning, 54*(3), 399–436. https://doi.org/10.1111/j.0023-8333.2004.00260.x

Martin, N. A., & Brownell, R. (2010a). *Expressive One-Word Picture Vocabulary Test* (4th ed.). Gander Publishing.

Martin, N. A., & Brownell, R. (2010b). *Receptive One-Word Picture Vocabulary Test* (4th ed.). Gander Publishing.

Meara, P. (1997). Towards a new approach to modelling vocabulary acquisition. In N. Schmitt & M. McCarthy (Eds.), *Vocabulary: Description, acquisition and pedagogy* (pp. 109–121). Cambridge University Press.

Melka, F. (1997). Receptive versus productive aspects of vocabulary. In N. Schmitt & M. McCarthy (Eds.), *Vocabulary: Description, acquisition, and pedagogy* (pp. 84–102). Cambridge University Press.

Miller, J. F. (1981). *Assessing language production in children: Experimental procedures*. University Park Press.

Montgomery, J. K. (2008). *MAVA: Montgomery Assessment of Vocabulary Acquisition (MAVA)*. Super Duper Publications.

Nation, L. (2001). *Learning vocabulary in another language*. Cambridge University Press.

Newcomer, P. L., & Hammill, D. D. (2019a). *Test of Language Development–Primary* (5th ed.). Pro-Ed.

Newcomer, P. L., & Hammill, D. D. (2019b). *Test of Language Development–Intermediate* (5th ed.). Pro-Ed.

Peña, E. (1993). *Dynamic assessment: A non-biased approach for assessing the language of young children*. Retrieved from ProQuest Dissertations and Theses. (Order No. 9316518).

Peña, E. (2000). Measurement of modifiability in children from culturally and linguistically diverse backgrounds. *Communication Disorders Quarterly, 21*(2), 87–97.

Peña, E., Iglesias, A., & Lidz, C. S. (2001). Reducing test bias through dynamic assessment of children's word learning ability. *American Journal of Speech Language Pathology, 10*(2), 138–154. https://doi.org/10.1044/1058-0360(2001/014)

Pearson, D., Hiebert, E., & Kamil, M. (2007). Vocabulary assessment: What we know and what we need to learn. *Reading Research Quarterly, 42*(2), 282–296. http://doi:10.1598/RRQ.42.2.4

Petersen, D. B., Tonn, P., Spencer, T. D., & Foster, M. E. (2020). The classification accuracy of a dynamic assessment of inferential word learning for bilingual English/Spanish speaking school-age children. *Language, Speech, and Hearing Services in Schools, 51*(1), 144–164. https://doi.org/10.1044/2019_LSHSS-18-0129

Qian, D. D. (2002). Investigating the relationship between vocabulary knowledge and academic reading performance: An assessment perspective. *Language Learning, 52*(3), 513–536. https://doi.org/10.1111/1467-9922.00193

Schmitt, N. (2010). *Researching vocabulary.* Palgrave Macmillan.

Schmitt, N. (2014). Size and depth of vocabulary knowledge: What the research shows. *Language Learning, 64*(4), 913–951. https://doi.org/10.1111/lang.12077

Stahl, K. A., & Bravo, M. A. (2010). Contemporary classroom vocabulary assessment for content areas. *The Reading Teacher, 63*(7), 566–578. https://doi.org/10.1598/RT.63.7.4

Vygotsky, L. S. (1978). *Mind in society: The development of higher psychological processes.* Harvard University Press.

Wallace, G., & Hammill, D. (2002). *Comprehensive Receptive and Expressive Vocabulary Test* (2nd ed.). Pro-Ed.

Watkins, R. V., & DeThorne, L. S. (2000). Assessing children's vocabulary skills: From word knowledge to word learning potential. *Seminars in Speech and Language, 21*(3), 235–246. https://doi.org/10.1055/s-2000-13197

Wiig, E. (2004). *WABC: Wigg Assessment of Basic Concepts.* Pro-Ed.

Wiig, E. H., Semel, E., & Secord, W. A. (2013). *Clinical Evaluation of Language Fundamentals* (5th ed.). NCS Pearson.

Williams, K. T. (2018). *The Expressive Vocabulary Test* (3rd ed.). NCS Pearson.

World Health Organization (WHO). (2001). *International classification of functioning, disability and health (ICF).* Author.

Appendix 7–1

An Overview of Current Standardized Tests That Evaluate Vocabulary Across Age Groups

(Table created by Claire Small and Sarah Larsen)
begins on following page

Title	Author(s)/ Date	Target Population	Purpose
Assesses Word Retrieval Ability			
Boston Naming Test (BNT)	Kaplan, Goodglass, & Weintraub, (1983)	5:0+	Designed to assess word retrieval abilities through confrontation naming. Patients must verbally respond.
Test of Adolescent/ Adult Word Finding– 2nd Edition (TAWF-2)	German (2016)	12 to 80	Assesses speed/ accuracy during word retrieval of nouns, verbs, and categories.
Test of Word Finding– 3rd Edition (TWF-3)	German (2015)	4:6 to 12:11	Assesses speed and accuracy when naming nouns; sentence completion; speed and accuracy when naming verbs; naming objects and categories.

Materials/Tasks	Receptive/ Expressive	The Proportion of Word Classes
■ Confrontation naming task with 60 line drawings ■ Stimuli increases in difficulty (e.g., from simple, high-frequency words to low-frequency words that are more phonemically complex)	Expressive	**60 concrete nouns:** animals, household objects, food, historical objects, measuring tools, and so forth —includes more low-frequency nouns
■ Picture naming: nouns ■ Sentence completion naming ■ Picture naming: verbs ■ Picture naming: word groups ■ Includes a comprehension check to assess the knowledge of missed words ■ Imitation of syllable shapes	Receptive/ Expressive	**nouns:** 24 **sentence completion naming (nouns):** 13 **verbs:** 19 **word groups:** 23 *Uses the same target words for each receptive/expressive test, but uses different stimuli books for each one.
■ Picture naming (nouns & verbs), ■ Sentence completion naming (nouns) ■ Picture naming (categories) ■ Comprehension check (missed items)	Expressive/ Receptive	**Nouns:** 87 **Verbs:** 41 **Categories:** 53

continues

Title	Author(s)/ Date	Target Population	Purpose
Assesses Semantic Knowledge			
The Pyramids and Palm Trees Test	Howard & Patterson (1992)	18 to 80	Assesses semantic relations. Provides information about the presence and nature of semantic impairment (i.e., modality-specific or modality-independent) related to concrete targets.
Assess Lexical Learning and Knowledge			
Communicative Development Inventories– (CDI)	Fenson, Marchman, Thal, Dale, Reznick, & Bates (2007)	Level I: 8 to 18 months Level II: 16 to 30 months Level III: 30 to 37 months	Provides a checklist of vocabulary words comprehension/ production, and includes a check-list and list of questions about word combi-nations. Helps screen children to determine if they have a developmental language delay.

Materials/Tasks	Receptive/ Expressive	The Proportion of Word Classes
■ Presented with a given item, the target and the distractor (picture or orthographic representation) ■ Individual must identify the 2 items that share a category (i.e., properties or shared associations)	Receptive	**52 concrete and relatively common nouns:** animals, household objects, etc.
It uses a checklist of words and morphemes. The parent must determine if the child understands or uses those words within their daily lives. It provides a checklist for word combinations and to determine if certain words were used in different tenses (e.g., past, present).	Expressive & Receptive	The test contains a large majority of concrete nouns. The level III contains more abstract nouns (e.g., tomorrow) and some adverbs, adjectives, & prepositions (e.g., why, empty, because, etc.)

continues

Title	Author(s)/ Date	Target Population	Purpose
Comprehensive Receptive and Expressive Vocabulary Test–2nd Edition (CREVT-2)	Wallace & Hammill, (2002)	Receptive = 4:0 to 17:11 Expressive = 5:0 to 17:11	Purpose is to identify deficiencies in expressive vocabulary and determine discrepancies between expressive/ receptive vocabulary skills.
Expressive Vocabulary Test–3rd Edition	Williams (2018)	2:6 to 90+	It measures expressive vocabulary knowledge and word retrieval skills.

Materials/Tasks	Receptive/ Expressive	The Proportion of Word Classes
Receptive: Uses real pictures and asks the individual to identify multiple names for each object- providing nouns and adjectives. (e.g., *plumage* & *talon* for the same picture of a bird). Breaks the images up into categories (e.g., animals, food, etc.). Expressive: Asks the individuals to define a word (uses words that are concrete and have one meaning and uses words that have multiple meanings).	Expressive & receptive	Receptive: almost all nouns, but a few adjectives were provided (e.g., translucent, vertical) Expressive: nouns (29) - some nouns have multiple meanings (e.g., sash could mean a scarf, ribbon, or a part of a window)
Based on visual stimuli, the individual needs to provide a one-word response. It asks the individual to label images or provide a synonym of the target word.	Expressive	Record Form A *Approximately ■ **131 Nouns:** includes nouns to describe categories (e.g., fruit, drinks), abstract nouns (e.g., sight, directions), & concrete nouns (e.g., rose, lamb) ■ **24 Verbs** ■ **33 Adjectives** ■ **1 Preposition** ■ **1 Adverb** Record Form B *Approximately ■ **135 Nouns** ■ **28 Verbs** ■ **25 Adjectives** ■ **2 Adverbs**

continues

Title	Author(s)/ Date	Target Population	Purpose
Expressive One Word Picture Vocabulary Test–4th Edition (EOWPVT-4)	Martin, & Brownell, (2010a)	2:0 to 80+	Assesses the client's word retrieval abilities through verbal naming (i.e., objects, actions, concepts).
Montgomery Assessment of Vocabulary Acquisition (MAVA)	Montgomery (2008)	3:0-12:11	Designed to assess children's oral language skills through listening and speaking vocabulary. Assess vocab across all three tiers.
Peabody Picture Vocabulary Test–5th Edition (PPVT-5)	Dunn (2019)	2:6 to 90+	Measures receptive vocabulary knowledge (i.e., nouns, verbs, and attributes).

Materials/Tasks	Receptive/ Expressive	The Proportion of Word Classes
■ Asks to identify the correct target word through the use of colored illustrations (190 pictures). ■ The test begins with words that are more concrete/frequently used and ends with words that are more esoteric/ less frequently encountered.	Expressive	*Approximately ■ **160 Nouns:** only 2 abstract nouns (i.e., *feelings/ emotions & directions*) ■ **8 Verbs** ■ **22 concepts/ categorizing** (e.g., "What word describes all of these?"—*animals;* "What are all these things used for?"—*measuring*)
■ Stimuli targets single words (verbs, nouns, adjectives) ■ Receptively: point to the corresponding image in a field of four ■ Expressively: name the image in a field of four	Expressive & Receptive	**Expressive:** *Approximately* **Nouns: 144** **Verbs: 17** **Adjectives: 12** **Receptive:** **Nouns: 98** **Verbs: 36** **Adjectives: 33** **Prepositions: 3**
■ Asks to identify the target word given 4 choices (color illustrations).	Receptive	*Approximately **158 Nouns:** abstract nouns first appear beginning in age 12 vocabulary (*time*). **30 Adjectives** **52 Verbs:** present progressive

continues

Title	Author(s)/ Date	Target Population	Purpose
Receptive One Word Picture Vocabulary Test–4th Edition (ROWPVT-4)	Martin, & Brownell (2010b)	2:0-80+	Assesses receptive language using a developmental sequence of vocabulary acquisition.
Receptive, Expressive, and Social Communication Assessment	Hamaguchi & Ross-Swain (2015)	5:0 to 12:11	Assesses expressive, receptive, and social communication skills. Both expressive and receptive language subtests target language at the word, sentence, and narrative level.

Materials/Tasks	Receptive/ Expressive	The Proportion of Word Classes
■ Asks to identify the target word given 4 choices (color illustrations).	Receptive	*Roughly ■ **130 nouns** ■ **30 verbs** ■ **30 adjectives**
Receptive Language assessment includes: comprehension of vocabulary, comprehension of oral directions, comprehension of stories and questions, comprehension of basic morphology and syntax, executing oral directions. Expressive Language assessment includes: expressive labeling of vocabulary, expressive skills for describing and explaining, narrative skills, expressive use of basic morphology and syntax. Social Communication Includes subtests in the following areas: Comprehension of Body Language and Vocal; Emotion; Social and Language Inference Situational Language Use. Requires participants to match images to emotions.	Expressive & Receptive	**Expressive labeling** **Nouns: 15** **Verbs: 4** **Adjectives: 13** **Categories: 9** **Comprehension of Vocabulary** **Nouns: 17** **Verbs: 11** **Adjectives: 20**

continues

Appendix 7–1. *continued*

Title	Author(s)/ Date	Target Population	Purpose
The Word Test 3 –Elementary	Bowers, Huisingh, LoGiudice, & Orman, (1990)	7:0 to 11	Test of expressive vocabulary . Assesses the individual's ability to recognize & express critical semantic attributes. They need to be able to categorize, define, inquire verbal reasoning, and select appropriate words based on their knowledge of semantic attributes.
Wigg Assessment of Basic Concepts WABC (1)	Wiig (2004)	Two-tests 2:6 to 5:11 And 5:0 to 7:11	This test assesses a child's understanding and use of basic concepts (e.g., numbers, colors, etc.).

Materials/Tasks	Receptive/ Expressive	The Proportion of Word Classes
Tasks include: (1) associations, (2) synonyms, (3) semantic absurdities, (4) Antonyms, (5) definitions (6) multiple definitions	Expressive	**Association:** 14 nouns (1 abstract) **Antonyms:** Adjective: 11 Verbs: 3 Nouns: 1 Prepositions: 1 **Synonyms:** Adjective: 5 Verbs: 8 Prepositions: 1 Nouns: 1 **Definitions:** Nouns: 8 Adjectives: 4 Verbs: 3 **Multiple Definitions:** Provide multiple definitions of 1 word (i.e., words that can be used as different word classes)
Evaluates the child's knowledge and use of basic concepts through an interactive picture book. Basic concepts include color, shape, size, weight/volume, distance, time/speed, quantity/completeness, location/direction, condition, sensation, emotion/evaluation.	Expressive & Receptive	Level 1: **Nouns: 5** **Verbs: 7** **Adjectives: 34 Adverbs: 4** **Prepositions: 9** Level 2: **Nouns: 2** **Verbs: 0** **Adjectives: 42** **Preposition: 7** **Adverbs: 6** Both Tests contain mostly abstract words and adjectives to describe concepts (e.g., apart, none, different, together). Was also extremely difficult to accurately distinguish between different word classes (e.g., adverbs vs. preposition vs. noun)

continues

Title	Author(s)/ Date	Target Population	Purpose
Test of Language Development– Primary: 5th Edition	Newcomer & Hammill, (2019a)	4:0 to 8:11	Measures comprehensive language skills.
Test of Language Development– Intermediate: 5th Edition	Newcomer & Hammill (2019b)	8:0 to 17:11	Measures comprehensive language skills.

Materials/Tasks	Receptive/ Expressive	The Proportion of Word Classes
Subtests in the following areas: ■ Picture Vocabulary ■ Relational Vocabulary ■ Oral Vocabulary ■ Syntactic Understanding ■ Sentence Imitation ■ Morphological Completion Supplemental Subtests: ■ Word Discrimination ■ Word Analysis ■ Word Articulation	Expressive & Receptive	**Expressive Labeling** **Comprehension of Vocabulary**
Subtests in the following areas: ■ Picture vocabulary ■ Word ordering (i.e., for declarative & interrogative sentences) ■ Relational vocabulary ■ Multiple meanings	Expressive & Receptive	It includes a high percentage of Tier Two and Three vocabulary (e.g., *patient predator, aquatic vertebrate, culinary apparatus, female bovine*). It includes different verb tenses such as irregular past tense (e.g., *stole, grew, saw*). It includes words that sound the same, but have multiple meanings (e.g., cent, sent, scent) It includes words within different semantic categories (e.g., animals, religions, tools, currencies, etc.).

continues

Title	Author(s)/ Date	Target Population	Purpose
Test of Early Language Development (TELD-4)	Hresko, Reid, & Hammill, (2018)	3:00 to 7:11	It measures language skills in the areas of semantics, syntax, and morphology.

Materials/Tasks	Receptive/ Expressive	The Proportion of Word Classes
Uses pictures and manipulatives to measure language comprehension and expression. Not all test items require the use of pictures or objects. The test incorporates questions (e.g., "What is the girl doing?") and commands (e.g., *"stand up and touch your nose"*).	Receptive & Expressive	Includes different parts of speech: **Concrete nouns** (*bug, shoes, hat, island*) **Abstract nouns** (*faith*) **Prepositions** (*up, down, around, beside, above, on, under*) **Adjectives** (*red, best, first, last, confused*) **Conjunctions** (*because, since, but*) **WH- words** (*who, what, where*) **Pronouns** (*I, they, he she, your*) **Verbs** (*running, stand, skip, eating, repair*) **Adverbs** (*quickly, slowly, rapidly*)

8

APPROACHES TO FACILITATE VOCABULARY LEARNING AND WORD RETRIEVAL IN CHILDREN

Lei Sun

Chapter Objectives

1. Explain what words are appropriate for intervention based on a child's needs.
2. Identify important ingredients in effective vocabulary intervention.
3. Describe when, why, how, and to whom to use different vocabulary intervention approaches.

The Importance of Vocabulary Intervention for Children with Underdeveloped Vocabulary

According to Beck, McKeown, and Kucan (2002), children typically add 2,000 to 3,000 new words a year. It is impossible for children to learn that many words through direct instruction; thus, wide reading, and engaging in reading for an extended period of time on a regular basis (Fisher et al., 2010), can promote the significant increase in vocabulary breadth and depth. In Chapter 3, we discussed several cognitive and linguistic limitations commonly reported in children with developmental language disorders (DLD). We also learned that children with DLD have a slower *fast mapping* ability than their peers; therefore, they require not only more exposure to new words but also explicit teaching. As discussed in Chapter 4, *the Matthew effect* refers to *good readers who read more and become better readers.* On the other hand, children with poor vocabulary knowledge tend to read less, so they acquire new words much slower than typically developing (TD) children, which in turn limits their vocabulary growth. Moreover, if a child is not given the opportunity for wide reading or is not motivated in reading materials slightly above their reading level, the child cannot learn new words. Children with broader and more in-depth vocabulary knowledge tend to read more complex texts, which in turn facilitates their vocabulary growth (Sedita, 2005). Effective reading creates an upward spiral that leads to better reading fluency, stronger reading comprehension, and more extensive world knowledge.

TD children are able to analyze all the meanings of a word and find the meaning that is suitable for the context, whereas children with DLD have difficulty using guide words and identifying the correct definition. Therefore, using a dictionary is not an effective strategy to help children with DLD learn new words. As Laufer and Goldstein (2004) and Pignot-Shahov (2012) pointed out that word knowledge is multifaceted; thus, the connection between word form and meaning is only the tip of the iceberg. Considering it is not possible to directly teach 2,000 new words a year, Biemiller and Boote (2006) claimed that teaching 400 words per school year is a reasonable goal for children with DLD. This finding leads to two challenging questions: What words should we teach? How do we effectively teach vocabulary?

Word Selection

Selecting target words is a relatively subjective process. Most of the time, it is based on a speech-language pathologist's professional judgment and the client's needs. SLPs often select words that are functional to the client based on the assessment results.

This practice aligns well with evidence-based practice (EBP) as target selection should be based on the client's value, clinician's expertise, and best available research. Research studies recommend choosing Tier Two words for vocabulary instruction. Stahl and Nagy (2006) suggested that instructors should consider the following three categories of words (p. 97).

1. High-frequency vocabulary
   High-frequency words are Tier One words that can often be found in oral and written language across genres. These words are fundamental words that children may know.
2. High utility-literate vocabulary
   High utility-literate words are Tier Two words that frequently occur in texts (primarily in written language). These words are usually acquired through schooling instead of the conversation such as Tier One words.
3. Key content area vocabulary
   Key content area words are Tier Three words that are specific and important to a subject or domain.

High-Frequency Words

High-frequency words (Tier One word) can be easily acquired without direct instruction. However, most children with DLD may struggle with acquiring these Tier One words and experience even more difficulty in learning Tier Two words. In this case, SLPs may continue to work on high-frequency words and gradually expand their vocabulary repertoire. Two open access resources below can help SLPs and teachers identify high-frequency words.

- Dolch words or sight words developed by William Dolch (1948) (https://mrsperkins.com).
- New General Service List developed by Charles Browne, Brent Culligan, and Joseph Phillips (2013) (http://www .newgeneralservicelist.org).

Although the lists of high-frequency words were initially developed for English language learners, these are also beneficial and fundamental for children with DLD. The Educator's Word Frequency Guide authored by Susan Zeno, Stephen Ivens, Robert T Millard, Raj Duvvuri, and Ernst Rothkopf (1995) is another resource for obtaining high-frequency words.

High-frequency words are usually short and can be used in a good variety of contexts. Because these words frequently occur in a given language, these are usually easy to learn and retrieve. Nation (2010, cited in Pignot-Shahov, 2012) and Stahl and Nagy (2006) claimed that learning the 2,000 most frequent words is beneficial for learners because these high-frequency words cover 75% to 80% of words in the text. On the other hand, low-frequency words (i.e., Tier Three words) only make up 5% of the text (Nation, 2010, cited in Pignot-Shahov, 2012). Thus, it is strategically beneficial to select high-frequency words in therapy for children with DLD.

Tier Two Words

Tier Two words are words learned by most TD learners between fourth and eighth grade. Children usually have some knowledge of these words but lack precision and specificity (Steele & Mills 2011). Tier Two words are primarily found in written language across a variety of texts and contexts. Beck et al. (2002, p. 19) listed three criteria for identifying Tier Two words because there is no consensus about the definition for these words. Even though these criteria are suggested for teachers, it is also applicable to school-based SLPs when collaborating with teachers on developing vocabulary intervention.

1. Importance and utility: Words used by mature users that frequently appear across texts in both written and oral language and across domains. An example Beck et al. (2002) included in their book is that when a child has learned the words "salesperson" or "clerk," potential Tier Two words for intervention are "merchant, broker, vendor." Another example is when a child can use the word "happy" accurately, the more advanced word choices (Tier Two) are "delighted, cheerful, merry."
2. Instructional potential: Words that can be connected to other words and concepts. Words that can enhance the richness of a child's word knowledge should be selected.

Beck et al. (2002) claimed that Tier Two words present "more precise or more complex forms of familiar words," not just synonyms (p. 17). For example, "appreciate, acknowledge, respect" for "know, value" or "comment, mention, remark" for "say, talk about."

3. Conceptual understanding: Similar to the point mentioned above, selecting Tier Two words can increase the precision and specificity of word knowledge.

In addition to Tier Two words, Biemiller (2012) also suggested the inclusion of academic words using the "Academic Word List (AWL)" developed by Averil Coxhead (2000). Coxhead (2000) created a list of 570 root words and 3,000 derived words based on the words that frequently occur in school texts. The academic word list can be accessed at http://www.uefap.com/vocab/select/awl.htm

It is important to keep in mind that the top 2,000 words account for 75% of the words in the text, and AWL covers about 10% of the words in the text. The rest are either low-frequency words or technical words associated with specific disciplines (Stahl & Nagy, 2006).

Important Elements Needed for Effective Vocabulary Instruction

Although almost all principles and strategies of successful vocabulary instruction are developed for teachers, these principles can still be applied to vocabulary intervention for children with DLD or children with below-average vocabulary knowledge. The principles of effective vocabulary instruction suggested by Stahl and Nagy (2006) are (1) including both definitional and contextual information of the target word, (2) requiring a student's active participation in learning, and (3) providing multiple exposures in meaningful contexts. Graves (2006) further suggested that instructors should review, rehearse, and remind students about words used in various contexts as well as allocate time for elaboration and extended word learning. Along the same line, the National Reading Panel (NICHD, 2000) also recommends components for rich and effective vocabulary instruction.

1. Include direct instruction of new words.
2. Provide multiple exposures to new words.
3. Include new words in meaningful and various contexts.
4. Go beyond definition and specific context. McKeown (2019) suggests that word knowledge needs to become decontextualized for learners to develop the flexibility to learn words in new contexts.
5. Do not rely on a single vocabulary instruction. Incorporate multiple instructional methods to promote optimal learning, such as teaching definition along with using contextual clues.

Beck, McKeown, and Kucan (2002) also recommended several components for effective vocabulary instruction. Powerful vocabulary instruction:

1. Involves both definitions and contexts instead of including only one of these;
2. Activates the student's prior knowledge;
3. Compares and contrasts word meanings; and
4. Engages student's active participation by manipulating meanings, inference making, searching for applications, and multiple exposures.

In summary, regardless of the vocabulary level, children benefit from (1) explicit vocabulary instruction, (2) frequent exposures across multiple contexts, and (3) integration of definitional and contextual information from the content areas (Pollard-Durodola, et al., 2016).

Approaches to Facilitate Vocabulary Learning

In this section, we will discuss the commonly implemented strategies and approaches that promote lexical acquisition. As suggested by Steele and Mills (2011), vocabulary instructions designed for TD children are applicable to children with DLD or learning difficulties, such as direct and explicit instructions on word meaning (Jitendra et al., 2004). Stahl and Vancil (1986) suggested that explicit instruction should include finding a synonym or antonym, using new words to create sentences, comparing words, tying to personal experience, and multiple exposures. Based on their systematic review, various vocabulary instructions are effective for children with learning disabilities to gain word knowledge, including but not limited to direct instruction (e.g., giving definition), cognitive strategy instruction (e.g., semantic mapping, semantic feature analysis), and key word strategy. These strategies are mostly designed for school-age children or readers but can be modified for non-readers and preschoolers by incorporating more pictures and pre-selecting materials based on the child's present level. We will further discuss these strategies in this section.

Naturalistic Language Stimulation Techniques for Young Children and Children With Limited Verbal Output

In Chapter 3, we discuss extensively about how TD children develop their language naturally. Promoting the use of different types of gestures, gestures and words combinations, and expanding a child's phonetic inventory and syllable shapes can facilitate lexical development in young children. We also identify additional support that children with DLD would need for developing their general language skills, such as maximal repetitions, practice in various contexts, elaboration, and discussion of the new words. When working with young children, SLPs could apply indirect language stimulation techniques, such as self-talk, parallel talk, expansion, and extension. Below are the descriptions and examples of these commonly used techniques for promoting lexical development.

1. Self-talk: The adult or clinician narrates their actions while the child is present.

    Example: *"I am putting soap on my hands . . . I am washing my hands with cold water."*

2. Parallel talk: The adult or clinician narrates the actions of the child

    Example: *"You are putting soap on your hands . . . you are scrubbing your hands with soap and water."*

3. Expansion: Expands the child's utterance by using an adult language form without adding new information

    Example: The child says, *"wash hands"* and the adult responds with, *"yes, you are washing your hands."*

4. Extension: Extends the child's utterance by using an adult language form and adding new information.

    Example: The child says, *"wash hands"* and the adult responds with, *"you are washing your hands because they are dirty."*

Based on the child's present level, Milieu Teaching (MT) can be implemented with children at the prelinguistic stage (Prelinguistic Milieu Teaching [PMT]) and children who have a mean length of utterance (MLU) between 1 and 3.5 (Enhanced Milieu Teaching [EMT]) (Fey et al., 2006; Hancock & Kaiser, 2006; Yoder & Warren, 2002). Milieu Teaching is not designed especially for lexical development, but it can be used to facilitate overall language development. Through modeling and highlighting the target words, MT can effectively help young children learn these words in a natural environment (e.g., play, daily routines). The core elements of MT include the following (Hancock & Kaiser, 2002).

1. Model: Adults provide a model of desired responses and correct the child's responses as needed. For example, Child: "dog" (when pointing to a big dog not a small dog) Adult: "BIG dog" (emphasize the adjective "BIG").
2. Mand-Model: Adult provides a prompt (mand) for a target behavior. For example, Adults can ask questions like "What do you want?" "Which one?" "Do you want CAR or BABY?" If the child does not respond, adults provide a model.
3. Time delay: Adults provide a stimulus and then wait for a short period of time before the child loses interest. The goal is to elicit a child-initiated response. For example, adults can hold an inflated balloon and wait for the child to initiate a request like "FLY balloon" "GO balloon." If the child does not initiate a request, adults can provide a mand-model.
4. Incidental teaching: Adults move things out of the child's reach. The purpose of the environmental arrangement is

to create opportunities for the child to communicate their needs and wants. Once the child initiates the request, adults expand the child's remark to a complete form. For example, adults put the child's favorite toys in a tightly closed container, leave the toys on a shelf that the child cannot reach, or give the child a puzzle board without puzzle pieces.

The goal of PMT is to establish routines for communication and increase the frequency of vocalization, gaze, gesture, and combinations of these modalities (Fey et al., 2006). EMT operates under a similar framework with more advanced goals to increase the rate, diversity, complexity and independence of a child's communication. Through modeling and expanding the child's language use in communicative contexts and routines as well as arranging the environment, adults utilize a child's interests and everyday contexts to promote communication (Kaiser & Roberts, 2013). SLPs are encouraged to visit Vanderbilt KidTalk (http://kidtalk.vkcsites.org) to learn more about the efficacy of EMT and available resources for parents.

Kaiser and Roberts (2013) also strongly advocate for incorporating EMT principles into parent coaching. Parent coaching is commonly used in early intervention because it is a family-centered, naturalistic, and collaborative process (Stoner, Meadan, & Angell., 2013). Parents can be trained by SLPs to become effective co-interventionists to promote the implementation of strategies to be consistent, monitored, and individualized to address the child's needs. Kaiser and Roberts (2013) suggested following a "Teach-Model-Coach-Review" approach to ensure the fidelity of a parent-coaching program. During the coaching phase, parents practice implementing the strategies while simultaneously receiving support from SLPs. During the review phase, SLP and parents should review a recorded session together and discuss the effectiveness of the implemented strategies as well as any changes observed from the child.

In conclusion, the naturalistic teaching techniques to be incorporated into early lexical intervention should include (1) using the activities of a child's interest, (2) giving a child the opportunity to communicate, (3) taking advantage of language-rich daily routines, (4) responding positively to a child's attempt to communicate, and (5) encouraging a child to talk in new or different ways (Dunst, Raab, & Trivette, 2012; Dunst, Trivette, & Raab, 2013).

Shared Book Reading and Dialogic Reading

As discussed in Chapter 4, incidental word learning or fast mapping is a primary way for young children to build lexical knowledge through daily routines (e.g., conversation, play, and watching TV). However, the results of several studies show that incidental learning (e.g., only hearing the new words) has limited to no effect on learning new words (Ard & Beverly, 2004; Blewitt et al., 2009; Coyne et al., 2007). Through incidental learning only, kindergarteners who are at risk of reading difficulties were found to develop limited lexical knowledge (Justice et al., 2005). This is because extended mapping (a.k.a. slow mapping) is also required for developing precise lexical knowledge and flexibility to use words in diverse contexts. Thus, book reading provides a rich context for extended mapping. Studies have shown that young children learn new words through either self-reading or being read to, and book reading is effective in teaching vocabulary to both preschool and young school-age children (Pollard-Durodola et al., 2016; Silverman, 2007; Silverman & Crandell, 2010). In this subsection, we will review two instructional approaches that promote lexical acquisition, including shared book reading and dialogic reading.

Shared Book Reading

Shared book reading (SBR) is one of the natural approaches for younger children to acquire new words. It is an interactive book reading method in that both adults and children actively engagein book reading through discussing pictures, words, events, and characters in the book (Pollard-Durodola et al., 2016). SBR also provides a rich context for children to learn Tier Two words and decontextualized language. It not only bridges oral and written language naturally but also paves the way for young children to develop print awareness, learn sight words, acquire background knowledge, know phonological and orthographic features of the words, and gain knowledge of genre-specific rules (e.g., story grammar for narratives).

As discussed before, children with DLD tend to learn new words more slowly and have difficulty making associations among words. These children need more than twice as many trials as their TD peers to understand and use a new word (Gray, 2003). Thus, implementing SBR along with embedded and elaborated instruction is warranted.

SBR with Embedded and Extended Instruction. The following steps are suggested to SLPs when implementing SBR as a context to introduce new words (modified, based on Kaderavek and Justice's suggestions in 2002).

1. **Book Selection**
   - Selecting an appropriate book for SBR is based on the child's present level. Start with short stories and gradually increase the length and complexity based on the child's progress.
   - For preschool children, SLPs can consider starting with interactive picture books, such as lift-the-flap books or sound books.
   - Give the child 2 to 3 books to choose from.
2. **Target Word Selection**
   - Select words that the child does not know and appear several times throughout the book.
   - The number of target words should depend on the child's present level. SLPs can start with few words (e.g., three to five targets) and then gradually increase the number.
3. **Teach One New Concept at a Time**
   - If teaching new words is the focus of a session, leave other treatment objectives/goals (morphemes or sentence structure) to the next session. Children with DLD need more time to learn and consolidate information; thus, including several treatment objectives/goals in one session may compromise learning.
   - SLPs could continue to model the correct language use for other treatment objectives by manipulating intonation without explicit teaching. For example, highlight the plural in the sentence "The mouse has

TWO cookIES" or highlight the third person singular and subject-verb agreement in the same sentence "The mouse HAS two cookies."

4. **Active Participation**
   - During SBR, SLP and the child can take turns flipping the pages. Allow the child to have some control of the book.
   - Make sure to spend ample time on each page to talk about the story, discuss the target words and pictures, and add explanation and elaboration.

5. **Provide Ample Time for Information Processing**
   - Due to slow information processing speed, it is important to give the child extra time to process and reflect on information.
   - Ask the child what the target word means, explain it, and encourage the child to use the word/sentence naturally through open-ended questions to avoid merely repetition.

6. **Asking Questions and Making Comments**
   - During SBR, SLPs should make comments about the pictures and characters and ask questions to verify the child's comprehension accordingly. Ard and Beverly (2004) indicated that commenting during the book reading is more effective than asking questions only.
   - Asking too many questions may overwhelm the child.
   - Make sure to start with low-demand/literal questions (e.g., who, what, where) and gradually introduce high-demand/inferential questions (e.g., how, why, what/how do you think?) depending on the child's response (Kleeck et al., 2006). Blewitt et al. (2009) reported that asking questions, from easy to difficult ones, during book reading is beneficial to word learning.
   - Beck and McKeown (2001) also suggested that giving students time to reflect on story content is more important than getting the correct answers.

7. **Keep SBR Interactive and Fun**
   - Keep book reading activity fun, natural, and interactive rather than just for teaching targets. Make sure the reading book activity is not a daunting and intimidating task to the child.

■ Follow the child's lead and modify comments/questions based on the child's response.

8. **Use Follow-Up Activities to Review the Target Words**

■ Use the story context to support the child's explanation of word meaning.

■ Depending on the child's present level, follow-up activities can incorporate definitional information (e.g., synonyms, antonyms) and encourage the child to retell the story after reading the book several times.

■ A book used several times in SBR can always be brought back later for different purposes such as working on narrative skills (e.g., story retell, story generation) and word recognition since the child is familiar with the story.

■ Knowing the story plot can free up the cognitive resources for the child to focus on learning new words.

Supporting Evidence for SBS. The effectiveness of SBR with embedded and extended instruction has been supported by abundant research (Ard & Beverly, 2004; Blewitt et al., 2009; Coyne et al., 2007; Pollard-Durodola et al., 2016). Several studies have shown that conducting SBS in an interactive and extended way can be effective for TD children to learn new words, such as making comments, asking questions, adding explanation and elaboration, and asking children to explain their own definitions (Cain, 2007; Coyne, McCoach, & Kapp, 2007). Biemiller and Boote (2006) also found that combining repetitive book reading and explanations of words significantly help young school-age students gain word meaning. Additionally, at-risk kindergarteners made significant gains when adults elaborated on word meanings during book rearing (Justice et al., 2005).

It should be noted that children with DLD may still need additional support for consolidating word knowledge. Based on the study of Coyne et al. (2007), adding simple definitions of words during book reading only resulted in partial word learning. This is due to their limitation in processing semantic and phonological information and fragile semantic representations (Alt & Plante, 2006; McGregor et al., 2002). Therefore, SLPs are encouraged to explain the target words explicitly and promote a deeper level of understanding by using extended interactive activities. Increasing exposures of new words and making semantic information explicit for children could promote word learning (Nash & Donaldson, 2005).

Silverman (2007) suggested that actively engaging young school-age children in the analysis of word meanings through SBR was more effective than merely relating words to story context or personal experience. Young school-age children tend to focus on pictures and use their background knowledge to understand text instead of using text information (Beck & McKeown, 2001). Thus, directing their attention to phonological and orthographic features of words is beneficial for learning new words and concepts.

The effect of book reading on word learning was not only found in narrative text but also informational text. Leung (2008) reported that children who immediately retold the story after book reading can provide a better explanation of word meanings of target words. Therefore, they supported the effectiveness of book retelling on learning new words and complex concepts even for informational text. A similar finding was also reported by Pollard-Durodola et al. (2016). The effects of incorporating informational text in an intensive SBR program was also found in preschool children. They stated that explicit and thematic intervention combined with multiple exposures can increase a child's ability to make word associations and define new words. Pollard-Durodola et al. (2016) recommended that opportunities should be provided to children for talking about words, concepts, and life that are related to the book.

In summary, SBR is an evidence-based, effective, and powerful approach for TD children and children with DLD to learn new words. Effective SBR intervention should include active discussion using open-ended questions, elaboration and explanation, offering multiple exposures of target words, and interactive talk before, during, and after book reading (Pollard-Durodola et al., 2016).

Dialogic Reading

Dialogic reading (DR) refers to an adult and a child having a dialogue around the book that they are reading, and DR and SBR share similar techniques and procedures to promote language development through book-reading activities. DR is more frequently implemented by teachers while SLPs utilize SBR techniques more commonly. DR requires adults using prompts, feedback, and scaffolding to facilitate a child's lexical development (Whitehurst et al., 1988). DR follows more established procedures and uses more structured techniques than SBR. We will overview these techniques below and highlight the principles of dialogic reading. PEER is the acronym for the fundamental principles of dialogic reading, including (1) **prompt** the child to say something about the book, (2) **evaluate** the child's response, (3) **expand** the child's response and (4) **repeat** prompts to ensure the child's learning.

Dialogic reading can be achieved at two levels. In Level I, the focus is to introduce new vocabulary to the child, and the following steps should be implemented during book reading activities (Flynn, 2011, p. 10; Zevenbergen & Whitehurst, 2003, p. 171).

1. Ask simple "What" questions about the story, e.g., "What is this?" "What do you call this?"
2. Follow the child's remark with questions related to the object's attributes and function, e.g., "What color is it?" "What do you do with it?"
3. Repeat what the child says to reinforce the child's verbalization.
4. Help the child as needed through modeling.
5. Praise and encourage the child's attempt to talk about the book.
6. Follow the child's interests and encourage the child to talk more about a part of the story or a picture in the book.
7. Ensure that book reading is fun for the child. Continue the book reading activity when the child shows interest and end the activity when the child shows boredom.

Once the child is able to successfully label a minimum of 75% of the new words in a book, adults can proceed to Level II. The steps of Level II include (1) asking open-ended questions to prompt a more elaborative response. For example, adults can ask, "What do you see on this page?" "Tell me more," (2) expanding the child's remark by adding one to two words to the child's response. For example, when the child says, "car go," adults can say "The car goes fast!" (3) having the child repeat the expanded phrase. For example, ask the child "Can you say it by yourself ?" (4) promoting generalization of newly learned words. For example, when the child is able to use the newly learned words in expanded sentences, adults can encourage the child to relate the story to their personal experiences through conversation, such as asking "Have you ever been to ___?" "Have you ever seen ___?" to prompt the child to talk about related experiences (Flynn, 2011, p. 10).

Five types of prompts can be used in dialogic reading, including (Zevenbergen & Whitehurst, 2003, p. 173).

1. **Completion Prompts:** Adults ask fill-in-the-blank questions. Using the book "If You Give a Mouse a Cookie" as an example, a fill-in-the-blank question can be "What did the mouse draw with?" "The mouse drew with ___."
2. **Recall Prompts:** Adults ask questions about the book that the child just read. For example, "What was the mouse eating?" "What did he need with his cookie?"
3. **Open-Ended Prompts:** Adults ask the child about the pictures in the book. For example, "What is happening in this picture?"
4. **Wh-Prompts:** Adults ask various Wh questions and How questions to talk about pictures in the book and teach new words. For example, "Where is the mouse?" "Good, he is in the bathroom. Tell me what you see in the bathroom."
5. **Distancing Prompts:** Adults ask the child to relate the pictures and new words to something beyond the book. Through distancing prompts, children can connect their personal experiences and books to promote the generalization of newly learned knowledge and words. For example, adults can encourage the child to talk about their experience of having a pet hamster, such as "What does your hamster like to eat or drink?" "What do you do to keep you hamster clean?" "What does your hamster like to do?"

SBR and DR are both effective approaches to facilitate vocabulary development, but SLPs should keep in mind that dialogic reading was developed for TD children. Vocabulary instruction designed for TD children may not be suitable for children with learning difficulties. Thus, the protocols and procedures of DR must be modified for children with DLD or other special needs, such as difficulty in learning vocabulary. For example, SLPs may need to select fewer target words based on the child's present level and word knowledge and provide more prompts and support depends on the child's response.

Visual/Graphic Organizers

According to Leonard (1998), words are organized and stored based on associated phonological, morphological, and semantic information (cited in Zens, Gillon, & Moran, 2009). Therefore, learning new words in a systematic way (e.g., based on their features, categories, and associations) may facilitate word storage and promote word retrieval. Visual (or graphic) organizers can visually display the connections between concepts (or words) and promote learning words in a more systematic fashion. Additionally, visual organizers are an effective instructional tool because they reduce processing demands by making the concepts clear and less complicated.

The main purpose of visual organizers is to highlight the relationship between concepts while supporting a student's knowledge growth and retention (Baxendell, 2003; Nichols & Ruply, 2004; Shoari & Farrokhi, 2014; Taylor et al., 2009). Studies show that using visual organizers is more effective than traditional vocabulary instruction (e.g., using dictionary and providing definitions, offering context clues) when teaching English language learners (Al-Hinnawi, 2012; Shoari & Farrokhi, 2014). Jitendra et al. (2004) supported the effectiveness of utilizing categorizing methods to organize related words and concepts based on the similarities and differences. When implementing visual organizers, SLPs should collaborate with school teachers because the ultimate goal is for students to use visual organizers for different purposes independently.

Baxendell (2003) stated that visual organizers are not effective if these are not clear or straightforward to the learners. Thus, three elements/principles are recommended for developing and implementing visual organizers effectively (p. 47).

1. Consistent: Establish a routine and use a standard set of visual organizers across content areas and tasks.
2. Coherent: Provide clear labels for the relationship between concepts in visual organizers. Limit the number of covered concepts to minimize distractions.
3. Creative: Create visual organizers for different purposes (e.g., learn new words, develop in-depth word knowledge), tasks (e.g., writing, story retell, vocabulary instruction), stages (e.g., before, during, after reading), and formats (e.g., group or individual).

Different Types of Visual Organizers

Visual organizers can have different forms and names can be used across content areas and purposes (e.g., reading, writing, learning new concepts). Steele and Mills (2011) recommended four visual organizations for vocabulary interventions, including semantic map, semantic feature analysis table, four square, and Venn diagram.

The concept of using **semantic maps** and **semantic feature analysis tables** is similar. Both types of visual organizers emphasize semantic relatedness and associations of words and concepts. During the extension activities, clinicians can implement systematic word review by explicitly emphasizing semantic features of target words and semantic associations between the target words and words known by the children. Figure 8–1 is an example of a **semantic map** adapted from Steele and Mills (2011, p. 365). Three other examples of semantic maps are in Chapter 4. Table 8–1 is an example of a **semantic feature analysis table** adapted from Steele and Mills (2011, p. 365). More elaborated discussion on semantic feature analysis is in Chapter 4.

In the study of Zipoli et al. (2011), the results showed that systematically reviewing words and emphasizing semantic relatedness (e.g., synonyms, functions, superordinates, attributes) can facilitate word learning in children who are at risk for language and literacy difficulties. Their 18-week vocabulary

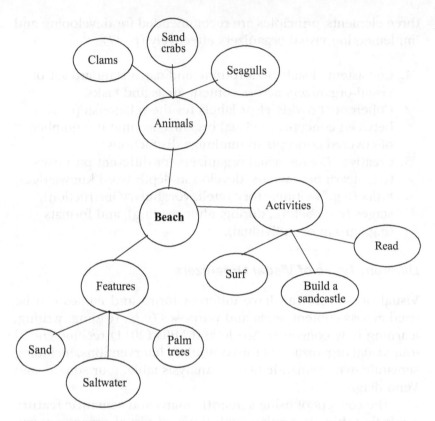

Figure 8–1. Semantic mapping using "beach" as an example.
Source: Adapted from Steele and Mills (2011, p. 365).

Table 8–1. Example of Semantic Feature Analysis

	Lives in ocean	Lives in sand	Has fins or flippers	Can fly	Has claws
Seagulls				+	
Sharks	+		+		
Crabs	+				+
Sea Lions	+		+		
Sand Crabs		+			+

Source: Adapted from Steele and Mills (2011, p. 365).

program targeting word knowledge systematically may facilitate word knowledge development by stimulating word consciousness (awareness and interest in words and word meanings). They concluded that emphasizing semantic features and word associations can deepen and consolidate word knowledge.

Another type of visual organizers is called "**four square**" which was proposed by Stahl and Nagy (2006). The steps of developing and using this organizer are listed below.

1. Fold a piece of paper twice to create four sections.
2. SLPs write the target word in the upper left section and verbally provide the definition of the word without writing it down. Make sure the child understands the meaning of the word.
3. Ask the child to provide three examples that are related to the target word and write them down in the upper right section. Review and discuss the related examples with the child.
4. Ask the child to provide three examples that are not related to the target word and write them down in the lower right section. Review and discuss the non-related examples with the child.
5. Lastly, ask the child using their own words to define the target word and write it down in the lower-left corner. Table 8–2 is a four square example adapted from Steele and Mills (2011, p. 365).

Venn diagrams are another type of visual organizer and can be used for comparing and discussing the similarities and differences between two (or more) words/concepts. Stahl and Nagy (2006) suggested using Venn diagrams to sort/categorize words. For example, SLPs can identify two categories (e.g., sea animal versus land animal, tools versus furniture, fruits versus vegetables) and ask the child to sort pictures or words based on its semantic categories. Through this sorting and categorizing process, children can develop more precise word knowledge and semantic representations that they may only have partial knowledge. For example, a child may only know that both seals and sea lions are sea animals, but does not know the similarities and differences between the two. Figure 8–2 is an example of a Venn diagram adapted from Stahl and Nagy (2006, p. 89). In this example, children are asked to compare the similarities and differences between sneakers and high heels.

All the visual organizers discussed above can be used in either individual or group sessions and can be modified for

Table 8–2. Example of Four Square

Target Word: **Comfortable**	Three examples that are <u>related to</u> the word • Soft blanket • Bed • Pajamas
Their words to define: "When someone's physical self feels at ease or when external objects help create a state of relaxation."	Three examples that are <u>not related</u> to the word • Concrete • High heels • Insects

Source: Adapted from Steele and Mills (2011, p. 365).

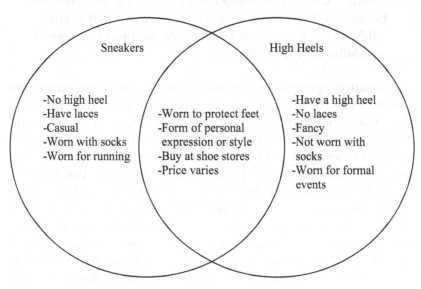

Figure 8–2. Venn diagram using "sneakers" and "high heels" as an example.

using in different content areas. Because there is no standard protocol for the implementation of visual organizers, SLPs can modify or adjust them based on a student's strengths and needs. One recommendation to keep in mind is carefully balancing the number of new words and known words when using visual organizers.

Definitions and Context Clues

Utilizing definitional and contextual information can be useful for learning words. The use of dictionary (definitional information) and contextual clues is one of traditional word instruction strategies that has been commonly implemented. However, several limitations have been reported regarding the use of dictionary and contextual clues. First, active participation is needed for successful word learning, but using dictionary and context clues can be passive. Secondly, using a dictionary successfully requires multiple skills, such as using guidewords and finding the correct definition. Thirdly, using context clues can also be challenging because a student has to integrate different types of information to infer the word meaning (Bryant et al., 2003), and the student may not be able to use contextual clues to derive precise word meanings (Graves, 2006). Lastly, context clues may be misleading or add confusion if the clues are not used effectively (Stahl & Nagy, 2006). Because of these limitations, it is important to provide clear instructions and training to students on how and when to use definitional and contextual information effectively.

When training students using **definitional information**, it is recommended to incorporate student-friendly definitions instead of using the information directly from a dictionary or asking the student to look up the definition independently (Steele & Mills, 2011). It is important to discuss the words that are related to the target word to facilitate lexical learning. Thus, clinicians can incorporate synonyms, antonyms, examples from the student's personal experiences or school content, and non-examples that contain words similar to the target word but have different use in context (Stahl & Nagy, 2006). For example, for the target word "skeptical," SLPs can ask the child to think of a synonym (e.g., doubt) and antonym (e.g., confident, convinced) and then have the child share a personal example (e.g., feel skeptical when watching a magic show) along with a non-example (pessimistic about a situation but does not necessarily feel skeptical). Subsequently, the clinician and the child engage in discussion about the similarities and differences between the target word (skeptical) and its related words (e.g., unsure, suspicious, iffy, disbelieve) to enrich and deepen lexical knowledge. Additionally, clinicians should consider keeping the definition broad enough to cover shades of word meanings and then presenting the words in different contexts for discussion (McKeown, 2019).

When training students using **context clues**, the following steps are suggested: (1) Pause when you find an unknown word. (2) Read the surrounding words and sentences to look for context clues. (3) Use the clues to infer the meaning of the unknown word. (4) Test your inference to see if it makes sense (Graves, Schneider, and Ringstaff, 2017). Nash and Snowling (2006) showed that children with poor vocabulary knowledge can benefit from using context clues when this method is explicitly taught.

Additional considerations for SLPs are listed below when training students using definitional information and context clues.

1. **Curriculum-based intervention.** SLPs should consider incorporating materials from content areas for training. However, it is important to keep in mind that the goal of speech and language services is to help the students develop and implement effective strategies.
2. **Use broad definitions.** When explaining the word meaning to the student, SLPs should use broad definitions rather than narrow definitions for capturing the shades of meaning. This can help children go beyond the specific context in which the target word appears. Students can understand the word meaning may change depending on the context.
3. **Active participation.** Encourage students to use their own words to explain the meaning of the target word. It should be noted that SLPs need to consider the student's present level since giving a definition is a metalinguistic skill.

4. **Connect to prior knowledge.** Activate students' prior knowledge and help them make a connection between what they have learned and what they are learning.
5. **Think aloud.** SLPs can verbally explain their own thought process when using context clues to infer the meaning of the target word. This is a powerful method to train students on how to infer word meaning by explicitly explaining our own problem-solving process.
6. **Encourage self-reflection.** Closely monitor the student's progress by engaging in active discussion and encouraging the student to reflect on their own learning. For example, asking the student some questions after practice, such as what type of context clue is effective or ineffective? Why? What other strategies can I use to infer the meaning? What makes a word inferring process successful or unsuccessful?

In conclusion, it is important to promote children's active engagement in learning the use of definitional and contextual information. Interactive and direct teaching is most beneficial for facilitating vocabulary development (Bryant et al., 2003). Additionally, it is important to keep in mind that children with language disorders have limitations in information processing speed and capacity, so SLPs should keep the number of new words manageable for these children. Lastly, it is also helpful to give them exposure to new words multiple times in various contexts to promote generalization.

Emphasize Both Semantic and Phonological Features

Semantic-based and phonological-based interventions are the two main types of vocabulary interventions. The main goal of semantic-based vocabulary intervention is to improve semantic awareness of words. Semantic vocabulary intervention focuses on word meanings and strengthens the relationship among words via discussing word function, location, attribute, and category (Lowe et al., 2018). In therapy, SLPs can ask children to identify and distinguish different semantic features. For example, SLPs can pose stimulus questions to elicit responses, such as "What do you do with ____?" "Where can you find ____?" "What parts does ____ have?" "What does ___ look like?" Semantic vocabulary therapy can help children develop semantic representations and deepen word knowledge by differentiating between words that have similar properties. On the other hand, phonological-based vocabulary intervention focuses on developing the awareness of phonemes and syllables at the word level (Lowe et al., 2018). In therapy, children are trained to identify and distinguish different phonological features. For example, SLPs can pose stimulus questions to elicit responses, such as "What does ____ sound like?" "How many syllables?" "Can you say a word that rhymes with ____ ?" "What sound does it begin with?" Phonological-based vocabulary therapy can help children develop phonological representations.

Incorporating both semantic and phonological features in vocabulary intervention can be more beneficial to children with language disorders than using either one alone because these children tend to have weak semantic and phonological representations. Research studies also support the effectiveness of a curriculum approach that **combines semantic and phonological methods** (Parsons et al., 2005; St. John & Vance, 2014). In Parsons et al.'s study, two elementary schoolers with DLD engaged in various word learning activities, such as playing games to enrich their semantic knowledge of new words. Then, the newly learned words were written in a notebook called "word bank book." The two children were asked to list two semantic features and one phonological feature for each word. The results showed that the combined approach was effective for both children with DLD.

St. John and Vance (2014) examined the effects of a daily word-learning program in kindergartners who have poor language skills. Their program includes both semantic-based and phonological-based activities at different learning phases, such as developing attribute webs and multiple-meaning trees. Figure 8–3 is the daily word-learning program used in St. John and Vance's study (2014). The instructor also used clarifying cue cards listed in Figure 8–4 for clarification purposes. Their findings support the positive effect of a vocabulary program that combined semantic and phonological methods.

Wright et al. (2018) also investigated the effects of the combined semantic and phonological approach on children with

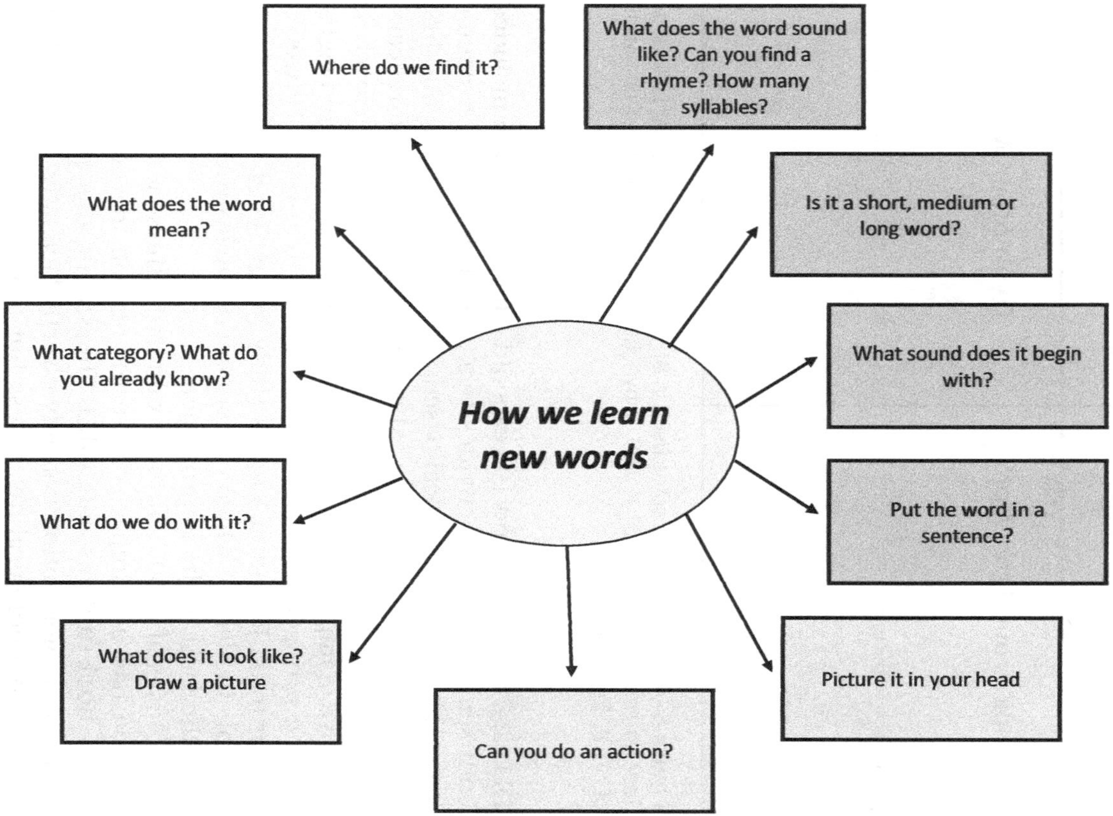
How we learn new words
Where do we find it?
What does the word sound like? Can you find a rhyme? How many syllables?
What does the word mean?
Is it a short, medium or long word?
What category? What do you already know?
What sound does it begin with?
What do we do with it?
Put the word in a sentence?
What does it look like? Draw a picture
Can you do an action?
Picture it in your head

Figure 8–3. The daily word learning program used in St. John and Vance, *Child Language Teaching and Therapy, 30*(3), p. 260, copyright © 2014. Adapted by Permission of SAGE Publications, Ltd.

Recall Your Memory?	**Study the Structure**
• Have you seen this word before? • Do you remember what it means?	• What sound does the word start with? • Is it a long or short word?
Look Around the Word	**Try Another Word**
• How is the word used? • Consider the context	• Can you think of another similar word? • Is there another word you could use instead?

Figure 8–4. Clarifying cue cards used in St. John and Vance, *Child Language Teaching and Therapy, 30*(3), p. 260, copyright © 2014. Adapted by Permission of SAGE Publications, Ltd.

DLD age between 7 and 19 years old. The intervention included both semantic-based activities (e.g., word definition, semantic features) and phonological-based activities (e.g., spelling, first sound) along with multiple exposures, repetitions, and rehearsals. They found that the combined intervention approach is effective in improving word knowledge of both nouns and verbs, but the stronger effect is found on nouns than verbs. However, similar to St. John and Vance's study, Wright et al. (2018) were not able to identify which component of the instruction contributed the most to the improvement.

Zens et al. (2009) further examined if the sequence of intervention had any impact on treatment gain in young elementary school students with DLD. They found that phonological awareness intervention not only directly facilitates the development of phonological awareness but also indirectly promotes semantic learning. When phonological awareness intervention is provided first followed by semantic intervention, children may use processing capacities more efficiently to learn other information about the new words. Therefore, they suggested that children may make greater gain when implementing phonological awareness intervention before the semantic-based intervention. Another study was conducted by Lowe et al. in 2018 to investigate the effect of a vocabulary intervention program on adolescents with language disorders. Their treatment program was called Word Discovery, and it aimed to make phonological and semantic information explicit and highlight the association between the two. Their results showed that the efficacy of the semantic-only or phonological-only intervention is either limited or inconclusive. However, the phonological-semantic combined intervention offers much stronger efficacy data to support its clinical use. Because the Word Discovery program emphasizes both phonological and semantic information, it is beneficial to students with weakness in either phonological representations or semantic representations. Therefore, a structured program that includes deliberate verbal repetition, visual support, and orthographic input is effective for students with language disorders to develop word knowledge.

In summary, a phonological-semantic combined intervention can strengthen both semantic and phonological representations of the words. However, it is important to keep in mind that an individualized intervention approach may be needed for children with WFD who have adequate semantic representations but only struggle with phonological representations (e.g., not being able to retrieve phonological forms). We will discuss the intervention options and efficacy studies that focus on this population in the next section "Intervention Suggestions for Children with WFD."

Analyze Word Parts/Increase Morphological Awareness

Analyzing word parts is a commonly implemented vocabulary instruction approach for mainstream students. Helping students understand the patterns of words is beneficial and can facilitate lexical development (McKeown, 2019). However, it should be noted that analyzing word parts is more appropriate for students in upper elementary level and beyond. This is because analyzing word parts/morphological awareness is a metalinguistic skill which requires students to think analytically beyond word meaning.

Many words in the English are made up of word parts, including prefixes, roots, and suffixes. Understanding the process of how the word parts are added together can help students determine the meaning of the word as a whole. A typical word parts lesson may include the following steps (Baumann et al., 2003; Graves et al., 2017).

1. **Identify Word Parts.** Have the student determine if a new, unknown word can be broken into smaller word parts and try to identify these word parts. Then, have the student use different colors to mark prefixes, roots, and suffixes. Kirby and Bowers (2012) also recommend the use of word sums and word matrices by asking students to construct a matrix based on the roots. Figure 8–5 is an example based on Kirby and Bowers's article (2012, p. 2).
2. **Understand the Meanings of Each Part.** Discuss the meaning of each part with the student, including the meaning of prefix, root word, and suffix.
3. **Derive Word Meaning.** Have the student combine the word parts to derive and infer the meaning of this unknown word.
4. **Evaluation.** Try to put the word back into the context and have the student evaluate if the inferred meaning makes sense. It is essential to teach students to be aware of possible variations and to be flexible during the meaning solving-process (McKeown, 2019).

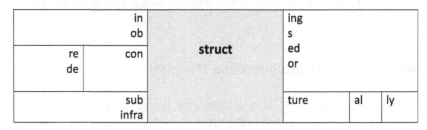

Figure 8–5. Word sums and word matrices using the root "struct" (Kirby & Bowers, 2012, p. 2).

Gibson and Wolter (2015) recommended two activities for word part analysis, including word sorting and word building tasks. In a **word sorting** task, SLPs can ask the student to group words together based on their structures and then discuss similarities and differences in word function, meaning, sound, and spelling. For example, in a word sorting task for developing derivations, SLP can have students group words based on their inflectional morphemes (e.g., plural -s, third-person singular -s, possessive 's). Then, SLPs can discuss the different changes related to these derivations, such as no change, spelling change, sound change, or change in both spelling and sound. More specifically, SLPs can have the student group words with plural -s together and discuss how spelling and sound change because of adding plural -s and how words ending with plural -s are different from words ending with third-person singular -s.

The other activity is a **word building** task. Three groups of word parts (i.e., prefixes, roots, and suffixes) are provided to the student. SLPs encourage the student to create as many words as possible; words can be both real and pseudo words. This is a process allowing the student to use word parts to construct new words. Then, SLPs implement a "think aloud" approach to model a word-building process and encourage the student to talk about word meaning and their own thought process. Lastly, SLPs can end this task by having the student create sentences using the newly created words. During the word building process, visual aids (e.g., blocks representing different word parts), flipbooks/flip charts, and graphic organizers should be used to make the process explicit and fun.

When teaching word parts to students, it is recommended to follow a sequence (Graves & Sales, 2013; Graves et al., 2017). It is essential to keep in mind that children with language deficits continue to struggle with inflectional morphemes (Wolter & Green, 2013). Thus, the recommended sequence starts by analyzing compound words (e.g., cowboy, sunflower) and inflections (e.g., plural -s, regular past tense -ed, third person singular), then moving to identifying derivational prefixes and suffixes (e.g., un-, in-, re, pre-, -able, -ive, -ment), and finally Latin and Greek roots (e.g., auto, micro, pho, bio, aud, port, mar, acid). Analyzing Latin roots can be more challenging because of the lack of consistency and transparency phonologically and orthographically

(McKeown, 2019). Lastly, SLPs can encourage students to find morphologically complex words from class materials. Students can compile these words in a notebook and add word parts (prefixes, roots, suffixes) as they encounter them.

A Mixed Vocabulary Intervention Program

Word learning is a multifaceted process that requires various linguistic information and cognitive functions to support the learning process. Thus, SLPs can consider combining several approaches when facilitating vocabulary development in children with language disorders. Murphy and colleagues (2017) examined the effects of a vocabulary enrichment program in a group of adolescents from socioeconomic disadvantaged backgrounds. This program consists of sessions that teach students using a wide variety of learning strategies, such as parts of speech, word part analysis, word map, semantic and phonological features, use of a dictionary, and definitional information. Their findings support the effects of implementing a mixed vocabulary program that combines different strategies on word learning.

Intervention Suggestions for Children with WFD

As discussed above, the intervention approaches for word finding difficulty (WFD) can be divided into two major categories: semantic-based and phonological-based intervention. German et al. (2012) recommended that a tailored intervention is needed for children with WFD because their retrieval breakdowns can be the result of different types of lexical processing difficulty. In other words, children with WFD know what word they intend to say but cannot access correct phonological forms due to either weak semantic-lexical-phonological or blockage during activation spreading (German, 2009).

Phonological-Based Lexical Intervention

The phonological-based lexical approach aims to enhance the phonological representations of the words through phonological awareness activities and phonemic cues. The underlying theoretical rationale is that WFD result from the "inadequate or underspecified" phonological representations despite these children having adequate semantic representations (Bragard et al., 2012). McGregor (1994) reported the effects of the phonological-based intervention on two children with WFD. Children were first asked to produce the first sound of the object and then determine the number of syllables of the target words. McGregor (1994) stated that enhancing phonological representations not only makes the activation of the target word easier but also reduces the competition strength of the competing words. Therefore, phonological awareness activities, such as rhyming and alliteration, may help children differentiate similar sounding words, which further enhance the access to phonological forms. Best (2005) also supported the effects of the phonological-based intervention on five children who struggled with word finding. The study results show that children with WFD have difficulty in storing phonological information and accessing phonological forms for production. Therefore, using phonemic cues (e.g., the first sound) would make the target word more salient than other competing words. Best (2005) explained that this bottom-up approach can strengthen the lexical-phonological connection and also enhance the link between the conceptual structure and lemma.

German (2002) also supported the effects of using phonological-based intervention to improve word retrieval abilities based on her report of two 8-years-old children with WFD. German's intervention involved three steps. First, the children worked on syllable segmenting tasks as a metalinguistic reinforcement activity and then used the word or cues given by the clinician to think of phonemic neighbors that share sound parts with the target word, such as bent to vent, flip to flipper, goat to oat. The final step is a rehearsal task requiring the children to verbalize the target word at word and sentence level. German (2002) reported the reduction of naming errors on treated words, the generalization of word retrieval at the sentence level, maintenance of treatment gains, and increasing the children's confidence in word retrieval after the phonological-based intervention. Therefore, similar to Best's claim (2005), German suggested that the breakdown of word retrieval may happen at the connection between lemma and lexeme connection or the lexeme selection level because these children have difficulty accessing the phonological form of the target word.

Semantic-Based Lexical Intervention

The semantic-based lexical approach aims to addresse inadequate semantic representations through strengthening the connection between the conceptual structure and lemma. It also intends to specify and consolidate the target word by enhancing its semantic network development (e.g., the knowledge of antonym and synonym) (Bragard et al., 2012). According to McGregor et al. (2002), semantic errors may result from fragile semantic representations, lexical gaps due to lack of storage of the word, and difficulty accessing phonological forms. Ebbels and colleagues (2012) conducted a randomized control trial study to examine a semantic-based lexical intervention in 15 children with language impairments and WFD between age 9 to 15 years old. During the intervention, they asked children to sort pictures based on their semantic categories, discuss semantic attributes, and use attributes and categories as cues in word games. They reported significant improvement in word-finding abilities after only four hours of semantic-based intervention. Additionally, the improvement was generalized to untrained words and was maintained over five months after the intervention. Therefore, they recommended that enriching semantic representations through discussing attributes could help distinguish between the target word and competing neighbors, which in turn can facilitate word retrieval (Ebbels et al., 2012).

Combined Phonological and Semantic-Based Intervention

Easton and colleagues (1997) examined the combined approach on four 10-year-old children with specific language impairment (SLI) and WFD. Children were trained to use semantic and phonemic elaboration strategies. During semantic elaboration sessions, children were required to think of the category that the target word belong to, its synonym, and function. During phonemic elaboration sessions, children were asked to identify the onset phoneme or cluster, think of a rhyming word, and then count the number of syllables. Easton et al. (1997) reported that this combined approach was effective for children who experience word learning and word-finding difficulties, and the improvement was maintained at least nine weeks after the intervention. German et al. (2012) also recommended a combination of teaching semantic and phonological features of words to improve word-finding ability. Teaching both word meanings and word forms through metalinguistic activities and rehearsal can improve children's word retrieval ability. Along the same line, Bragard et al. (2012) supported the use of combined intervention, and their findings showed that three out of four children had fewer speech errors after the intervention and were able to maintain the trained words six months after the intervention. Additionally, all children in their study showed improvement on giving definitions of words and giving attributes associated with the target words. Bragard et al. (2012) reminded SLPs not to assume the cause of WFD based on the naming errors and the importance of tailoring intervention based on a child's response to intervention. Also, it is important for clinicians not to make clinical decisions based solely on word-finding characteristics and "surface-level errors" since these children may benefit from both phonological-based and semantic-based intervention. More recently, Best and colleagues (2018) conducted a randomized control trial to examine the effects of a word-finding program. They encouraged children with WFD to generate semantic or phonological features of the target word and then asked children to use attributes to aid their word finding during barrier games. The findings revealed that children in the intervention group named more than four times as many treated words than the control group. They reported that repeated exposure through practice not only makes the target words more fine-grained and specified but also reduces the activation of competing words.

Discourse-Based Intervention for WFD

The literature on the effects of a discourse-based intervention targeting WFD in children is sparse. Stiegler and Hoffman (2001) developed a discourse-based treatment program to address the word-finding characteristics identified in their study. For example, when there was a naming delay longer than 30 seconds, the clinician encouraged the child to use circumlocution to facilitate word retrieval processes. Questions like "Can you describe it?" "Can you talk a little more about it?" can be used. Another example is how to respond when the child uses substitution. SLPs prompted the child that the response was not precise enough and asked the child to think of other words. Questions such as "What do you mean by "bird"?" when the child used "bird" instead of "ostrich." These strategies are intended to help these children recognize a WFD moment, being aware of a communication breakdown, and go through the word-finding process with the clinician's immediate and appropriate feedback without creating frustration and anxiety. Clinicians can consider using the following techniques in Stiegler and Hoffman's study (2001) during a client's discourse production (pp. 290–291).

1. Request more information (e.g., Can you describe it for me?).
2. Ask for clarification (e.g., What do you mean?).
3. Provide confirmation (e.g., I see).
4. Give the child the first phoneme of the target word. If not successful, provide the target word. This should be used as a last resort according to Stiegler and Hoffman (2001).
5. Wait until the child finishes a sentence before providing any feedback. Avoid interrupting the child's sentence production to avoid creating anxiety.

The outcome of this discourse-based intervention was promising since all three children showed fewer word-finding difficulty after treatment. It is noteworthy that different types of discourse may create different cognitive and linguistic demands. For example, picture description is less demanding than story retelling or story generation, and an expository task can be more cognitively and linguistically demanding than a narrative task. Also, children may show more word-finding difficulty when the text is getting longer, and the picture description is getting more complex.

A case study reported by Marks and Stokes (2010) took a different approach to address WFD in a narrative-based intervention in an 8-year-old boy. They measured naming accuracy and word-finding characteristics at both word and sentence levels before and after eight, one-hour therapy across three weeks. Different from Stiegler and Hoffman's study (2001), they created stories and sentences around the target words to elaborate on word meanings. The child was asked to retell the story, imitate sentences containing the target words, and generate his own stories using 3 to 4 target words. The naming accuracy improved and was maintained only for treated words after the treatment. Thus, Marks and Stokes (2010) emphasized the importance of incorporating a clear context for word learning, such as providing definitional and contextual information at the sentence level and giving children the opportunity to use target words in discourse.

Considerations for Managing WFD in Children

German and colleagues (2012) suggested that SLPs select target words by starting with common sound sequences (e.g., words with high neighborhood density, such as pat and jet) and gradually move to rare sound sequence (e.g., shovel and jelly). Additionally, target words should be selected from words that children have difficulty with, curriculum, and home and recreation contexts. Most researchers suggested selecting words known to the students based on their interests, daily life, and school needs to promote generalization and maintenance (Best et al., 2018; Bragard et al., 2012; German, 2002).

German (1992) also offered principles for designing a treatment session targeting word-finding ability (pp. 41–46).

1. Enhance a child's word retrieval by teaching retrieval strategies, enriching semantic representations, and strengthening phonological representations.
2. Identify appropriate and effective retrieval strategies for a child based on their linguistic profile and error patterns.
3. Use target words relevant to the child across different contexts.
4. Promote generalization from single word level to discourse (e.g., narrative) by embedding target words in sentences and discourse.

5. Encourage rehearsal of words in isolation, sentence, and discourse. Keep in mind the concept of "use it or lose it." Retrieval can enhance both storage and retrieval strength.
6. Teach self-applicable retrieval strategies and encourage the child using these strategies independently.
7. Create carryover activities to promote generalization and maintenance across settings.
8. Encourage the use of self-monitoring and self-correction by being aware of their own strengths and weaknesses in word production. Support children to identify the situations and contexts that may impede or facilitate word retrieval.

Chapter Summary

Building vocabulary knowledge, both in breadth and depth, is vital for communication and learning. Words are the building blocks for language learning and use. Therefore, promoting vocabulary development is one of the important treatment goals. In this chapter, we review the procedures and efficacy studies of several vocabulary instructions designed for preschool and school-age children (with or without language disorders) as well as for children with word finding difficulty. The strategies we reviewed could be modified to address the special needs in children with language disorders. For example, for children who are at the prelinguistic stage, combining play therapy and SBR can be used for teaching high-frequency words and the words that are important to the child. For children who need to add words to their toolbox, emphasizing the connections among meaning (features), sound, and word is crucial. Explicit teaching (e.g., pointing out, discussion, elaboration) along with repetition and multiple exposures is necessary. It is not uncommon to target many words in one session. However, having too many targets in one session may do more harm than good due to the limitations in information processing capacity and speed in children with language or learning disability. Hence, clinicians should consider keeping the number of targets manageable for the child, providing abundant repetitions and exposures in meaningful contexts, giving the child ample time to process, and encouraging the use of newly learned words.

Incorporating phonological awareness into vocabulary instruction can be beneficial. Also, gradually adding Tier Two words through book reading and utilizing graphic organizers during follow-up activities can facilitate word learning and retention process. For children who function at the lower elementary level, SLPs can introduce word part analysis for compound words and inflections, use graphic organizers, and teach students to use contextual and definitional information to infer word meaning.

For children with WFD, it is essential for SLPs to understand the child's linguistic profile and error patterns to explore what works and what may not work for them. It is important not to structure the therapy based solely on word-finding characteristics. The error patterns may give clinicians some idea about where the breakdown is in the word retrieval process, but it does not mean that a child who makes more semantic errors only benefits from the semantic-based lexical intervention. Another ingredient to facilitate the word learning process is actively retrieving the newly learned words during the learning process. Leonard and colleagues (2019) suggested the incorporation of repetitive word retrieval during the word learning process because asking a child to repetitively retrieve newly learned words during the learning process facilitates word retention. Therefore, clinicians are encouraged to add retrieval opportunities throughout a child's word learning process because these opportunities help children learn. Additionally, word form (phonological representations) takes longer to learn than word meaning. Therefore, it should be noted that a child may not have complete representations of the word meaning and form even though the child seems to know a word (Leonard et al., 2020; Leonard et al., 2019).

In regard to target word selection, Tier Two and academic words should be included as a child grows older. For children who function at the upper elementary level, SLPs should increase the complexity of word parts analysis by adding derivations, using more challenging words (e.g., abstract nouns, mental verbs) in graphic organizers, and encouraging the development of self-evaluation. It is important to keep in mind that an intervention is not effective if clinicians do not modify the strategies based on a student's present level, response, and needs. It i also vital to consider a child's zone of proximal development in order to give the child room for growth without overwhelming them.

Discussion Questions

1. Discuss explicit and implicit teaching methods for facilitating lexical learning in toddlers and children who are at the prelinguistic stage or have limited lexicon.
2. Compare and contrast the advantages and disadvantages of lexical learning strategies for school-age children. Discuss how strategies can be modified for preschool and school-age children who struggle with lexical learning.
3. How do you select words for therapy? What factors do you consider? Are there any changes to your target word selection method after reading this chapter?
4. Explain different strategies to tackle word-finding difficulty. What is the rationale behind each intervention approach?

References

Al-Hinnawi, A. (2012). The effect of the graphic organizer strategy on university students' English vocabulary building. *English Language Teaching, 5*(12), 62–69. https://doi.org/10.5539/elt.v5n12p62

Alt, M., & Plante, E. (2006). Factors that influence lexical and semantic fast mapping of young children with specific language impairment. *Journal of Speech, Language, and Hearing Research, 49*(5), 941–954. https://doi.org/10.1044/1092-4388(2006/068)

Ard, L., & Beverly, B. (2004). Preschool word learning during joint book reading: Effect of adult questions and comments. *Communication Disorders Quarterly, 26*(1), 17–28. https://doi.org/10.1177/1525740 1040260010101

Baumann, J. F., Edwards, E. C., Boland, E. M., Olejnik, S., & Kame'enui, E. J. (2003). Vocabulary tricks: Effects of instruction in morphology and context on fifth-grade students' ability to derive and infer word meanings. *American Educational Research Journal, 40*(2), 447–494. https://doi.org/10.3102/00028312040002447

Baxendell, B. W. (2003). Consistent, coherent, creative: The 3 C's of graphic organizers. *Teaching Exceptional Children, 35*(3), 46–55. https://doi.org/10.1177/004005990303500307

Beck, I. L., & McKeown, M. G., (2001). Text talk: Capturing the benefits of read-aloud experiences for young children. *The Reading Teacher, 55*(1), 10–20.

Beck, I., McKeown, M., & Kucan, L. (2002). *Bringing words to life: Robust vocabulary instruction* (2nd ed.). Guilford Press.

Best, W. (2005). Investigation of a new intervention for children with word-finding problems. *International Journal of Language & Communication Disorders, 40*(3), 279–318. https://doi.org/10.1080/136 82820410001734154

Best, W., Hughes, L., Masterson, J., Thomas, M., Fedor, A., Roncoli, S., . . . Kapikian, A., (2018). Intervention for children with word finding difficulties: A parallel group randomized control trial. *International Journal for Speech-Language Pathology, 20*(7), 708–719. https://doi .org/10.1080/17549507.2017.1348541

Biemiller, A. (2012). Teaching vocabulary in the primary grades: Vocabulary instruction needed. In J. Baumann & E. Kame'enui (Eds.), *Reading vocabulary: Research to practice* (2nd ed.). Guilford Press.

Biemiller, A., & Boote, C. (2006). An effective method for building meaning vocabulary in primary grades. *Journal of Educational Psychology, 98*(1), 44–62. https://doi.org/10.1037/0022-0663.98 .1.44

Blewitt, P., Rump, K. M., Shealy, S. E., & Cook, S. A. (2009). Shared book reading: When and how questions affect young children's word learning. *Journal of Educational Psychology, 101*(2), 294–304. https://doi.org/10.1037/a0013844

Bragard, A., Schelstraete, M., Snyers, P., & James, D. (2012). Word-finding intervention for children with specific language impairment: A multiple single-case study. *Speech, Language and Hearing Services in Schools, 43*(2), 222–234. https://doi.org/10.1044/0161-1461 (2011/10-0090)

Browne, C., Culligan, B., & Phillips, J. (2013). *New general service list.* http://www.newgeneralservicelist.org

Bryant, D. P., Goodwin, M., Bryant, B. R., & Higgins, K. (2003). Vocabulary instruction for students with learning disabilities: A review of the research. *Learning Disability Quarterly, 26*(2), 117–128. https:// doi.org/10.2307/1593594

Cain, K. (2007). Deriving word meanings from context: Does explanation facilitate contextual analysis? *Journal of Research in Reading, 30*(4), 347–359. https://doi.org/10.1111/j.1467-9817.2007.00336.x

Coxhead, A. (2000) A new academic word list. *TESOL Quarterly, 34*(2), 213–238. http://doi.org/10.2307/3587951

Coyne, M. D., McCoach, D. B., & Knapp, S. (2007). Vocabulary intervention for kindergarten students: Comparing extended instruction to embedded instruction and incidental exposure. *Learning Disability Quarterly, 30*(2), 74–88. https://doi.org/10.2307/30035543

Dolch, E. (1948). *Problems in Reading*. Garrard Press.

Dunst, C. J., Raab, M., & Trivette, C. M. (2012). Characteristics of naturalistic language intervention strategies. *Journal of Speech-Language Pathology and Applied Behavior Analysis, 5*(3-4), 8–16. http://citeseerx.ist.psu.edu/viewdoc/download? doi=10.1.1.475.1839&rep=rep1&type=pdf#page=11

Dunst, C., Trivette, C., & Raab, M. (2013). An implementation science framework for conceptualizing and operationalizing fidelity in early childhood intervention studies. *Journal of Early Intervention, 35*(2), 85–101. https://doi.org/10.1177/1053815113502235

Easton, C., Sheach, S., & Easton, S. (1997). Teaching vocabulary to children with word finding difficulties using a combined semantic and phonological approach: An efficacy study. *Child Language Teaching and Therapy*, 13(2), 125–142. https://doi.org/10.1177/026565909701300202

Ebbels, S.H., Nicoll, H., Clark, B., Eachus, B., Gallagher, A.L., Horniman, K. . . . Turner, G. (2012), Effectiveness of semantic therapy for word-finding difficulties in pupils with persistent language impairments: A randomized control trial. *International Journal of Language & Communication Disorders*, 47(1), 35–51. https://doi.org/10.1111/j.1460-6984.2011.00073.x

Fey, M., Warren, S., Brady, N., Finestack, L., Bredin-Oja, S., Fairchild, M., . . . Yoder, P. (2006). Early effects of responsivity education/prelinguistic milieu teaching for children with developmental delays and their parents. *Journal of Speech, Language, and Hearing Research*, 49(3), 526–547. https://doi.org/10.1044/1092-4388(2006/039)

Fisher, D., Ross, D., & Grant, M. (2010). Building background knowledge in physical science. *The Science Teacher*, 77(1), 23–26.

Flynn, K. S. (2011). Developing children's oral language skills through dialogic reading: Guidelines for I\implementation. *TEACHING Exceptional Children*, 44(2), 8–16. https://doi.org/10.1177/004005991104400201

German, D. J. (1992). Word-finding intervention for children and adolescents. *Topics in Language Disorders, 13*(1), 33–50. https://doi.org/10.1097/00011363-199211000-00006

German, D. (2009). Child word finding. *The ASHA Leader, 14*(2). https://doi.org/10.1044/leader.FTR2.14022009.10

German, D. J. (2002). A phonologically based strategy to improve *word finding* abilities in children. *Communication Disorders Quarterly, 23,* 179–192.

German, D. J., Schwanke, J. H., & Ravid, R. (2012). Word finding difficulties: Differentiated vocabulary instruction in the speech and language room. *Communication Disorders Quarterly, 33*(3), 146–156. https://doi.org/10.1177/1525740111405840

Gibson, F., & Wolter, J. (2015). Morphological awareness intervention to improve vocabulary and reading success. *Perspectives on Language Learning and Education, 22*(4), 147–155. https://doi.org/10.1044/lle22.4.147

Graves, M. F. (2006). *The vocabulary book: Learning & instruction.* Teachers College Press.

Graves, M., & Sales, G. (2013). *Teaching 50,000 words: Meeting and exceeding the Common Core State Standards for vocabulary.* International Literacy Association. http://doi.org/10.1598/e-ssentials.8035

Graves, M., Schneider, S., & Ringstaff, C. (2017). Empowering students with word learning strategies: Teach a child to fish. *The Reading Teacher, 71*(5), 533–543. https://doi.org/10.1002/trtr.1644

Gray, S. (2003). Word-learning by preschoolers with specific language impairment: What predicts success? *Journal of Speech, Language, and Hearing Research, 46*(1), 56–67. https://doi.org/10.1044/1092-4388(2003/005)

Hancock, T. B., & Kaiser, A. P. (2002). The effects of trainer-implemented enhanced milieu teaching on the social communication of children with autism. *Topics in Early Childhood Special Education, 22*(1), 39–54. https://doi.org/10.1177/027112140202200104

Hancock, T. B., & Kaiser, A. P. (2006). Enhanced milieu teaching. In R. McCauley & M. Fey (Eds.), *Treatment of language disorders in children* (pp. 203–236). Paul H. Brookes.

Jitendra, A., Edwards, L., Sacks, G., & Jacobson, L. (2004). What research says about vocabulary instruction for students with learning disabilities. *Exceptional Children, 70*(3), 299–322. https://doi.org/10.1177/001440290407000303

Justice, L. M., Meier, J., & Walpole, S. (2005). Learning new words from storybooks: An efficacy study with at-risk kindergartners. *Language, Speech and Hearing Services in Schools, 36*(1), 17–32. https://doi.org/10.1044/0161-1461(2005/003)

Kaderavek, J., & Justice, L. M. (2002). Shared storybook reading as an intervention context. *American Journal of Speech-Language Pathology*, *11*(4), 394–406. https://doi.org/10.1044/1058-0360(2002/043)

Kaiser, A., & Roberts, M. (2013). Parent-implemented enhanced milieu teaching with preschool children who have intellectual disabilities. *Journal of Speech, Language, and Hearing Research*, *56*(1), 295–309. https://doi.org/10.1044/1092-4388(2012/11-0231)

Kirby, J. R., & Bowers, P. N. (2012). Morphology works. *What Works? Research into Practice*. http://www.edu.gov.on.ca/eng/literacynumeracy/inspire/research/WhatWorks.html

Laufer, B., & Goldstein, Z. (2004). Testing vocabulary knowledge: Size, strength, and computer adaptiveness. *Language Learning*, *54*(3), 399–436. https://doi.org/10.1111/j.0023-8333.2004.00260.x

Leonard, L. B. (1998) Children with specific language impairment. *Language, speech, and communication*. The MIT Press.

Leonard, L., Deevy, P., Karpicke, J., Christ, S., & Kueser, J. (2020). After initial retrieval practice, more retrieval produces better retention than more study in the word learning of children with developmental language disorder. *Journal of Speech, Language, and Hearing Research*, *63*(8), 2763–2776. https://doi.org/10.1044/2020_JSLHR-20-00105

Leonard, L., Karpicke, J., Deevy, P., Weber, C., Christ, S., Haebig, E., . . . Krok, W. (2019). Retrieval based word learning in young typically developing children and children with developmental language disorder I: The benefits of repeated retrieval. *Journal of Speech, Language and Hearing Research*, *62*(4), 932–943. https://doi.org/10.1044/2018_JSLHR-L-18-0070

Leung, C. B. (2008). Preschoolers' acquisition of scientific vocabulary through repeated read-aloud events, retellings, and hands-on science activities. *Reading Psychology*, *29*(2), 165–193. https://doi.org/10.1080/02702710801964090

Levelt, W. J. (1989). *Speaking: From intention to articulation*. MIT Press.

Lowe, H., Henry, L., Muller, L., & Joffe, V. (2018). Vocabulary intervention for adolescents with language disorder: A systematic review. *International Journal of Language and Communication Disorders*, *53*(2), 199–217. https://doi.org/10.1111/1460-6984.12355

Marks, I., & Stokes, S. (2010). Narrative-based intervention for word-finding difficulties: A case study. *International Journal of Language Communication Disorders*, *45*(5), 586–599. https://doi.org/10.3109/13682820903277951

McGregor, K. K. (1994). The use of phonological information in a word-finding treatment for children. *Journal of Speech and Hearing Research*, *37*, 1381–1393.

McGregor, K., Newman, R., Reilly, R., & Capone, N. (2002). Semantic representation and naming in children with specific language impairment. *Journal of Speech, Language, and Hearing Research,* *45*(5), 998–1014. https://doi.org/10.1044/1092-4388(2002/081)

McKeown, M. G. (2019). Effective vocabulary instruction fosters knowing words, using words, and understanding how words work. *Language, Speech, and Hearing Services in Schools, 50*(4), 466–476. https://doi.org/10.1044/2019_LSHSS-VOIA-18-0126

Murphy, A., Franklin, S., Breen, A., Hanlon, M., McNamara, A., Bogue, A., & James, E. (2017). A whole class teaching approach to improve the vocabulary skills of adolescents attending mainstream secondary school, in areas of socioeconomic disadvantage. *Child Language Teaching and Therapy, 33*(2), 129–144. https://doi.org/10.1177/0265659016656906

Nash, M., & Donaldson, M. L. (2005). Word learning in children with vocabulary deficits. *Journal of Speech, Language, and Hearing Research, 48*(2), 439–458. https://doi.org/10.1044/1092-4388(2005/030)

Nash H., & Snowling, M. (2006). Teaching new words to children with poor existing vocabulary knowledge: A controlled evaluation of the definition and context methods. *International Journal of Language and Communication Disorders, 41*(3), 335–354. https://doi.org/10.1080/13682820600602295

Nation, I.S.P. (2010). *Learning vocabulary in another language.* Cambridge University Press.

National Reading Panel (U.S.), & National Institute of Child Health and Human Development (U.S.). (2000). *Report of the National Reading Panel: Teaching children to read: An evidence-based assessment of the scientific research literature on reading and its implications for reading instruction: Reports of the subgroups.* National Institute of Child Health and Human Development, National Institutes of Health.

Nichols, W., & Rupley, W. (2004). Matching instructional design with vocabulary instruction. *Reading Horizons: A Journal of Literacy and Language Arts, 45*(1), 55–71. https://scholarworks.wmich.edu/reading_horizons/vol45/iss1/4/

Parsons, S., Law, J., & Gascoigne, M. (2005). Teaching receptive vocabulary to children with specific language impairment: A curriculum-based approach. *Child Language Teaching and Therapy, 21*(1), 39–59. https://doi.org/10.1191/0265659005ct280oa

Pignot-Shahov, V. (2012). Measuring L2 receptive and productive vocabulary knowledge. *Language Studies Working Papers, 4,* 37–45.

Pollard-Durodola, S. D., Gonzalez, J. E., Simmons, D. C., Kwok, O., Taylor, A. B., Davis, M. J., . . . Simmons, L. (2016). The effects of an intensive shared book-reading intervention for preschool children at risk for vocabulary delay. *Exceptional Children, 77*(2), 161–183. https://doi.org/10.1177/001440291107700202

Sedita, J. (2005). Effective vocabulary instruction. *Insights on Learning Disabilities, 2*(1) 33–45.

Sheng, L., & McGregor, K. (2010). Lexical semantic organization in children with specific language impairment. *Journal of Speech, Language, and Hearing Research, 53*(1), 146–159. https://doi.org/10.1044/1092-4388(2009/08-0160)

Shoari, E., & Farrokhi, F. (2014). The effects of graphic organizer strategy on improving Iranian EFL learners' vocabulary learning. *Research in English Language Pedagogy, 2*(1), 71–82. https://www.semantic scholar.org/paper/The-Effects-of-Graphic-Organizer-Strategy-on-EFL-Rasouli-Heravi/55f97373d09358d478992772dc7afc05384f91ef

Silverman, R. D. (2007). A comparison of three methods of vocabulary instruction during read-alouds in kindergarten. *The Elementary School Journal, 108*(2), 97–113. https://doi.org/10.1086/525549

Silverman, R. D., & Crandell, J. D. (2010). Vocabulary practices in pre-kindergarten and kindergarten classrooms. *Reading Research Quarterly, 45*(3), 318–340. https://doi.org/10.1598/RRQ.45.3.3

Sinatra, R., & Dowd, C. (1991). Using syntactic and semantic clues to learn vocabulary. *Journal of Reading, 35*(3), 224–229. https://doi.org/10.2307/40033183

Stahl, S., & Nagy, W. (2006). *Teaching word meanings.* Lawrence Erlbaum Associates.

Stahl, S., & Vancil, S. (1986). Discussion is what makes semantic maps works in vocabulary instruction. *Reading Teacher, 40*(1), 62–67.

Steele, S. C., & Mills, M. T. (2011). Vocabulary intervention for school-age children with language impairment: A review of evidence and good practice. *Child Language Teaching and Therapy, 27*(3), 354–370. https://doi.org/10.1177/0265659011412247

Stiegler, L. N., & Hoffman, P. R. (2001). Discourse-based intervention for word finding in children. *Journal of Communication Disorders, 34*(4), 277–303. https://doi.org/10.1016/S0021-9924(01)00051-X

St. John, P., & Vance, M. (2014). Evaluation of a principled approach to vocabulary learning in mainstream classes. *Child Language Teaching and Therapy, 30*(3), 255–271. https://doi.org/10.1177/026565 9013516474

Stoner, J., Meadan, H., & Angell, M., (2013). A model for coaching parents to implement teaching strategies with their young children with language delay or developmental disabilities. *Perspectives on Language Learning and Education, 20* (3), 112–119

Taylor, D. B., Myraz, M., Nichols, W. D., Rickelman, R. J., & Wood, K. D. (2009). Using explicit instruction to promote vocabulary learning struggling readers. *Reading & Writing Quarterly, 25*(2–3), 205–220. https://doi.org/10.1080/10573560802683663

Whitehurst, G. J., Falco, F. L., Lonigan, C. J., Fischel, J. E., DeBaryshe, B. D., Valdez-Menchaca, M. C., & Caulfield, M. (1988). Accelerating language development through picture book reading. *Developmental Psychology*, *24*(4), 552–559. https://doi.org/10.1037/0012-1649.24.4.552

Wilson, J., Aldersley, A., Dobson, C., Edgar, S., Harding, C., Luckins, J., . . . Pring, T. (2015). The effectiveness of semantic therapy for the word finding difficulties of children with severe and complex speech, language, and communication needs. *Child Language Teaching and Therapy*, *31*(1), 7–17. https://doi.org/10.1177/0265659014523299

Wolter, J. A., & Green, L. (2013). Morphological awareness intervention in school-age children with language and literacy deficits: A case study. *Topics in Language Disorders*, *33*(1), 27–41. https://doi.org/10.1097/TLD.0b013e318280f5aa

Wright, L., Pring, T., & Ebbels, S. (2018). Effectiveness of vocabulary intervention for older children with (developmental) language disorder. *International Journal of Language and Communication Disorders*, *53*(3), 480–494. https://doi.org/10.1111/1460-6984.12361

Yoder, P. J., & Warren, S. F. (2002). Effects of prelinguistic milieu teaching and parent responsivity education on dyads involving children with intellectual disabilities. *Journal of Speech, Language, and Hearing Research*, *45*(6), 1158–1174. https://doi.org/10.1044/1092-4388(2002/094)

Zeno, S., Ivens, S. H., Millard, R. T., Duvvuri, R., & Rothkopf, E. Z. (1995). *The educator's word frequency guide*. Touchstone Applied Science Associates.

Zens, N. K., Gillon, G. T., & Moran, C. (2009). Effects of phonological awareness and semantic intervention on word-learning in children with SLI. *International Journal of Speech-Language Pathology*, *11*(6), 509–524. https://doi.org/10.3109/17549500902926881

Zevenbergen, A. A., & Whitehurst, G. J. (2003). Dialogic reading: A shared picture book reading intervention for preschoolers. In A. van Kleeck, S. A. Stahl, & E. B. Bauer (Eds.), *Center for Improvement of Early Reading Achievement, CIERA. On reading books to children: Parents and teachers* (pp. 177–200). Lawrence Erlbaum Associates.

Zipoli, R. P., Jr., Coyne, M. D., & McCoach, D. B. (2011). Enhancing vocabulary intervention for kindergarten students: Strategic integration of semantically related and embedded word review. *Remedial and Special Education*, *32*(2), 131–143. https://doi.org/10.1177/0741932510361262

Appendix 8–1

Examples of Therapy Plans

Shared Book Reading Lesson Plan (Created by Claire Small and Sarah Larsen)
Targeted population: Preschoolers with DLD
Book title: *If You Give a Mouse a Cookie* by Laura Joffe Numeroff
Objectives: By _____, the client will use five target verbs (e.g., a*sk, see, finish, drink, give)* during an unstructured activity (e.g., shared book reading) with 90% accuracy when given minimal prompting, as measured by clinician data. By _____, the client will use nouns (i.e., Tier One vocabulary) during shared book reading with 80% accuracy and minimal cues, as measured by clinician data.
Therapy Materials: (need to provide some pictures, figures) ■ The book ■ Props for story retell: *stuffed or printed animal mouse, boy, cookie, milk, straw, napkin, mirror, scissors, broom, pillow, blanket, book, crayons, paper, pen, tape*
Session Plan: *Preselect approximately 4 to 5 words to target during EACH book reading. Targets will vary depending on the child's present level of functioning and vocabulary size. 1. Select only 4 to 5 words to target in each session. The targets can be incorporated into follow-up vocabulary activities such as play, narrative building, and games. 2. Always review the targets from the previous session to ensure word retention. Revisit the previous targets while introducing new targets. If the child needs more time with the previously taught words, reduce the number of new words you plan to introduce in the second read.

Step 1: Introduce the book and check for background knowledge. Examples of questions:

1. *"Has mom or dad ever given you a cookie?"*
2. *"Do you like cookies? What kind?"*
3. *"What do you like to drink when you eat a cookie?"*
4. *"Show me how you would ask for a cookie."*
5. *"Do you think a mouse is a good pet? Why?"*

Following the introduction, give the book to the child and allow them to open it

Step 2: Begin reading the book at a good pace. During the book reading, pause to incorporate open-ended questions and allow the child to make comments. Examples: *"What happened?" "What do you think the mouse will need next?"*

1. Ask 1 to 2 questions per page as needed to avoid cognitive overload.
2. When reading the story, try to be animated and make it fun and interesting.
3. Highlight the target words by alternating intonation and using exaggeration.
4. Keeping the same questions and the same sentence structure throughout the book can enhance comprehension and learning.

Step 3: Have the child retell the story using the provided props, based on the child's present level. The child may refer to the pictures in the book as a reference.

Step 4: During the discussion and carryover, make sure to discuss the story and attempt to incorporate the words outside of the therapy room. Example of questions:

1. *The mouse cleaned up his mess that he made. Do you clean up your messes at home? How do you clean them up?*
2. *How do you do your hair in the morning before school?*
3. *When you're hungry what do you do?*
4. *What type of snacks do you have in your refrigerator?*

continues

Appendix 8–1. *continued*

Management of Unexpected Responses:

If the child responds with a word that has a similar meaning but not the target word, then try the following.

*Example: The child looks at the glass of milk and says *juice* instead of milk

1. Point to the image and ask the child to label the object again (e.g., "*Wait, can you tell me what that is?*").
2. If still incorrect, provide a phonemic cue (e.g., "It's not juice, it's mmm-").
3. If still incorrect, provide a closed set (e.g., "Is it juice or milk?").
4. Discuss the two meanings:
   a. *What color is milk? What color is juice?*
   b. *Where does milk come from? Where does juice come from?*
   c. *Have you ever had milk? Do you like juice or milk better?* (Connect this with personal experience.)

If the child responds with an irrelevant word, the following examples may be used.

*Example: The child responds with *drawer* instead of refrigerator.

1. Have them discuss the meaning of the incorrect word.
   a. *Can you tell me what a drawer is?*
2. Compare the meaning of their word to the meaning of the target word.
   a. *Good, this is a refrigerator. What does a refrigerator do? Does a drawer do that?*

If the child does not want to read the book, what can I do?

If the child refuses to read the book, begin using the props/pictures to tell the story and teach the vocabulary. Once the child is engaged, attempt to switch over to the book. Tell them "*We have to open the book to find out what is next!*" If they want to keep playing with the props, have them continue acting out the story as you read the book.

If the child is completely uninterested in the story, allow them to choose between two books. (Use *If You Give a Mouse a Cookie* or an alternative book.)

Data Collection for Progress Monitoring (Possible Targets) Across Multiple Readings:

Prepositions: in, with, on

Nouns: mouse, cookie, glass, milk, straw, napkin, mirror, mustache, broom, hair, house, room, box, blanket, pillow, story, picture, crayons, paper, pen, refrigerator, tape,

Verbs: give*, ask*, finish*, want*, look, see, need, trim, cut, drink, eat, sweep, clean, take, read, draw, write, sleep, sign, hang (*repeated many times throughout the story)

Adjectives: thirsty, hungry, sleepy, tired,

Pronouns: He, him

continues

Appendix 8–1. *continued*

Prepositions	
In	
On	
With	
Nouns	
Mouse	
Cookie	
Glass	
Refrigerator	
Straw	
Mirror	
broom	
Verbs	
Give	
Ask	
Finish	
See	
Drink	
Eat	
want	
Adjectives	
Thirsty	
Tired	
Hungry	
Pronouns	
Him	
He	

NR = no response P = prompted + = Independent - = Incorrect

Graphic Organizer Lesson Plan	
Target Population	High school students with DLD
Objective	By _____, the client will explain the meaning of unknown words by using graphic organizers, such as a four-square, during structured language tasks with 75% accuracy when given minimal prompting, as measured by clinician data.
Therapy Materials	■ Use a current event or reading excerpt from classroom material (e.g., history lesson on the Bill of Rights). ■ Four-square graphic organizer:

Four Square	
Target Word:	Examples:
Definition (own words):	Nonexamples:

Session Plan	1. Introduce the topic that the child will be reading about and check for background knowledge.
	  a. What is the Bill of Rights?
	  b. How is the Bill of Rights related to the Constitution?
	  c. How does the Bill of Rights impact your daily life?
	2. Prior to reading, have the child scan the passage for unknown words. When an unknown word is identified, collaborate with the child to complete the four-square graphic organizer. Provide them the definition and encourage them to document the definition in their own words (e.g., *declaration, citizens, political institutions, legislative, rights, pursuant, press, grievances, capital, prosecutions, enumeration, etc.*).

continues

Appendix 8–1. *continued*

Session Plan *continued*	3. After all the new words have been identified and defined using the four-square graphic organizer, have the child read the passage.
	4. Review new words at the end of the session (target 4 to 5 each session) and ask the student to define each word and use it in a novel sentence.
	5. Provide the student with several copies of the graphic organizer and encourage them to use this graphic organizer in the classroom. Or, encourage them to document unfamiliar words encountered in the classroom in the "target word" section to be discussed in an upcoming session.
Management of Unexpected Responses	**If the student responds with a word that has a similar meaning but not the target word, try the following.**
	▪ In student friendly terms, define the two words and prompt the student to discuss how the two words are the same and how they are different. Try using both words in a sentence and discuss how it changes the meaning of the utterance.
	If the student responds with an irrelevant word:
	▪ Ask the student what the irrelevant word means.
	▪ Reread the sentence and paragraph and explain how the irrelevant word fits in the context.
	▪ Discuss the difference between the irrelevant word and the target word, and ask why the target word fits better in the context.
	▪ Ask the student to define the target word again using their words.
	▪ If they are unable to, provide them with a student friendly definition.
	▪ Ask the student to reflect on how the use of the two words would change the meaning of the sentence. If the student is unable to do this task, then model using the "think aloud" strategy.

Data Collection	See attached template below:

Key

+/-	Correct/Incorrect
P/I	Prompted/Independent

Content-Specific Targets	Word Definition — Example: "To make a formal announcement to a group of people."	+/- (+ / -)	P/I	Use of word in a sentence — Example: "The student made a declaration to his parents about his college acceptance."	+/- (+ / -)	P/I
Declaration						
Citizens						
Enumeration						
Legislative						
Rights						
Pursuant						
Press						
Grievances						
Capital						
Prosecutions						

continues

Amendment I

Congress shall make no law respecting an establishment of religion or prohibiting the free exercise thereof, or abridging the freedom of speech or of the press, or the right of the people peaceably to assemble and to petition the government for a redress of grievances.

Amendment II

A well-regulated Militia being necessary to the security of a free State, the right of the people to keep and bear Arms shall not be infringed.

Amendment III

No soldier shall, in time of peace, be quartered in any house without the consent of the owner, nor in time of war but in a manner to be prescribed by law.

Amendment IV

The right of the people to be secure in their persons, houses, papers, and effects against unreasonable searches and seizures shall not be violated, and no warrants shall issue but upon probable cause, supported by oath or affirmation, and particularly describing the place to be searched and the persons or things to be seized.

Amendment V

No person shall be held to answer for a capital or otherwise infamous crime unless on a presentment or indictment of a grand jury, except in cases arising in the land or naval forces, or in the militia, when in actual service in time of war or public danger; nor shall any person be subject for the same offense to be twice put in jeopardy of life or limb; nor shall be compelled in any criminal case to be a witness against himself, nor be deprived of life, liberty, or property without due process of law; nor shall private property be taken for public use without just compensation.

Amendment VI

In all criminal prosecutions, the accused shall enjoy the right to a speedy and public trial by an impartial jury of the state and district wherein the crime shall have been committed, which district shall have been previously ascertained by law, and to be informed of the nature and cause of the accusation; to be confronted with the witnesses against him; to have compulsory process for obtaining witnesses in his favor; and to have the assistance of counsel for his defense.

Amendment VII

In suits at common law, where the value in controversy shall exceed twenty dollars, the right of trial by jury shall be preserved, and no fact tried by a jury shall be otherwise reexamined in any court of the United States than according to the rules of the common law.

Amendment VIII

In suits at common law, where the value in controversy shall exceed twenty dollars, the right of trial by jury shall be preserved, and no fact tried by a jury shall be otherwise reexamined in any court of the United States than according to the rules of the common law.

Amendment IX

The enumeration in the Constitution of certain rights shall not be construed to deny or disparage others retained by the people.

Amendment X

The powers not delegated to the United States by the Constitution, nor prohibited by it to the states, are reserved to the states respectively, or to the people.

Context Clues	
Target Population	School-age child with DLD
Objective	By _____, the student will use context clues to correctly describe the meaning of target words in 8/10 trials with minimal cues, as measured by clinician data.

Therapy Materials	■ Reading material used in the classroom
	  ■ 9th grade curriculum example: *Lord of the Flies* by William Golding
	  ■ 5th grade curriculum example: The French and Indian War

Session Plan	1. Identify the reading material to be used in session. Check for background knowledge by discussing how the material is being used in class
	2. Identify unknown words:
	  a. Have the student scan the page for unknown words prior to reading.
	  b. If the student stumbles on a word while reading, (that was not identified earlier as unknown) pause and discuss.
	3. Identify context clues
	  a. Have the student read the sentence and circle the unknown word.
	  b. Have them identify the nouns/verbs that they already know by underlying them. Make sure the student underlines only relevant words that provide context for the unknown word.
	  c. Ask them to consider how these words may help them discover the meaning of the novel word.
	4. Discussing new words: As Stahl and Nagy (2006) suggest, use synonyms, antonyms, examples from personal experiences or school content, nonexamples that contain words similar to the target word but have different use in context, and discussion of words related to the target word. Model these skills using the "think aloud" strategy.

continues

Appendix 8–1. *continued*

Session Plan *continued*	a. Example of the think aloud strategy for the word *lagoon*: "Okay, based on the context I know that the boy is climbing down the rock toward something, I think it may be a body of water. Another word similar to lagoon would be pond, let's see what happens when I replace the word *lagoon* with *pond*: *The boy with fair hair lowered himself down the last few feet of rock and began to pick his way toward the pond.* That sentence makes sense! Have you ever seen a pond or a lagoon?
	5. After unfamiliar words have been identified, read the passage. Target 4 to 5 words per session. At the end of the session, review all new words and ask the student to provide a definition and use it in a sentence.
Management of Unexpected Responses	**If the student highlights irrelevant contextual information:**
	■ Ask them to define all the known words they've underlined and consider how the meaning of the words might be related to the word in question.
	For example, have the student identify the following words as context clues: *The boy with fair hair lowered himself down the last few feet of rock and began to pick his way toward the **lagoon**.*
	■ Good, you've selected 5 words that serve as context clues. What does the word "fair" mean? Is "fair" describing the boy or the lagoon? Yes, the word "fair" is describing the boy's light hair. This helps give us an image of the boy but doesn't really help us uncover the meaning of *lagoon*. The other words "lowered," "rock," "pick," and "toward" all help us determine the meaning of *lagoon*.
	If the student responds with a word/definition that has a similar meaning but not the target word:
	■ In student friendly terms, define the two words and prompt the student to discuss how the two words are the same and how they are different.

Manage-ment of Unexpected Responses *continued*	Try using both words in a sentence and discuss how it changes the meaning of the utterance. **If the student responds with an irrelevant word/ definition:** ■ First, ask the student to define the word. If they are unable to, provide them with a student-friendly definition. Ask the student to reflect on how the use of the two words would change the meaning of the sentence. If the student is unable to do this, model using the "think aloud" strategy.
Data Collection	

Data collection grid:

Key		Target	Underline appropriate context words		Defines underlined words		Forms hypotheses about meaning of target		Use it in a novel sentence	
+/-	Correct/incorrect		+/-	P/I	+/-	P/I	+/-	P/I	+/-	P/I
P/I	Prompted/Independent									

continues

Appendix 8–1. *continued*

<u>(9th Grade Literature)</u> Excerpt from *Lord of the Flies*:

THE BOY WITH FAIR HAIR LOWERED HIMSELF down the last few feet of rock and began to pick his way toward the **lagoon**. Though he had taken off his school sweater and trailed it now from one hand, his grey shirt stuck to him and his hair was **plastered** to his forehead. All round him the long scar smashed into the jungle was a bath of heat. He was **clambering** heavily among the creepers and broken trunks when a bird, a vision of red and yellow, flashed upwards with a witch-like cry; and this cry was echoed by another.

...

The shore was **fledged** with palm trees. These stood or leaned or reclined against the light and their green feathers were a hundred feet up in the air. The ground beneath them was a bank covered with **coarse** grass, torn everywhere by the **upheavals** of fallen trees, scattered with **decaying** coconuts and palm **saplings**. Behind this was the darkness of the forest proper and the open space of the scar. Ralph stood, one hand against a grey trunk, and screwed up his eyes against the shimmering water. Out there, perhaps a mile away, the white surf slinked on a coral reef, and beyond that the open sea was dark blue. Within the irregular arc of coral the lagoon was still as a mountain lake—blue of all shades and shadowy green and purple. The beach between the palm terrace and the water was a thin stick, endless apparently, for to Ralph's left the perspectives of palm and beach and water drew to a point at infinity; and always, almost visible, was the heat.

Excerpted from *Lord of the Flies* by William Golding. Copyright 1959 by William Golding. Perigee Books.

<u>(5th Grade History) The French and Indian War: The Differences Between New France and American Colonies</u>

"Unlike the English, most French **colonists** could not become farmers, so they had no **desire** to take land from the Indians. The king of France did not allow the French colonists the rights the English colonists had. The people who went to New France were **expected** to work as the king told them. He was not interested in family life or farm life. He was interested in the **valuable** fur trade. So while the English brought their families, most French colonists were unmarried men. As they moved about trading and trapping furs, they often lived with the Indians instead of building their own homes.

France was a Catholic country, and no one was **allowed** to go to New France **except** Catholics. The French sent Catholic **missionaries** (priests) to the Native Americans." (Moore, 2015, pp. 93–94)

Moore, J. H. (2015). *The history of our United States in Christian perspective* (4th ed.). A Beka Book.

continues

Appendix 8–1. *continued*

Semantic & Phonological Aspects	
Target Population	School-age children with DLD
Objective	■ When presented with a vocabulary word (i.e., noun) the student will identify seven attributes (i.e., function, first sound, rhyme, spelling, category, attributes, and location) with 80% accuracy and moderate prompting, as measured by clinician data. ■ When presented with a vocabulary word (i.e., verb) the student will identify seven attributes (i.e., who does the action, what is needed for the action, where the action takes place, first sound, rhyme, spelling, attributes) with 80% accuracy and moderate prompting, as measured by clinician data.
Therapy Materials	■ Selection of 4 to 5 vocabulary words (nouns or verbs) ■ Select words using tiers of vocabulary or through collaborating with the student's teacher to include curriculum-based vocabulary. ■ Worksheet of semantic and phonological aspects
Session Plan	1. Review vocabulary from the previous session. Ask the child to describe several semantic and phonological features of the word (e.g., *What does it do? What does it look like? What is the first sound? What does it rhyme with?*). 2. Introduce the concept of semantic features (i.e., describing what we know about a word) and phonological awareness (i.e., make sure they understand the concept of rhyming). 3. For each new word, complete the chart below. Use the relevant chart depending on if the target is a noun or a verb. 4. At the end of the session, have the child write all new words in their word journal to show their teacher/stakeholders.

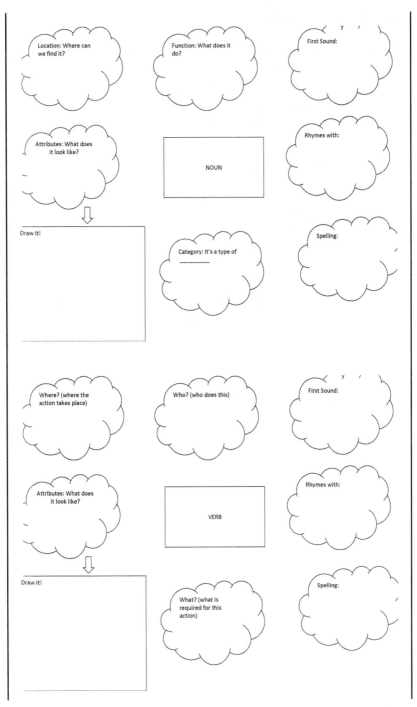

continues

Appendix 8–1. *continued*

Manage-ment of Unexpected Responses	**If the student responds with a feature that is incorrect or not specific enough:** ■ Ask the student to explain how their response relates to the target word. ■ Discuss how their response is unrelated to the target. ■ Ask them to select a better/more specific feature to describe the target word. ■ Ask them to compare that response to the previous response and discuss why the latter is more appropriate. *Example: If they say the function of the target word "hammer" is "to smash" then say: ■ What does it mean to smash something? How does a hammer smash? ■ A hammer doesn't always break the object. ■ Is there a word that better describes the function of a hammer? ■ Yes, hit/build is a much better response. How is hit/build different from smash?

Data Collection

Key

+/-	Correct/incorrect
P/I	Prompted/Independent

Target	Function		Location		Attributes		Category		Spelling		Rhyme		First phoneme	
	+/-	P/I	+/-	P/I	+/-	P/I	+/-	P/I	+/-	P/I	+/-	P/I	+/-	P/I

continues

Appendix 8–1. *continued*

Analyze Word Parts & Increase Morphological Awareness	
Target Population	School-age children with DLD
Objective	By _____, the student will explain the meanings of words containing target morphemes (e.g., un-, re-) following structured language tasks in 8/10 trials with minimal cues as measured by clinician data.
Therapy Materials	■ Laminated word cards ▪ Words that include the prefixes: *un, re* ▪ Example words: <table><tr><td>***un-***</td><td>***re-***</td></tr><tr><td>Unhappy Uneducated Untrue Unfinished Unload</td><td>Review Reinvestigate Restart Revisit Retrace</td></tr></table>
Session Plan	1. Introduce the concept of morphemes by discussing prefixes and suffixes. Demonstrate how a word can be deconstructed into smaller parts that alter its meaning using an example word of appropriate level. 2. Spread the laminated word cards out face up on the table and have the student use an EXPO® marker to delineate the prefix from the root word on each card. Ask the student to separate the words into two groups based on the prefix used. 3. Discuss the meaning of each prefix. Ask the student to consider how each prefix alters the meaning of the word. Model using the "think aloud" strategy if necessary. Additionally, prompt the student to compare the difference in meaning between the two prefixes: how are they the same or different?

Session Plan *continued*	4. Can the student think of any other words that contain this prefix? If they are unable to think of a word, have them create a silly word that includes a real root word to describe the meaning when combined with the prefix.

Management of Unexpected Responses	**If the student is unable to infer the meaning of word:**
	
	■ First, ensure the student understands the meaning of the root word.
	
	■ Next, have them the combine the definition of the prefix with the root word and discuss the meaning
	
	   ■ For example, What does *not-educated* mean? What does *again-investigate* mean?
	
	If the student is unable to differentiate the meanings of the two prefixes:
	
	■ Have them compare the meanings of the two words with the same root and different prefixes (nonwords are okay)
	
	   ■ What is the difference between *unused* and *reused?* What is the difference between *undo* and *redo?*

continues

Appendix 8–1. *continued*

Data Collection

Key	
+/-	Correct/incorrect
P/I	Prompted/Independent

Target Prefix	Groups prefix +/-	P/I	Explain how prefix changes meaning +/-	P/I	Define real word or silly word +/-	P/I
Un-						
Re-						

Mixed Vocabulary Intervention Program	
Target Population	School age children (upper elementary and beyond) with DLD
Objective	By _____, the client will independently use strategies (e.g., word part analysis, dictionary, word map, etc.) to explain the meanings of unknown words and give an example by using the unknown word with 75% accuracy, as measured by clinician data.
Therapy Materials	■ Short Story "The Detective and the Lost Dog" ■ Parts of Speech Diagram ■ Printed or online list of English roots (prefixes & suffixes) ■ http://www.prefixsuffix.com/rootchart.php ■ Dictionary (printed or online) ■ Word map worksheet ■ Semantic and phonological aspects worksheet
Session Plan	A mixed vocabulary intervention approach goes beyond the semantic and phonological meaning of words. Children will expand their vocabularies by "learning strategies, such as parts of speech, word part analysis, word map, semantic and phonological information, use of dictionaries, and definitional information" (Chapter 8). Once children learn multiple different strategies, they can apply these strategies to help them comprehend and acquire new vocabulary words.
	Part 1 (Parts of Speech)
	1. Begin by reading through the short story. While reading through the short story, the child should underline each unfamiliar word. 2. The child will look at each word and determine the role in each sentence (i.e., parts of speech). They will determine if it is a noun, verb, pronoun, and so forth.

continues

Appendix 8–1. *continued*

Session Plan *continued*	3. The student can refer to the parts of speech diagram for support if needed. 4. Example: *"He was a **reliable** detective who always got the job done."* Answer: Reliable is an adjective because it describes the noun (detective).

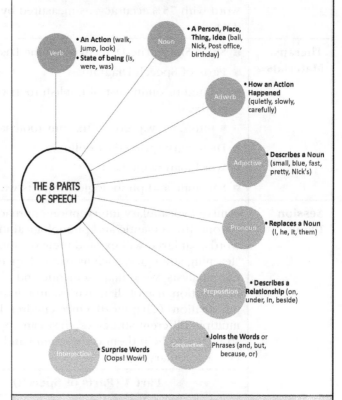

THE 8 PARTS OF SPEECH

- **Verb** — • An Action (walk, jump, look) • State of being (is, were, was)
- **Noun** — • A Person, Place, Thing, Idea (ball, Nick, Post office, birthday)
- **Adverb** — • How an Action Happened (quietly, slowly, carefully)
- **Adjective** — • Describes a Noun (small, blue, fast, pretty, Nick's)
- **Pronoun** — • Replaces a Noun (I, he, it, them)
- **Preposition** — • Describes a Relationship (on, under, in, beside)
- **Conjunction** — • Joins the Words or Phrases (and, but, because, or)
- **Interjection** — • Surprise Words (Oops! Wow!)

Part 2 (Word Part Analysis)

1. For words that have multiple prefixes and suffixes, the child should practice identifying the meaning by breaking up the word into different parts

2. Example: *"It seemed **incomprehensible** that this gentleman took Janet's dog . . . "*

Session Plan
continued

3. The child should refer to a word roots dictionary in order to accurately understand each prefix or suffix.

   a. Breaking the word up: *in - comprehen - sible*

   b. **in** = not

   c. **comprehen** = to understand

   d. **ible** = not able to do something; turns a verb into an adjective (descriptive)

   e. **Incomprehensible** = not able to understand something

   f. Conclusion: the sentence means that they cannot understand why the gentleman would take Janet's dog.

Part 3 (Word Map) & Part 4 (Dictionary & Definition Information)

1. Children will identify unfamiliar words and use the worksheet to define the word.

2. They will begin by looking the word up in a dictionary. Make sure the child knows how to use a dictionary.

   a. Tell them to open the dictionary to the corresponding first letter, and then look for the second letter, then the third, until they locate the word.

   b. Look at the top two definitions along with examples.

   c. Use the definition in the sentence to see if it fits.

3. They will write out the dictionary definition of the word on the worksheet.

4. They will then write out the definition of the word in their own words.

5. They will then use the word to generate a sentence.

6. Finally, they will draw an illustration of the word.

7. Example from the story: *"They quickly ran up to the door, but Mrs. Hayfield yelled, "Go away!" Janet and Detective Jones thought that Mrs. Hayfield was being very **suspicious**."*

continues

Appendix 8–1. *continued*

**Session
Plan**
continued

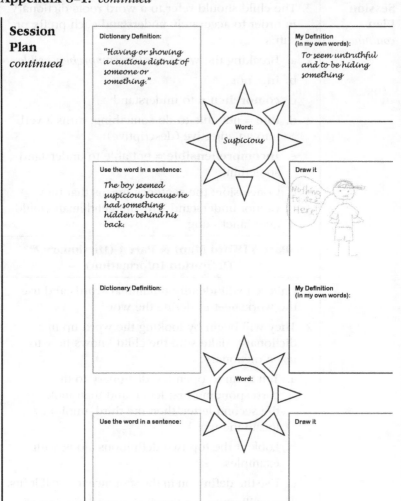

Part 5 (Semantic and Phonological Information)

*See previous activity that uses a worksheet to
identify semantic and phonemic aspects of words
(e.g., *rhyming, who, what, where, draw it, etc.*).

Session Plan *continued*	**Comprehension Check**
	1. After the child has identified all of the unfamiliar words and used a strategy to understand each word, ask the child to reread the story on their own.
	2. After reading the story, ask the child specific questions about the story to ensure they understand the new words. The student will have a hard time answering the questions if they do not understand the meaning of each word in the text.
	3. Allow the child to refer to the story text if needed.
	4. Example questions below: a. <u>True or false:</u> Criminals never get caught when Detective Jones is on the case. *"There was not one **criminal** who could **evade** their **capture** when he was on the case."* b. <u>True or false:</u> The twins that robbed 12 banks looked the exact same. *"These **identical** twins had robbed 12 banks across the country . . . "* c. <u>True or false:</u> If they didn't find the dog soon he might have fallen asleep. *" . . . if he wasn't found soon, he could **perish**."* d. <u>True or false:</u> It was possible that Mrs. Hayfield took the dog because she is such a nice person. *"Because Mrs. Hayfield was such a nice lady, it seemed **incomprehensible** that she took Janet's dog."* e. <u>True or false:</u> Detective Jones did not think that they were going to find Spot. *" . . . Detective Jones **reassured** her that they were going to find Spot."*

continues

Appendix 8–1. *continued*

Data Collection

Target Word	Strategy used	Defines the word in their own words (+/-)	Provides an Example	Prompted or Independent (P/I)
Brisk				
Impressive				
Incomprehensible				
Suspicious				
Evade				
Perish				
Reassure				
Decline				

List of Strategies	
1.! Parts of Speech	4.! Semantic & Phonological Information
2.! Word Part analysis	5.! Use of a Dictionary
3.! Word map	6.! Definitional Information

The Detective and the Lost Dog
Author: Sarah Larsen

On a **brisk** Saturday morning, Detective Jones sat on his porch and looked across the **horizon** while he **sipped** his warm coffee and stroked his dog's floppy ears. He had finally **retired** after working for **numerous** years as a detective for the Los Angeles Police Department (LAPD). During his time on the force, he received many **impressive** awards. He was a **reliable** detective who always got the job done. There was not one **criminal** who could **evade** their **capture** when he was on the case. Capturing the Robinson twins during a **massive** bank robbery was one of his greatest **accomplishments**. These **identical** twins had robbed 12 banks across the country, but their time robbing banks came to an end when Detective Jones caught them red handed.

As Detective Jones **reflected** on his time at LAPD, he began to miss the exciting adventures that he **encountered** every day. Then, he looked up and saw his neighbor, Janet running straight towards him. She was yelling, "Detective Jones, Detective Jones! You have to help me!" She said that her new puppy, Spot went missing and she needed him to help **locate** him. She said that her dog was in danger and if he wasn't found soon, he could **perish**. Although this was not a typical case for detective Jones, he agreed to help Janet find her puppy. After all, he had a lot of time on his hands and he was always up for a **challenge.**

They began by planning multiple different **routes** to start searching the neighborhood for the dog. They split up and knocked on every neighbor's door and asked if they had seen Spot. Some neighbors were helpful and even **offered** to help look for the missing puppy. However, some neighbors **declined** to help by slamming their doors shut. Just when Janet felt like giving up, Detective Jones **reassured** her that they were going to find Spot. Detective Jones had never **failed** during a case before and he was not going to start now. At that moment, they saw tiny footprints in Mrs. Hayfield's flower garden. Janet said, "Hey, those look like Spot's footprints!" They quickly ran up to the door, but Mrs. Hayfield yelled, "Go away!" Janet and Detective Jones thought that Mrs. Hayfield was being very **suspicious.**

continues

Appendix 8–1. *continued*

Because Mrs. Hayfield was such a nice lady, it seemed **incomprehensible** that she took Janet's dog. However, they were **confident** that she was hiding something. So, detective Jones and Janet began creating a **strategy** to help rescue Spot.

TO BE CONTINUED . . .

A list of 5th grade vocabulary words was adapted from https://www.flocabulary.com/5th-grade-vocabulary-word-list/

9

TREATMENT FOR LEXICAL RETRIEVAL IN NEUROGENIC LANGUAGE DISORDERS

Pei-Fang Hung

Chapter Objectives

1. Describe commonly implemented treatment approaches for word finding difficulties secondary to neurogenic language disorders.
2. Compare and contrast semantic-based and phonological-based lexical treatment approaches.
3. Identify the factors for choosing appropriate lexical treatment for a client with neurogenic word finding difficulty.

Introduction

People with aphasia and other related neurogenic communication disorders commonly experience word-finding difficulties
(WFDs). As discussed in Chapter 2, successful verbal production of words requires three types of information: (1) conceptual-semantic information, (2) lexical representation of the target
word, and (3) phonological representation of the target word.
Word-finding difficulties in aphasia and related neurogenic
communication disorders often stem from incomplete, weak,
or unsuccessful activation of the intended word at the semantic-lexical and/or lexical-phonological levels while they have preserved semantic knowledge at the conceptual level. For example,
when insufficient distinguishing semantic features are activated
(e.g., animals that can be pets, have four legs, fur, etc.), other
lexicons (e.g., "*dog*" or "*hamster*") that share similar features
may be selected instead of the intended target word ("*cat*"). In
other words, distinguishing and unique semantic features are
required to make the target word win the competition during the
selection/activation process. In this chapter, we review several
commonly implemented lexical treatment approaches that aim
to improve word retrieval in individuals with aphasia or other
related neurogenic communication disorders. This chapter is not
a comprehensive review of all treatment approaches for neurogenic word retrieval disorders.

Response Elaboration Training (RET)

Response Elaboration Training (RET) is a "loose training"
approach that aims to facilitate verbal production of words in
individuals with aphasia and other related neurogenic communication disorders. This approach was developed under the inspi-
ration of the Incidental Teaching approach (Hart, 1981; Hart &
Risley, 1974). Positive treatment effects have been reported for
persons with different types and severities of aphasia (Wambaugh, Nessler, & Wright, 2013). For example, Wambaugh and

Martinez (2000) examined effects of RET in three individuals with chronic aphasia and apraxia. Their results indicated that all three participants showed improved verbal production in picture description tasks and the personal recount condition.

Treatment Procedures of RET

As implemented in Kearn's studies (1985, 1997), the procedures of RET are summarized below.

- The clinician will begin the session by presenting a visual stimulus to the client (e.g., a picture of a man riding a bike). The clinician will ask the client to describe the picture.
- Based on the client's response, the clinician will provide reinforcement, as well as shape and model their response.
  - For example, if the client responds with *"Man bike."* The clinician might say, *"Yes, the man is on a bike."*
- Then the clinician will use WH-questions (i.e., *who, what, when, where, why, how*) to cue the client and elicit an elaborated response.
  - For example, the clinician might ask the client, *"What is he doing on the bike?"* or *"Why is he on the bike?"* After asking the question, the client might respond with, *"man riding."*
- The clinician will reinforce the client's attempt and elaborate the response by modeling the original response + the elaborated response.
  - For example, *"Great! The man is riding the bike."*
- The clinician will ask the client to repeat the clinician's combined model.
  - For example, *"Can you say, the man is riding the bike?"* The client might respond with, *"man ride bike."*
- The clinician will then elicit a delayed imitation of the combined model.
  - For example, *"You're right! The man is riding the bike."*

Lexical Retrieval Cueing Treatments

Historically, in clinical practice, speech-language pathologists provide different types of cues to individuals with WFD to elicit target responses and to promote successful communication exchanges. The commonly provided types are semantic cues (e.g., describing the function of the target word), phonological cues (e.g., the first sound), and orthographic cues (e.g., writing or spelling out the target word). These cues can be implemented as needed or systematically. This type of treatment program is commonly referred to as cueing hierarchies. We will review a few cueing treatment programs that were implemented and reported by researchers (e.g., Meteyard & Bose, 2018; Wambaugh, 2003).

Semantic Cueing Treatment

The semantic cueing treatment starts by presenting a target picture to the client with WFD. When the client cannot spontaneously name the target word, the clinician can provide different types of semantic cues to facilitate word retrieval. The first type of semantic cue is the **function** of the target word, such as "*saying meow*" for the target word "cat". The second type of semantic cue is the **category** of the word, such as "*it is a pet animal*" for the target word "cat". The third type of semantic cue is a **sentence completion phrase** that requires the client to fill in with the target word, such as "____ *love eating fish*" for the target word "cat". The last type of semantic cue is **synonym and antonym**, such as "*feline*" for the target word "cat". The client is expected to achieve certain accuracy established by the clinician, such as 80% accuracy, independently (without cues).

Phonological Cueing Treatment (PCT)

The procedures are practically the same for semantic cueing treatment and phonological cueing treatment. The only difference is the types of cues implemented in the therapy. In phonological cueing treatment, only phonological cues/prompts are provided to clients. The first type of phonological cue is presenting an **initial phoneme** cue (first sound), such as "*it starts with the sound /k/*" for the target word "cat". The initial phoneme cue can also be modified to the initial syllable for multisyllabic words, such as "*/kæl/*" for the target word "California". The second type of phonological cue is providing **a word that rhymes** with the target word, such as "*it rhymes with tat*" for the target word "cat". The last type of phonological cue is offering both **rhyming words and first sound** cues.

Research Evidence That Supports the Efficacy of Cueing Treatment

Meteyard and Bose conducted a study in 2018 to compare the effects of phonological cues to semantic cues in ten individuals with moderate to severe aphasia. Their results show that shorter and high imaginable words were named more accurately, and phonological cues were slightly more effective than semantic cues. They stated that phonological information can facilitate the mapping from the conceptual level to lexical and phonological levels and concluded that phonological cues were more effective than semantic cues in improving naming accuracy, regardless of the locus of lexical breakdown.

Clinicians are encouraged to give a test drive on different types of cues and combination of cues and carefully monitor clients' response to different cues and focus on what type and/ or what combination of cues works best for clients. Although strengthening the activation and the connection between the levels throughout the lexical access process may facilitate word retrieval, giving too many cues at once may overwhelm clients. Therefore, gradually increasing the number of cues and carefully monitoring clients' responses to different cues and different combinations of cues is crucial and essential. It is not uncommon to have individuals with neurogenic communication disorders experience altered or declined cognitive function. Therefore, giving an appropriate number of cues at an optimal pace and providing clients more time to process information can be beneficial. Table 9–1 provides examples of semantic, phonological, and orthographic cues that can be used in lexical retrieval cueing

Table 9–1. Examples of Semantic, Phonological, and Orthographic Cues (Target Word: Coffee)

Semantic Cues	Phonological Cues	Orographic Cues
The function of the target word: You drink it at breakfast.	The initial phoneme (first sound): It starts with /k/.	Write the first letter: [C]
The category of the target word: It is a type of hot beverage.	A word that rhymes with the target word: It rhymes with "toffee."	Spelling the word aloud: "C-O-F-F-E-E"
A sentence completion phrase: Pour me a cup of ____.	Both the rhyming word and first sound	Write the whole word: [COFFEE]

treatments. The use of orthographic cues will be discussed later in the chapter.

Semantic Feature Analysis (SFA)

Ylvisaker and Szekeres (1985) introduced a semantic-based lexical intervention called semantic feature analysis (SFA) that focuses on promoting the activation of semantic representations and strengthening the semantic-lexical connection (van Hees et al., 2013). The theoretical base of SFA is that words sharing more semantic features connect more closely together than words that do not share features (Boyle, 2010; Boyle & Coelho, 1995; Coelho et al., 2000). In other words, the more overlapping between two words, the stronger the connection becomes (e.g., apple and orange), and the connected word is more likely to be coactivated (Sheng & McGregor, 2010). Additionally, the more distinguishing and unique semantic features of the target concept are activated, the more likely the target lexical representation will be activated. The ultimate goal of SFA is to facilitate the activation of more strongly associated and unique features, which leads to successful activation of the intended word production.

Treatment Procedures of SFA

As implemented in the Boyle and Coelho (1995) study, clinicians start SFA therapy by presenting an SFA chart to a client with WFD. The target word is represented by either a line-drawing picture or a photograph in the center of the SFA chart and surrounded by six different semantic categories (a.k.a. attributes) related to the target word, including:

- group (e.g., *it is a* _____),
- use (e.g., *you use it to/for* _____),
- action (e.g., *what does it do?*),
- properties (e.g., *describe it*),
- location (e.g., *where do you find it?*), and
- association (e.g., *what does it make you think of?*).

An example of SFA charts is presented in Figure 9–1 (adapted from Boyle, 2010). The clinician encourages the client to name the target picture. Regardless of the success of naming

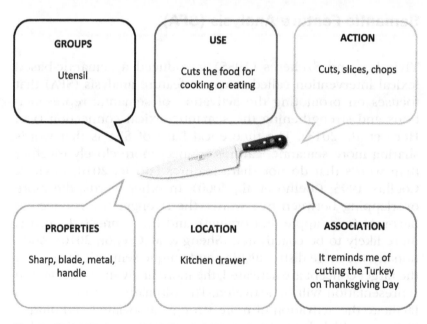

Figure 9–1. An example of SFA charts (Target Word: Knife). Adapted from Boyle, M. (2004) *Aphasiology, 28*(1), 1–24.

the picture, the client is required to use the SFA chart to verbally generate semantic features for the target picture, and the clinician writes down the features named by the client on the semantic chart. If the client cannot verbally name a feature spontaneously, the clinician can provide cues to elicit verbal production of features, such as using fill-in-the-blank or "wh" questions. If these cues still do not elicit responses, the clinician can provide verbal cues using binary-forced choices, such as "*is it long* or *short?*" The goal is to have the client complete the chart by providing features of all semantic attributes. After the chart is completed, the client is asked to name the target picture again. If the client still cannot name the picture successfully, the clinician names the picture, asks the client to repeat the target word, and then reviews all the features (Boyle & Coelho, 1995). Cues should be gradually faded as the client increasingly gains independence in generating features to facilitate word retrieval. It is advised that clients complete the SFA chart with minimal prompts in order to engage in a systemic and effective word retrieval process (Boyle, 2010). Appendix 9–1 provides a lesson plan example of SFA.

Modified Procedure of SFA

Because SFA does not have a standardized procedure and protocols, several modified procedures have been proposed and reported, such as:

- Modifying the modality of lexical production: For example, clients can either say or write the generated semantic features.
- Modifying the numbers of semantic categories (attributes): For example, only three instead of six semantic categories are listed on the SFA chart.
- Modifying the minimum number of generated responses for each sematic category: For example, one semantic feature versus three features per category.

Hashimoto and Frome (2011) examined the effects of all three aforementioned SFA modifications on an individual with moderate to severe Broca's aphasia with apraxia of speech. The sole participant showed increased naming accuracy of the trained items in naturalistic contexts, but naming accuracy declined over time after the treatment. Hashimoto and Frome (2011) concluded that reducing the number of semantic categories may be sufficient to improve naming accuracy; however, it may not be sufficient to maintain the treatment gain over time. Reducing the number of required semantic categories in the modified SFA may still promote the effectiveness of word retrieval. However, based on other studies (Coelho et al., 2000; Conley & Coelho, 2003; Rider et al., 2008), the number of semantic features generated by the clients is an important element of SFA intervention as recalling semantic features strengthens the semantic-lexical connections. Hence, it is highly recommended having the clients generate as many semantic features as possible to facilitate successful word retrieval.

Modified SFA for Verbs

Another modification to SFA is changing the word classes of targeted words. The original SFA and modifications discussed above are all targeting nouns or objects. Wambaugh and Ferguson (2007) and Wambaugh, Mauszycki, and Wright (2014) incorporated the concepts of argument structure and modified the six semantic categories to promote successful verb retrieval. Figure 9–2 is an example SFA chart for verbs (adapted from Wambaugh et al., 2014).

The modified treatment procedure for verbs is similar to the original SFA. Clinicians start the treatment by asking clients to name the target verb. Regardless of verb naming accuracy, the client is asked to complete the verb semantic chart from the top and then move to the bottom by verbally producing the semantic features. The modified semantic categories for verbs include subject, the purpose of action, part of body or tool used to carry out the action, description, location, and associated objects or actions. Clinicians write the responses produced by the client in the corresponding box on the chart. After all categories are filled, the client is asked to name the target verb again. If the client cannot correctly name the action word, the clinician reviews all the features with the client again.

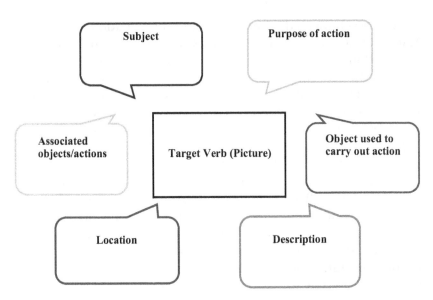

Figure 9–2. Verb SFA chart example. Adapted from Wambaugh, J., Mauszycki, S., and Wright, S. (2014).

Wambaugh et al. (2014) examined the effects of a modified SFA for verbs in four individuals with chronic anomia. Their results show three out of the four participants improved their verb naming accuracy after treatment and were able to maintain the gain up to six weeks after the treatment. However, generalization to untrained verbs was not found. In Webster and Whitworth's systematic review (2012), they suggested that word retrieval intervention for nouns can be effective for verbs, but the improvement on verb naming is less robust and limited. The effectiveness may be influenced by the individual's cognitive functions as well as the severity of lexical impairment. In other words, individuals with more severe lexical impairments may show less treatment gains.

Research Evidence That Supports the Efficacy of SFA

Several systemic reviews and meta-analysis studies showed that SFA is effective in improving the accuracy of picture naming (confrontation naming). However, generalization to untrained words and connected speech is limited (Efstratiadou et al., 2018; Maddy et al., 2014; Quique et al., 2019). In a recent systematic review done by Efstratiadou et al. (2018), the generalization to untrained words and connected speech was reported in approximately 40% of participants, whereas maintenance of trained words was reported in almost 60% of participants. SFA seems more effective for individuals with mild to moderate fluent aphasia (Boyle, 2010; Efstratiadou et al., 2018) and without non-verbal cognitive impairments (Boyle, 2010).

In Boyle's systematic review (2010), the author indicated that asking the client to generate features or to respond to the semantic features generated by the clinician resulted in improved noun naming across fluent and nonfluent aphasia with mild to moderate severity. However, SFA intervention that required clients generating semantic features rather than reviewing features generated by the clinicians can have a longer-lasting effect after the treatment.

Gravier and colleagues (2018) stated that the most important factor of promoting SFA's effectiveness is the number of semantic features generated by clients. This factor is also a good predictor for the improvement of trained words and untrained but semantically related words. Gravier et al.'s finding is also supported by Quique et al. (2019). Quique and colleagues' meta-analysis of SFA outcomes also concluded that the number of semantic features generated by clients during SFA treatment was a reliable predictor for improvement on both trained and untrained semantically connected words. In addition, they suggested that overtraining words, which means continuing the treatment procedure after reaching the established accuracy, may promote generalization.

Verb Network Strengthening Treatment (VNeST)

Verb Network Strengthening Treatment (VNeST) is a therapy approach that targets lexical retrieval by promoting retrieval of verbs and related argument structure. Retrieving and processing verbs can be more complex than nouns because syntactic information has to be incorporated when forming lexical concepts of verbs. (Wambaugh & Ferguson, 2007; Wambaugh, Mauszycki, & Wright, 2014). VNeST aims to strengthen the verb semantic network and its connection to argument structures by asking clients to generate pairs of agents (i.e., the entity that carries out the action of the verb) and patients (i.e., the entity that directly receives the action of the verb). An example of an agent-verb-patient pair is carpenter [agent] *cut (verb)* wood [patient]. The argument structure is the interface between semantics and syntax (Webster & Whitworth, 2012, p. 621). Increasing the activation of verbs and their argument structures facilitie the effectiveness of lexical retrieval and sentence production (Edmonds, 2016; Edmonds & Babb, 2011; Edmonds, Mammino, & Ojeda, 2014).

Treatment Procedures of VNeST

As implemented in Edmonds, Nadeau, and Kiran's study in 2009, clinicians start VNeST by selecting a list of transitive verbs which can accept one or more objects. Examples of appropriate transitive verbs are "push", "measure", and "cut". Write each verb on a 3×5" or 4×6" card and then create five stimulus cards saying the following words: [*who*], [*what*], [*where*], [*when*], and [*why*] respectively. The treatment steps are summarized below. Appendix 9–2 provides a lesson plan example of VNeST.

- Step 1: Set up. Present the verb card in the middle between the two stimulus cards saying [who] and [what] as the sequence of [who]-verb-[what]. Figure 9–3 illustrates an example of VNeST card arrangement.
- Step 2: Generating agents. Prompt the client to verbally generate three (3) agent examples for the target verb, such as [policeman], [cat], [children] for "chase." Write the responses on three cards, respectively, and add these below the [who] card.
- Step 3: Generating patients. Prompt the client to verbally generate three (3) complementary patient examples relative to Step 2, such as [thief], [mouse], [ball] for "chase." Write the responses on three cards respectively, and add them below the [what] card.

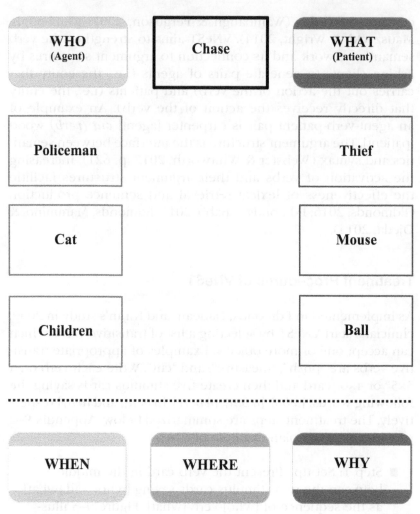

Figure 9–3. An example of VNeST cards arrangement (adapted from Edmonds & Babb, 2011).

- Step 4: Discussing agent/patient pairs. Have the client choose one agent/patient pair, such as [policeman/thief] to discuss and ask the client to answer wh-questions about the pair using the remaining three stimulus cards (*when, where, why*). For example, "*Why does a policeman chase a thief?*"
- Step 5: Semantic judgment. The clinician reads four (4) sentences that contain appropriate and inappropriate

agent/patient pairs with the target verb and have the client make a judgment if the sentence makes sense. The sentences should include at least one appropriate sentence, one with inappropriate agent role, one with inappropriate patient role, and one with the agent and patient switched (Edmonds, Nadeau, & Kiran, 2009).

■ Step 6: Generating agent/patient pairs. Without using the stimulus cards, ask the client to independently generate three (3) agent/patient pairs for the verb.

Research Evidence That Supports the Efficacy of VNeST

When generating thematic roles from a given verb, this process can simultaneously activate the relevant words and world knowledge (Edmonds et al., 2014; Edmonds, 2016; McRae et al., 2005). It is based on the theory that thematic roles co-activate other associated verbs (Ferretti, McRae, & Hatherrell, 2001; McRae et al., 2005). Verbs and the related argument structures are neurally coactivated, suggesting that the verb activates additional agents and patients and vice versa. Thus, repeated and simultaneous activations can strengthen the shared verb semantic network. When accessing the target verb, other semantically related verbs may also be activated due to spreading activation, such as [cut] vs. [trim], [slice], and [chop] (Edmonds et al., 2009; Webster & Whitworth, 2012). The activation of semantically related verbs could further facilitate the production of sentences that contains these verbs.

Edmonds, Nadeau, and Kiran (2009) reported the effects of VNeST in four individuals with moderate aphasia. They found that VNeST facilitated successful retrieval of agents and patients in sentences containing trained and semantically related but untrained verbs. In addition, generalization to connected speech was observed in three out of the four participants. Edmonds and Babb (2011) further examined the effects of VNeST in two individuals with moderate to severe aphasia. After VNeST, one of the two participants showed limited generalization, but both of them showed improvement on functional communication. They suggested that more treatment hours are needed for clients with severe aphasia in order to achieve a comparable treatment effect.

Phonological Component Analysis (PCA)

As discussed above, semantic-based interventions focus on strengthening the semantic-lexical connection to promote successful word retrieval. On the other hand, phonological-based interventions intend to strengthen the lexical-phonological connections (van Hees et al., 2013). Based on Coelho, McHugh, and Boyle's SFA treatment procedure (2000), Leonard et al. (2008) introduced a phonological-based intervention called Phonological Component Analysis (PCA). Instead of generating semantic features, individuals with WFD are required to verbally produce five phonological components associated with the target word.

Treatment Procedures of PCA

The procedures of PCA are similar to SFA that starts by presenting a chart to the client with WFD. The target word is represented by either a line-drawing picture or a photograph in the center of the PCA chart and surrounded by five different phonological components. First, the clinician asks the client to name the stimulus picture. Whether the client can correctly name the target picture or not, the clinician asks the client to verbally produce phonological components using the chart and writes the client's response on it. The five components are listed below.

1. Rhymes: "What does this rhyme with?"
2. First sound: "What sound does it start with?"
3. First sound associate: "What other word starts with the same sound?"
4. Final sound: "What sound does it end with?"
5. Number of syllables: "How many beats does the word have?"

   If the client cannot spontaneously produce phonological components, the clinician then provides up to an array of three choices for the client to pick from. The choices are presented on a card and read aloud by the clinician. For example, for the target word "*cat,*" the clinician could say "*bat, desk, mug*" to the client and have the client choose the word that rhymes with "*cat.*" After all components are successfully generated, the client is asked to name the target picture again. If the client could not successfully name the target word, the clinician would review all phonological components with the client and ask them to name the picture again. If the client still cannot name the picture successfully, the clinician provides the correct response and asks the client to repeat it. Figure 9–4 is an example of PCA charts and Appendix 9–3 provides a lesson plan example of PCA.

Research Evidence That Supports the Efficacy of PCA

The effects and efficacy of PCA have been supported by Leonard et al. (2008). Their results indicated that seven out of ten participants in their study showed noticeable improvement, and treatment effects were maintained for at least a month after treatment. In addition, five out of these seven participants were able to independently generate phonological components at least 50% of the time. They claimed that the key ingredient to the long-lasting treatment effects was the clients' active participation in therapy.

In 2013, van Hees et al. compared the effects of SFA and PCA in eight individuals with mild to moderate aphasia. Despite the locus of lexical impairment, seven out of the eight participants showed immediate post-treatment effect after PCA treatment while only 4 out of 8 participants showed improvement after SFA treatment. van Hees et al. (2013) indicated that SFA not only increases semantic specificity of the target words but also engages phonological processing. Similarly, PCA involves both phonological and semantic processing. Therefore, treatment planning should not be solely based on the types of lexical errors produced by the clients.

Phonomotor Treatment (PMT)

Phonomotor treatment (PMT) for word retrieval is a relatively new approach developed by Kendall and her colleagues (Kendall et al., 2019; Kendall & Nadeau, 2016; Kendall et al., 2015). PMT aims to strengthen the connection between lexical and phonological

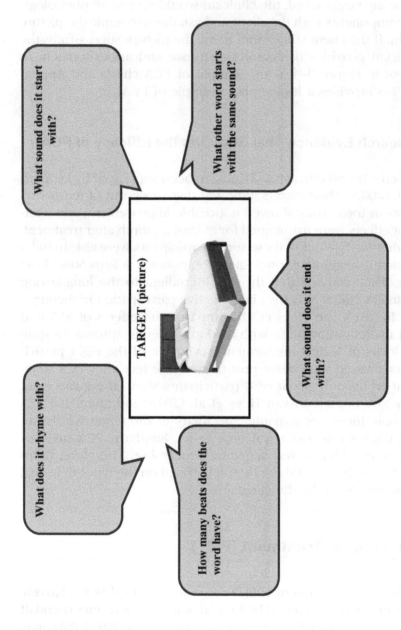

Figure 9–4. An example of PCA charts (Target Word: Bed). Adapted from van Hees, Angwin, McMahon, and Copland (2013).

representations by systematically training sounds and sound sequences. Kendall and her colleagues introduced the training of phonemes in one- to three-syllabic real words and nonwords through intensive and multimodal approaches, such as auditory, articulatory-motor, orthographic, visual, and tactile. Their theoretical base is that generalization may happen when the untrained items share similar phonological sequence with the trained items. For example, training words that rhyme with the target word (e.g., cat/kæt/) can enhance the production of rhyming words (e.g., hat/hæt/, bat/bæt/, rat/ræt/) because of the shared phonological sequence (e.g., /æt/). Kendall et al. (2015) stated using multimodal training can further strengthen phonological representation and improve phonological awareness.

Treatment Procedures of PMT

PMT is a bottom-up approach that focuses on articulation and phonetic encoding and is delivered across two stages. Stage One focuses on sounds in isolation and Stage Two trains sound combinations, such as consonant-vowel-consonant (CVC) and consonant-consonant-vowel-consonant (CCVC) combinations. In Stage One, the clinician asks the client to discriminate and identify the target sound or word in auditory perception tasks. In Stage Two, the client is asked to produce sounds in isolation and sound combinations in real and non-real words with the assistance of mouth pictures, mirrors, motor description, and clinician's verbal prompts. Appendix 9–4 is a simplified lesson plan example of PMA. The detailed training manual is available online (https://canvas.uw.edu/courses/1166215).

Research Evidence That Supports the Efficacy of PMA

Kendall et al. (2015) found that both naming accuracy of untrained nouns and treatment effects of trained nouns were maintained three months after PMT treatment in 26 individuals with chronic aphasia. Furthermore, Kendall et al. (2019) compared treatment effects between PMT and SFA in individuals with anomia. They discovered that naming accuracy of trained words and untrained words that shared features with the trained words improved after PMT. However, generalization to untrained words that do not share features with the trained words was not found. More research to support the generalization from trained to untrained words after PMT is warranted.

Semantic-Based Versus Phonological-Based Lexical Treatments

According to the lexical access models, naming errors may reflect the locus of the deficit. It is common to presume that phonological-based treatments benefit individuals with WFD who tend to make phonemic errors, and semantic-based treatments are more effective for clients who have more semantic errors. However, clinicians should not make clinical decisions solely based on the types of lexical errors and assume these errors are caused by a specific locus of deficits in word retrieval processes (Lorenz & Ziegler, 2009; Nickels, 2002). For example, semantic paraphasia may be the result of deficits at the lemma level, lexeme level, or the combination of both. Several areas of breakdown can also lead primarily to phonological errors. In addition, it is also possible that clients make both types of lexical errors and respond positively to both phonological-based and semantic-based treatments. Therefore, clinicians should avoid making clinical decisions solely based on types of lexical errors (Neumann, 2018; Nickels, 2002).

Lorenz and Ziegler (2009) investigated the relationship between the types of lexical errors and the outcome of semantic-based and phonological-based interventions in ten individuals with aphasia. Their findings revealed that the participants with semantic anomia benefited from phonological-based lexical treatment and the participants with phonological anomia improved after the semantic-based lexical treatment. Phonological-based treatment generated short-term, immediate, and word-specific improvement in most clients. No generalization to untrained words was observed after either treatment programs. They also stated that semantic-based treatments seemed to support a more conscious retrieval by strengthening the semantic level and the connection between semantic and lexical levels, which further facilitates the activation of the corresponding word forms and phonological representations. On the other hand, phonological-based treatments seemed to generate an automatic retrieval process that requires less cognitive engagement compared to semantic-based treatment. They concluded that both semantic- and phonological-based lexical treatment can strengthen the connection between semantical and phonological levels because both interventions address more than one level of lexical processing.

Neumann (2018) compared the effects between SFA and PCA on word retrieval in four individuals with aphasia. The finding showed that both interventions were effective for participants with mild anomia but not for participants with moderate anomia. She explained that both interventions provided the clients with the opportunity to process both semantic and phonological information. However, activating semantic elements seemed to result in longer-lasting improvement than activating phonological elements. She also suggested that activation of both semantic and phonological processes could strengthen the bidirectional connections between semantic-lexical and lexical-phonological levels. According to Wisenburn and Mahoney's meta-analysis (2009), semantic, phonemic, and combined treatments were effective in improving word finding even though sematic-based intervention seemed to yield better generalization to untrained words.

Target Selection Considerations

There is no standard protocol regarding word selection for therapy, and strategies for selecting target words/items remain unclear. When selecting target words for therapy, several factors should be considered, such as the severity of WFD and lexical factors, including word frequency, imageability, age of acquisition, word class, neighborhood density, context, and so forth. A comprehensive review of lexical factors that are related to word retrieval can be found in Chapter 5. In this section, our discussion will focus on selecting atypical words and personally relevant words for treatment.

Using Atypical Words and Complex Words

Selecting more complex or atypical words for word retrieval intervention is considered a relatively new approach. It is a top-down approach that activates and strengthens the semantic network via more complex, abstract, and low-frequency words. This approach is based on the theory that training items that are more complex can facilitate the generalization to less complex, untrained items (Kiran & Thompson, 2019). Kiran (2007) stated that prototypical features are commonly shared by more members in the lexical network because of the generic representation and commonality. Therefore, typical members in the network share more features with each other while atypical members share fewer features with other members. For example, typical members of the fish family [salmon] and [tuna] share more prototypical semantic features (e.g., *sea animal, scale,* and *fin*), whereas atypical members of the fish family [sting ray] and [seahorse] share fewer features (e.g., only *sea animal*).

The implementation of using atypical words (i.e., more complex, abstract, and low-frequency words) in lexical treatment to promote generalization to untrained typical words is supported by several studies (Kiran, 2007; Kiran & Thompson, 2003). Kiran and Thompson (2003) investigated the benefit of using atypical words in semantic-based treatment in individuals with fluent aphasia. They discovered that training atypical words (e.g., *scallions, artichoke*) resulted in improvement in untrained typical words (e.g., *carrot, cauliflower*) and intermediate words (e.g., *green beans, gourd*) in the same semantic category (e.g., [vegetables] in this example). On the other hand, no generalization from training typical words to atypical words was found. Kiran and Thompson (2003) claimed that training atypical words highlights unique and different semantic features within the same category which facilitate greater access to untrained and less complex words. Therefore, they encouraged clinicians to consider targeting atypical words when implementing semantic-based treatment to promote generalization. Kiran and Johnson (2008) also examined the generalization effects of treating atypical items in facilitating retrieval of untrained typical items. Their results revealed that generalization to untrained typical items was found in two out of the three participants.

However, it should be noted that selecting more complex, abstract, and low-frequency words for word retrieval intervention can be challenging to clients. Some clients may respond positively to the complexity approach, but some may not. Hence, it is important for clinicians to be aware that this type of approach may work better for people with mild word-finding difficulty than someone with severe anomia.

Using Personally Relevant Words

A relatively common target word selection approach is choosing personally relevant and generally frequent items. The rationale of selecting these words is to keep the treatment targets functional to clients and for promoting generalization. Renvall et al. (2013) defined personally relevant items as things or topics that clients are interested in and wish to use in communication. The generally frequent words are typically identified based on general public use. However, it is not easy to identify personally relevant and generally frequent words because personally chosen items can vary from one person (e.g., identified by clients themselves) to another (e.g., identified by spouses or other family members) and also vary from one context to another. Additionally, many high-frequency words identified via analyzing word databases can be unsuitable or too general to be used in lexical treatment, such as [the], [of], [do], and so forth.

Clinicians often choose concrete and imaginable words for treatment targets, but words that can help express feelings and opinions should also be considered. Renvall et al. (2013) highlighted that target word selection should be modified based on the stages of recovery and for addressing different communication needs. Palmer et al. (2017) surveyed 100 individuals with aphasia who representing different areas of the United Kingdom to identify important words/topics they wished to say. The top eight topics were *"food and drink," "nature and gardening," "entertainment," "places," "people," "house," "clothes,"* and *"travel."* Other identified topics included *"feelings and senses," "shopping," "weather,"* and *"personal care."*

Clinicians should also keep in mind that clients can respond differently to different categories. Therefore, when clients do not respond well to one category, other categories should still be attempted, especially personally relevant categories. Some clients respond more positively to personally relevant items or activities than other types of treatment materials. It can be more motivating to clients if treatment targets are commonly used in their daily life or relevant to their hobbies or favorite activities.

Word Retrieval at Discourse Level

The ultimate goal of lexical intervention for neurogenic communication disorders is not just to address impaired linguistic abilities but also to improve clients' overall communication effectiveness and quality of life. Therefore, generalizing treatment gains from lexical-based interventions to connected speech is important (Boyle, 2011). It has been reported in a few studies that lexical cueing treatments and other semantic-based treatment, such as SFA, can be modified to promote word retrieval in connected speech.

In Peach and Reuter's study (2010), SFA procedures were modified to facilitate clients' discourse production. They identified nouns and verbs that the two participants failed to retrieve in narrative and procedural discourse tasks. Then, the clinician used these words as targets for treatment following the SFA protocol. Their findings showed that treating retrieval errors occurring in the discourse resulted in increased verbal productivity and improved informativeness of the discourse. The treatment effect also generalized to untrained nouns and verbs. Peach and Reuter (2010) stated that discourse-based SFA can better address WFD in daily communication due to higher ecological validity.

In the Cameron and colleagues (2006) study, the authors modified the lexical cueing treatment program to address word finding difficulties in connected speech. They implemented both semantic cues and phonologic cues in story retelling activities instead of picture naming tasks to facilitate connected speech production in five individuals with aphasia. Their results showed that four out of five participants successfully produced more target words and more information units that convey accurate and relevant information about the trained stories. Thus, Cameron et al.

(2006) conclude that story context may not only facilitate word retrieval but also promote generalization to connected speech.

In the Boyle (2004) study, the author modified the SFA protocol and trained three individuals with aphasia to generate semantic features when they had difficulty retrieving words during story-telling tasks. The study results showed that all participants improved on retrieving trained and untrained nouns, and the treatment effect was maintained for one month after treatment. In addition, all three participants produced more correct information units during storytelling activities.

In summary, although the research evidence is still limited, targeting word retrieval at the discourse level could promote generalization to real-life conversations. Boyle (2011) indicated that discourse can facilitate overall process of word retrieval instead of just improving *"the ability to name specific items."* Therefore, clinicians could consider training clients to apply the practiced word retrieval techniques to their daily conversations by incorporating story context or discourse tasks. When experiencing word finding difficulties, instead of being frustrated and agitated, clients can utilize various cues (e.g., describing properties [semantic] or saying the first sound [phonological]) to facilitate word retrieval and promote communication success.

Writing and Word Retrieval

In the previous sections, our discussions focused on the use of semantic and phonological cues to improve word retrieval. In this section, we discuss the use of orthographic cues and incorporating writing modality to promote successful verbal production of words.

Using Orthographic Cues

Orthographic cues give information about the spelling of the word. Writing the whole word (e.g., [PHONE]), the first letter (e.g., [P]), or spelling the word aloud (e.g., [P-H-O-N-E]) can all be used to facilitate word retrieval. See Table 9–1 for the examples of orthographic cues. However, it should be noticed that regularity of orthographic-phonological conversion (OPC) of the target's initial letter can impact the effectiveness of orthographic cues (Lorenz & Nickels, 2007). An example of words starting with regular OPC of initial letter is the word [DOG]; the initial letter represents the initial phoneme /d/. On the other hand, an example of words starting with irregular OPC of initial letter is the word [HOUR]; the initial letter does not represent the initial phoneme /aʊ/.

Lorenz and Nickels (2007) examined the effects of using orthographic cueing alone in three individuals with chronic anomic aphasia. Their findings showed that letter cues are effective in improving naming even for the clients who did not benefit from phonological cues. Lorenz and Nickels (2007) suggested that the processing of orthographic cues may not rely on the same mechanism as phonological cues. Thus, they recommended that letter cues should be used to facilitate naming for those clients who show a limited response to phonological cues.

Greenwood and colleagues (2010) examined the effect of combining phonological and orthographic cues in supporting word retrieval in an individual with moderate WFD due to aphasia. Both forms of cues were presented. When the sole participant was not able to name the target word, the first phoneme and grapheme were given. If the participant was still not able to name the word, the first syllable was given and then followed by the whole word. The participant showed significant improvement in picture naming after the treatment, and generalization to untreated words was also noted. Additionally, there was a small but positive change of word retrieval in the participant's connected speech.

However, the effectiveness of orthographic cues is not fully supported by literature (Best et al., 2002; Howard & Harding, 1998). Researchers have pointed out that the effectiveness of orthographic cues is related to clients' ability of sounding out letters or reading nonwords (Best et al., 2002). As discussed above, clinicians should consider giving a test trial on different types of cues and combination of cues (e.g., semantic, phonological, and orthographic cues) and carefully monitor clients' responses to the cues to identify what combination of cues works best for clients.

Treatment Programs Incorporating Writing

Writing requires the selection of letterforms and the planning/ execution of motor movements. Additionally, this process requires successful phoneme-to grapheme conversion. There are several well-established treatment programs that aim to improve individuals' abilities to successfully retrieve target words and effectively communicate through writing, such as Anagram and Copy Treatment (ACT; Beeson, 1999), Copy and Recall Therapy (CART; Beeson et al., 2003), and Anagram, Copy, and Recall Treatment (ACRT; Helm-Estabrooks & Albert, 2004). However, these types of treatment programs are not suitable for all clients with WFD or neurogenic language disorders. Candidacy requirements include the ability to copy words, good single-word reading comprehension, relatively spared visual memory, and motivation (Helm-Estabrooks et al., 2014). Appendix 9–5 provides a lesson plan example of ACT and Appendix 9–6 is a lesson plan example of CART.

Using Other Communication Modalities to Promote Lexical Retrieval

In this section, we discuss the use of other communication modalities to promote successful verbal production of words, such as the use of gestures and drawing. Clinicians can systematically introduce other communication modalities by following well-established procedures or implement these communication modalities as needed to promote verbal production and communication effectiveness. One example of well-established procedures is Gestural Facilitation of Naming (GES); one example of a loose procedure is Promoting Aphasics' Communicative Effectiveness (PACE; Davis & Wilcox, 1985). PACE aims to increase the communicative effectiveness of individuals with aphasia through any communication modality (Davis, 2005). PACE is not a structured, impairment-based treatment program. Instead, PACE only proposes four treatment principles, including equal participation, new information, communication modality choice, and natural feedback for clinicians to follow. Clients are encouraged to use different communication modalities during PACE activities, such as gestures, drawing, writing, or facial expressions. Appendix 9–7 provides an example lesson plan of PACE.

Gestures and Word Retrieval

As discussed in Chapter 3, gestures and language, two symbolic systems, are strongly correlated and share common cognitive processes. Additionally, neuroimaging studies suggested that comprehension of symbolic gesture and language may be supported by overlapping brain areas (Xu et al., 2009). Different theoretical models (de Ruiter, 2000; Krauss et al., 2000; Rose & Douglas, 2008) suggest that gestures can either directly or indirectly assist lexical access and word retrieval.

Structured Treatment Procedures

Several gesture lexical treatment programs were proposed and discussed in aphasia literature. For example, the concept of Gestural Facilitation of Naming (GES) was proposed and discussed in several studies. (Attard et al., 2013; Marshall et al., 2012; Rose, 2006). The general procedures of GES are summarized below.

- Present the client with a picture card and model the spoken word and associated gesture of the target picture.
- Have the client imitate the gesture three times. If the client is unable to imitate or makes errors, provide hand-over-hand prompting until they can successfully produce the gesture.
- Have the client imitate the verbal production of the target. If the client is unable to imitate, have the client imitate each syllable of the word before imitating the entire word.
- Have the client imitate both the gesture and the verbal production of the target three times.
- After a brief pause (5 seconds), prompt the participant to provide the name and gesture for the target picture and repeat it 3 times. If they are unable to remember the name (verbal production) of the target, model both outputs for the client to repeat three times.

Raymer and colleagues (2006) proposed a treatment program called Gesture + Verbal Training (GVT), which is similar to GES. The clinician first modeled the target word and gesture and then asked the participants to produce the target word and gesture three times. Secondly, the clinician presented the gesture in isolation and asked the participants to imitate the gesture three times. Thirdly, the clinician presented the word and asked the participants to repeat it three times. Lastly, after a 5-second pause, the participant was promoted to show and tell what was in the picture. Raymer et al. (2006) examined the effects of GVT on word retrieval in nine participants with mild to severe anomia. Their findings showed that GVT was effective in improving word retrieval in most participants, thereby increasing their use of gestures. In addition, the improvement was found in both trained nouns and verbs. However, the generalization to unstrained words was found in gesture production but not in verbal production. They concluded that GVT increased the participants' awareness in using gestures to promote word retrieval and communication effectiveness.

Raymer et al. (2012) compared a gesture training program to errorless naming intervention in eight individuals with moderate to severe anomia. During the gesture training, they followed a similar procedure of GVT with some modifications listed in the Raymer et al. study (2006). They found that both errorless naming therapy and gestural training were effective in improving word retrieval. Their findings indicated that the participants used gestures as a means of compensatory communication after therapy.

However, Marshall et al. (2012) claimed that stand-alone pantomime (gesture) training did not promote word retrieval, and pantomime gestures are cognitively demanding for individuals with brain injury to learn. They reported that participants with severe aphasia responded better to verbal naming therapy than gesture therapy.

Using Gestures as Cues for Word Retrieval

Rose and Douglas (2008) examined the effects of gesture naming therapy alone, verbal naming therapy alone, and the combination of the two therapy programs on word retrieval in one individual with anomia. During the gesture training, the participant was asked to use a gesture before naming the target. The gestures were spontaneously generated by the participant, and the clinician elicited the response by saying, "*Show me how you could represent this object with your hands."* If the participant was unsuccessful, a correct gesture was modeled by the clinician. They found that the gesture training was equally effective as the verbal treatment and the combined treatment, and the improvement was maintained up to three months. They highlighted that the naming therapy should focus on the function and feature of the target words.

Carragher et al. (2013) examined the effect of the combination of semantic, phonological, orthographic, and gestural cues on facilitating verb retrieval in nine individuals with chronic nonfluent aphasia. The participants were presented with a visual organizer similar to the SFA chart with six components including the subject (who usually does it?), purpose (why does this happen?), how (what body part is used?), associations (what tools are necessary?), location (where does this usually happen?), and gesture (associated hand/arm gesture). The participants were required to generate features for each category, either verbally or nonverbally. They were instructed to use the gestures from the Makaton communication program (http://www.makaton .org) to communicate, and all gestures were modeled using one hand. All semantic features were discussed before the clinician asked the participant to name the target action word. Phonological and orthographic cues were provided until the participant was able to successfully name the action word. The participants then were required to repeat the verb three times, along with the gesture. Their findings showed that the multicomponent approach was effective for retrieving verbs regardless of the root problem of word finding difficulty (e.g., semantic-based or phonological-based). However, generalization to untreated verbs only occurred in the participants with less impaired verb retrieval.

What do we learn from the related research studies? Most studies we reviewed supported the efficacy of using gesture and verbal combined treatment to improve word retrieval for individuals with WFD. It should be noted that some clients may have limb apraxia, but the severity of limb apraxia does not always predict gesture gains (Marshall et al, 2012). Therefore, the diagnosis and severity of limb apraxia should not be used as a sole criterion to consider clients for gesture training. As suggested by Rose and Douglas (2008), clinicians can elicit a gesture either by asking clients to simply show how to present the target word using their hands or by following the well-established training protocols, such as GES or GVT. Box 9–1 lists tips for incorporating gestures in lexical treatment. In summary, gestures can be used to assist word retrieval by reactivating semantic representations or serve as a means of communication.

Box 9–1. Tips for Incorporating Gestures in Lexical Treatment

- Combine gestures with verbal treatment to improve word retrieval.
- Even if the client has limb apraxia, gesture training may still be an option.
- The clinician will need to consider the cognitive demands before teaching a client pantomime gestures.
- Clients can use gestures to assist with word retrieval or as a means of compensatory communication
- Utilize gestures and verbal treatment for best results in clients with anomia.
- Example of GES:
  - Step 1: The clinician presents the image (e.g., *toothbrush*) and models the target word and gesture three times.
  - Step 2: The client will reproduce the target word and gesture three times.
  - Step 3: The clinician models only the gesture without verbal production and asks the client to imitate the gesture three times.
  - Step 4: The clinician provides the target word without the gesture and asks the client to repeat the word three times.
  - Step 5: After 5 seconds, ask the client to show and tell what is in the picture (e.g., *toothbrush*).

*The client should respond by verbally naming the picture and providing the appropriate gesture.

Drawing and Word Retrieval

Compared to writing, drawing relies on the activation of the right hemisphere and non-linguistic system, so drawing can be a less cognitively and linguistically demanding task than writing for individuals with moderate to severe aphasia or other neurogenic language disorders. Drawing can bring people's attention to an object's structural and perceptual features, which facilitates the processing of semantic features (Gleichgerrcht et al., 2016; Hung & Ostergren, 2019). Thus, instead of introducing drawing as an alternative communication modality, clinicians can offer drawing as a type of cueing strategy to promote effectiveness of word retrieval.

Farias et al. (2006) found that the act of drawing significantly improved naming ability in comparison to writing because the action of drawing facilitated the use of non-lexical routes to access semantic knowledge via the right hemisphere. They also pointed out that the quality of drawing did not correlate with naming accuracy. In the study of Hung and Ostergren (2019), the authors also compared the effect of drawing and writing on facilitating noun retrieval. Their results showed that individuals with aphasia improved their naming ability when asked to draw the target picture rather than to write the name of the picture. They concluded that when people drew, they actively recalled the visual attributes of the object, which in turn deepens the semantic processing and facilitates the word retrieval process.

Furthermore, Kinney and colleagues (2020) reported that significant improvement was found when people with aphasia completed the SFA chart and drew the target object. However, significant improvement in naming accuracy was not observed when clients only completed the SFA chart or in drawing only conditions. Kinney et al. (2020) suggested that the incorporation of drawing strategy promoted improvement of confrontation naming.

To summarize, drawing can encourage clients with WFD to actively recall semantic features of the target/intended word, which promotes the effectiveness of word retrieval. Therefore, clinicians could consider incorporating drawing as a type of cueing strategy and encourage clients to actively recall semantic features instead of just using drawing as an alternative mode of communication. Box 9–2 lists tips for incorporating drawing in lexical treatment.

Box 9–2. Tips for Incorporating Drawing in Lexical Treatment

- Use the drawing instruments that are easiest for the client, such as pens, pencils, markers, crayons, and so forth.
- Encourage the client to draw and do not mind the quality of drawing.
- When the client experiences difficulty with drawing, clinicians may consider implementing the prompts listed below.
  - "Are you able to imagine the object in your head? If not, try closing your eyes."
  - "Start with the overall shape of the object."
  - "If you can't draw the object, what about drawing the context you usually see the object in?"
- The client can draw additional objects that are related to the target/context, such as drawing both *pepper* and *salt* for the target [salt]).
- Have the client describe the features of the object before, during, or after drawing it.
  - Use, group, location, properties, action association.
- Have the client connect the drawing to a personal experience. For example, the clinician can ask, "*Have you ever used [salt]? Why did you need to use it last time?*"

Conclusion

Word retrieval has been a hallmark deficit in a vast majority of neurogenic communication disorders regardless of type, severity, and time post onset. In this chapter, we reviewed several commonly implemented treatment approaches for word retrieval deficits along with the research evidence that supports the treatment effects and efficacy. Each treatment approach has its advantages and limitations. It is always critical to be aware of its strengths and weaknesses before implementing a specific treatment approach and to follow the protocol developed by the researchers in order to obtain the optimal effects of the treatment. However, it should also be noted that it can be challenging when applying well-controlled laboratory conditions to real-life clinical practice. The intention of presenting the variety of word retrieval treatment approaches is to expand your clinical toolbox with the most current research evidence. As advocated by ASHA, evidence-based practice should guide our clinical decisions and treatment selection. However, modifications to the treatment protocol may be necessary, based on the client's response to treatment and the scaffolding needed for improvement.

Discussion Questions

1. Describe the procedures of any two semantic-based lexical treatment approaches described in this chapter.
2. Describe the procedures of any two phonological-based lexical treatment approaches described in this chapter.
3. What are the similarities and differences between semantic-based and phonological-based lexical treatment approaches?
4. What are the considerations of selecting target words in lexical treatment activities for neurogenic communication disorders?
5. How do you promote generalization of treatment gains to a client's functional communication?

References

Attard, M. C., Rose, M. L., & Lanyon, L. (2013). The comparative effects of Multi-Modality Aphasia Therapy and Constraint-Induced Aphasia Therapy-Plus for severe chronic Broca's aphasia: An in-depth pilot study. *Aphasiology, 27*(1), 80–111.

Beeson, P. M. (1999). Treating acquired writing impairments: Strengthening graphemic representations. *Aphasiology, 13,* 767–785.

Beeson, P. M., Rising, K., & Volk, J. (2003). Writing treatment for severe aphasia: Who benefits? *Journal of Speech, Language, and Hearing Research, 46,* 1038–1060.

Best, W., Herbert, R., Hickin, J., Osborne, F., & Howard, D. (2002). Phonological and orthographic facilitation of word-retrieval in aphasia: Immediate and delayed effects. *Aphasiology, 16,* 151–168. https://doi.org/10.1080/02687040143000483

Boyle, M. (2004). Semantic feature analysis treatment for anomia in two fluent aphasia syndromes. *American Journal of Speech-Language Pathology, 13*(3), 236–249. https://doi.org/10.1044/1058-0360(2004/025)

Boyle, M. (2010). Semantic feature analysis treatment for aphasic word retrieval impairments: What's in a name? *Topics in Stroke Rehabilitation, 17*(6), 411–422. https://doi.org/10.1310/tsr1706–411

Boyle, M. (2011). Discourse treatment for word retrieval impairment in aphasia: The story so far. *Aphasiology, 25*(11), 1308–1326. https://doi.org/10.1080/02687038.2011.596185

Boyle M., & Coelho, C. (1995). Application of semantic feature analysis as a treatment for aphasic dysnomia. *American Journal of Speech-Language Pathology, 4*(4), 94–98. https://doi.org/10.1044/1058-0360.0404.94

Cameron, R. M., Wambaugh, J. L., Wright, S. M., & Nessler, C. L. (2006). Effects of a combined semantic/phonological cueing treatment on word retrieval in discourse. *Aphasiology, 20*(2-4), 269–285. https://doi.org/10.1080/02687030500473387

Carragher, M., Sage, K., & Conroy, P. (2013). The effects of verb retrieval therapy for people with non-fluent aphasia: Evidence from assessment tasks and conversation. *Neuropsychological Rehabilitation, 23*(6), 846–887. 10.1080/09602011.2013.832335

Coelho, C. A., McHugh, R. E., & Boyle, M. (2000). Semantic feature analysis as a treatment for aphasic dysnomia: A replication. *Aphasiology, 14*(2), 133–142. https://doi.org/10.1080/026870300401513

Conley, A., & Coelho, C. (2003). Treatment of word retrieval impairment in chronic Broca's aphasia. *Aphasiology, 17,* 203–211.

Davis, G. A. (2005). PACE revisited. *Aphasiology, 19*(1), 21–38.

Davis, G. A. & Wilcox, M. J. (1985). *Adult aphasia rehabilitation: Applied pragmatics.* Singular Publishing.

de Ruiter, J. P. (2000). The production of gesture and speech. In D. McNeill (Ed.), *Language and gesture.* Cambridge University Press.

Edmonds, L. (2016). A review of Verb Network Strengthening Treatment: Theory, methods, results, and clinical implications. *Topics in Language Disorders, 36*(2), 123–135.

Edmonds, L., & Babb, M. (2011). Effect of verb network strengthening treatment in moderate to severe aphasia. *American Journal of Speech-Language Pathology, 20*(2), 131–145. https://doi.org/10.1044/1058-0360(2011/10-0036)

Edmonds, L. A., Mammino, K., & Ojeda, J. (2014). Effect of Verb Network Strengthening Treatment (VNeST) in persons with aphasia: Extension and replication of previous findings. *American Journal of Speech-Language Pathology, 23*, S312–S329.

Edmonds, L. A., Nadeau, S. E., & Kiran, S. (2009). Effect of Verb Network Strengthening Treatment (VNeST) on lexical retrieval of content words in sentences in persons with aphasia, *Aphasiology, 23*(3), 402–424. https://doi.org/ 10.1080/02687030802291339

Efstratiadou, E. A., Papathanasiou, I., Holland, R., Archonti, A., & Hilari, K. (2018). A systematic review of semantic feature analysis therapy studies for aphasia. *Journal of Speech, Language, and Hearing Research, 61*(5), 1261–1278. https://doi.org/10.1044/2018_JSLHR-L-16-0330

Farias, D., Davis, C., & Harrington, G. (2006). Drawing: Its contribution to naming in aphasia. *Brain and Language, 97*(1), 53–63. https://doi.org/10.1016/j.bandl.2005.07.074

Ferretti, T. R., McRae, K., & Hatherell, A. (2001). Integrating verbs, situation schemas, and thematic role concepts. *Journal of Memory and Language, 44*, 516–547.

Gleichgerrcht, E., Kocher, M., Nesland, T., Rorden, C., Fridriksson, J., & Bonilha, L. (2016). Preservation of structural brain network hubs is associated with less severe post-stroke aphasia. *Restorative Neurology and Neuroscience, 34*(1), 19–28. https://doi.org/10.3233/RNN-150511

Gravier, M., Dickey, M., Hula, W., Evans, W., Owens, R., Winans-Mitrik, R., & Doyle, P. (2018). What matters in semantic feature analysis: Practice-related predictors of treatment response in aphasia. *American Journal of Speech-Language Pathology, 27*(1S), 438–453. https://doi.org/10.1044/2017_AJSLP-16-0196

Greenwood, A., Grassly, J., Hickin, J., & Best, W. (2010). Phonological and orthographic cueing therapy: A case of generalised improvement. *Aphasiology, 24*(9), 991–1016. https://doi.org/10.1080/0268 7030903168220

Hashimoto, N., & Frome, A. (2011). The use of a modified semantic features analysis approach in aphasia. *Journal of Communication Disorders, 44*(4), 459–469. https://doi.org/10.1016/j.jcomdis.2011.02.004

Hart, B. (1991). Pragmatics: How language is used. *Analysis and Intervention in Developmental Disability, 1*, 299–313.

Hart, B. M., & Risley, T. R. (1974). Using preschool materials to modify the language of disadvantaged children. *Journal of Applied Behavior Analysis, 7*, 243–256.

Helm-Estabrooks, N., & Albert, M. L. (2004). *Manual of aphasia therapy.* Pro-Ed.

Helm-Estabrooks, N., Albert, M. L., & Nicholas, M. (2014). *Manual of aphasia and aphasia therapy* (3rd ed.). Pro-Ed.

Howard, D., & Harding, D. (1998). Self-cueing of word retrieval by a woman with aphasia: Why a letter board works. *Aphasiology, 12*, 399–420. https://doi.org/10.1080/02687039808249540

Hung P. & Ostergren, J. (2019). A comparison of drawing and writing on facilitating word retrieval in individuals with aphasia. *Aphasiology, 33*(12), 1462–1481. https://doi.org/10.1080/02687038.2019.160 2861

Kearns, K. P., (1997). Broca's aphasia. In L. L. LaPointe (Ed.), *Aphasia and related neurogenic language disorders* (2nd ed., pp. 1–41). Thieme Medical Publishers.

Kendall, D., Moldestad, M., Allen, W., Torrance, J., & Nadeau, S. (2019). Phonomotor versus semantic treatment for anomia in 58 persons with aphasia: A randomized control trial. *Journal of Speech, Language, and Hearing Research, 62*(12), 4464–4482. https://doi.org/ 10.1044/2019_JSLHR-L-18-0257

Kendall. D., & Nadeau, S. (2016). The phonomotor approach to treating phonological-based language deficits in people with aphasia. *Topics in Language Disorders, 36*(2), 109–122. https://doi.org/10.1097/TLD .0000000000000085

Kendall, D., Oelke, M., Brookshire, C., & Nadeau, S. (2015). The influence of phonomotor treatment on word retrieval abilities in 26 individuals with chronic aphasia: An open trial. *Journal of Speech, Language, and Hearing Research, 58*(3), 798–812. https://doi.org/10 .1044/2015_JSLHR-L-14-0131

Kinney, J., Wallace, S., & Schreiber, J. (2020). The relationship between word retrieval, drawing and semantics in people with aphasia. *Aphasiology, 34*(2), 254–274. https://doi.org/10.1080/02687038.2019.160 2862

Kiran, S. (2007). Complexity in the treatment of naming deficits. *American Journal of Speech-Language Pathology, 16*(1), 18–29. https:// doi.org/10.1044/1058-0360(2007/004)

Kiran, S., & Johnson, L. (2008). Semantic complexity in treatment of naming deficits in aphasia: Evidence from well-defined categories. *American Journal of Speech-Language Pathology, 17*(4), 389–400. https://doi.org/10.1044/1058-0360(2008/06-0085)

Kiran, S., & Thompson, C. (2003). The role of semantic complexity in treatment of naming deficits. *Journal of Speech, Language, and Hearing Research*, *46*(4), 773–787. https://doi.org/10.1044/1092-4388(2003/061)

Kiran, S., & Thompson, C. (2019). Neuroplasticity of language networks in aphasia: Advances, updates, and future challenges. *Frontiers in Neurology*, *10*, 295. https://doi.org/10.3389/fneur.2019.00295

Krauss, R., Chen, Y., & Gottesman, R. (2000). Lexical gestures and lexical access: A process model. In D. McNeill (Ed.), *Language and gesture*. Cambridge University Press.

Leonard, C., Rochon, E., & Laird, L. (2008). Treating naming impairments in aphasia: Findings from a phonological components analysis treatment, *Aphasiology*, *22*(9), 923–947. https://doi.org/10.1080/02687030701831474

Lorenz, A., & Nickels, L. (2007). Orthographic cueing in anomic aphasia: How does it work? *Aphasiology*, *21*(6-8), 670–686. https://doi.org/10.1080/02687030701192182

Lorenz, A., & Ziegler, W. (2009). Semantics vs. word-form specific techniques in anomia treatment: A multiple single case study. *Journal of Neurolinguistics*, *22*(6), 515–537. https://doi.org/10.1016/j.jneuroling.2009.05.003

Maddy, K., Capilouto, G., & McComas, K. (2014). The effectiveness of semantic feature analysis: An evidence based systematic review. *Annals of Physical and Rehabilitation Medicine*, *57*(4), 254–267. https://doi.org/10.1016/j.rehab.2014.03.002

Marshall, J., Best, W., Cocks, N., Cruice, M., Pring, T., Bulcock, G., . . . Caute, A. (2012). Gesture and naming therapy for people with severe aphasia: A group study. *Journal of Speech, Language, and Hearing Research*, *55*(3), 726–738. https://doi.org/10.1044/1092-4388(2011/11-0219)

McRae, K., Hare, E., & Ferretti, T. R. (2005). A basis for generating expectancies for verbs from nouns. *Memory & Cognition*, *33*, 1174–1184.

Meteyard, L., & Bose, A. (2018). What does a cue do? Comparing phonological and semantic cues for picture naming in aphasia. *Journal of Speech, Language, and Hearing Research*, *61*(3), 658–674. https://doi.org/10.1044/2017_JSLHR-L-17-0214

Neumann, Y. (2018). A case series comparison of semantically focused vs. phonologically focused cued naming treatment in aphasia. *Clinical Linguistics & Phonetics*, *32*(1), 1–27. https://doi.org/10.1080/02699206.2017.1326166

Nickels, L. (2002). Therapy for naming disorders: Revisiting, revising, and reviewing, *Aphasiology*, *16*(10–11), 935–979. https://doi.org/10.1080/02687030244000563

Palmer, R., Hughes, H., & Chater, T. (2017). What do people with aphasia want to be able to say? A content analysis of words identified as personally relevant by people with aphasia. *PLoS ONE, 12*(3): e0174065. https://doi.org/10.1371/ journal.pone.0174065

Peach, R., & Reuter, K. (2010). A discourse-based approach to semantic feature analysis for the treatment of aphasic word retrieval failures, *Aphasiology, 24*(9), 971–990. https://doi.org/10.1080/026870 30903058629

Quique, Y., Evans, W., & Dickey, M. (2019). Acquisition and generalization responses in aphasia naming treatment: A meta-analysis of semantic feature analysis outcomes. *American Journal of Speech-Language Pathology, 28*(1S), 230–246. https://doi.org/10.10 44/2018_AJSLP-17-0155

Raymer, A., McHose, B., Smith, K., Iman, L., Ambrose, A., & Casselton, C. (2012). Contrasting effects of errorless naming treatment and gestural facilitation for word retrieval in aphasia, *Neuropsychological Rehabilitation, 22*(2), 235–266. https://doi.org/10.1080/09602011.20 11.618306

Raymer, A., Singletary, F., Rodriguez, A., Ciampitti, M., Heilman, K., & Rothi, L. (2006). Effects of gesture verbal treatment for noun and verb retrieval in aphasia. *Journal of the International Neuropsychological Society, 12*(6), 867–882. https://doi.org/10.1017/S1355 617706061042

Renvall, K., Nickels, L., & Davidson, B. (2013). Functionally relevant items in the treatment of aphasia (Part I): Challenges for current practice. *Aphasiology, 27*(6), 363–650.

Rider, J. D., Wright, H. H., Marshall, R. C., & Page, J. L. (2008). Using semantic feature analysis to improve contextual discourse in adults with aphasia. *American Journal of Speech-Language Pathology, 17*, 161–172.

Rose, M. (2006). The utility of gesture treatments in aphasia. *Advances in Speech-Language Pathology, 8*, 92–109.

Rose, M., & Douglas, J. (2008). Treating a semantic word production deficit in aphasia with verbal and gesture methods, *Aphasiology, 22*(1), 20–41. https://doi.org/10.1080/02687030600742020

Sheng, L., & McGregor, K. (2010). Lexical-semantic organization in children with specific language impairment. *Journal of Speech, Language, and Hearing Research, 53*(1), 146–159. https://doi.org/ 10.1044/1092-4388(2009/08-0160)

Silkes, J., Oelke, M., Allen, W., & Jendall, D. (2021, May 18). *Guide to phonomotor yherapy.* University of Washington. https://canvas.uw .edu/courses/1166215/pages/guide-to-phonomotor-therapy

van Hees, S., Angwin, A., McMahon, K., & Copland, D. (2013). A comparison of semantic feature analysis and phonological components analysis for the treatment of naming impairments in aphasia. *Neurophysiological Rehabilitation, 23*(1), 102–132. https://doi.org/10.10 80/09602011.2012.726201

Wambaugh, J. (2003). A comparison of the relative effects of phonologic and semantic cueing treatments, *Aphasiology, 17*(5), 433–441. https://doi.org/10.1080/02687030344000085

Wambaugh, J., & Ferguson, M. (2007). Application of semantic feature analysis to retrieval of action names in aphasia. *Journal of Rehabilitation Research & Development, 44*(3), 381–394. https://doi.org/10.1682/JRRD.2006.05.0038

Wambaugh, J., & Martinez, A. (2000). Effects of rate and rhythm control treatment on consonant production accuracy in apraxia of speech. *Aphasiology, 14*, 851–871.

Wambaugh, J., Mauszycki, S., & Wright, S. (2014). Semantic feature analysis: Application to confrontation naming of actions in aphasia. *Aphasiology, 28*(1), 1–24. https://doi.org/10.1080/02687038.2013.845739

Wambaugh, J., Nessler, C., & Wright, S. (2013). Modified response elaboration training: application to procedural discourse and personal recounts. *American Journal of Speech-Language Pathology, 22*(2), S409–S425. https://doi.org/10.1044/1058-0360

Webster, J., & Whitworth, A. (2012). Treating verbs in aphasia: Exploring the impact of therapy at the single word and sentence levels. *International Journal of Language and Communication Disorders, 47*(6), 619–636. https://doi.org/10.1111/j.1460-6984.2012.00174.x

Wisenburn, B., & Mahoney, K. (2009). A meta-analysis of word-finding treatments for aphasia, *Aphasiology, 23*(11), 1338–1352. https://doi.org/10.1080/02687030902732745

Xu, J., Gannon, P., Emmorey, K., Smith, J., & Braun, A. (2009). Symbolic gestures and spoken language are processed by a common neural system. *Proceedings of the National Academy of Sciences, 106*(49), 20664-20669. https://doi.org/10.1073/pnas.0909197106

Ylvisaker, M., & Szekeres, S. (1985, November). *Cognitive-language intervention with brain injured adolescents and adults.* Mini-seminar presented at the annual convention of the Illinois Speech-Language-Hearing Association.

Appendix 9–1
Lesson Plan Example for Semantic Feature Analysis (SFA)

(Created by Claire Small and Sarah Larsen)

Semantic Feature Analysis (SFA)	
Goal/ Objective	In 20 sessions, the client will generate at least two features per semantic attribute (category) for each target noun and correctly name the target word with 80% accuracy when given minimal prompting, as measured by clinician data.
Therapy Materials	■ SFA Chart ■ Picture cards (Theme: Things found in a kitchen) ■ *Refrigerator, stove, pan, sink, soap, trashcan, knives, towel, pot, spoon, oven, salt/pepper, can opener, blender, bowl, cutting board.*
Treatment Procedure	■ Present the topic of the photocards (e.g., things found in a kitchen). ■ Place a photocard at the center of the SFA chart. ■ Ask the client to name the picture. ■ If the client accurately names the picture, continue completing all of the features in the SFA chart in order to strengthen their semantic network. ■ Clinician can ask questions that are related to the features from the SFA chart in order to elicit responses (e.g., *Where can you find this object? Can you describe what it looks like? How does it feel? What category does this object belong in?*). ■ If the client is unable to name one of the features, the clinician can give them a binary-forced choice (e.g., *Is it sharp or soft? Do you find it in a kitchen or bathroom? Do you use it to cook or clean?*). ■ After the client completes all of the features, ask them to name the picture again. ■ If the patient is unable to name the picture, provide them with the name. ■ Ask them to repeat the name and review the features. ■ Continue to gradually fade prompts.

continues

Appendix 9–1. *continued*

Data Collection

Key	
+/−	Correct/incorrect
P/I	Prompted/Independent

Target Word	Accuracy (+/−)		Modality of Response	Prompted/Independent (I/P)	Semantic Features											
					GROUPS		USE		ACTION		PROPERTIES		LOCATION		ASSOCIATION	
					+/-	I/P	+/-	I/P	+/-	I/P	+/-	I/P	+/-	I/P	+/-	I/P

References | Boyle, M. (2004). Semantic feature analysis treatment for anomia in two fluent aphasia syndromes. *American Journal of Speech-Language Pathology, 13*(3), 236–249.

Appendix 9–2

Lesson Plan Example for Verb Network Strengthening Treatment (VNeST)

(Created by Claire Small and Sarah Larsen)

Verb Network Strengthening Treatment	
Objective	In 20 sessions, the client will generate 3 agent-patient pairs for the target verb during structured language tasks in 8/10 trials with minimal cues as measured by clinician data.
Therapy Materials	■ Laminated cards, including "WHO" and "WHAT" cards and blank cards ■ Expo marker ■ Target verb cards (10 verbs)

Treatment Procedure	1. Set up. Presents the verb card in the middle between the two stimulus cards saying [who] and [what] as the sequence of [who]-verb-[what].
	
	2. Client generates 3 agent examples for target verb
	
	  ■ Prompt the client to generate 3 agent roles (or "who") for the target verb.
	
	  ■ After the client identifies each agent role, write it on a card and add it to the "who" column.
	
	3. Client generates 3 complementary patient examples relative to Step 2
	
	  ■ Prompt the client to generate 3 "what" examples and fill in the cards with each response.
	
	4. Have the client answer questions about a particular pair.
	
	  ■ Have the client choose one agent/patient pair to discuss.
	
	  ■ Ask the client wh-questions about the pair (*when, where, why*).

Treatment Procedure *continued*	5. Semantic judgment task ■ Read 4 sentences that contain the target verb and appropriate/inappropriate agent-patient relationships. Have the client make a judgement if the sentence makes sense. ■ Clients should compose appropriate sentences, sentences with inappropriate agent roles, sentences with inappropriate patient roles, and sentences with the agent and patient roles switched. 6. Generating agent/patient pairs ■ Without using the cards, ask the client to independently generate 3 agent/patient pairs for the verb.
Prompting	■ *If the client is unable to produce 3 agent/patient pairs* ■ Provide the client with a card with appropriate options and foils and have them identify the appropriate agents and patients. ■ *When prompting for an agent role: Tell me **who** can [verb].* ■ *When prompting for a patient role: Tell me **what** can be [verb].*

continues

Appendix 9–2. *continued*

**Data
Collection**

Key	
+/–	Correct/incorrect
P/I	Prompted/ Independent

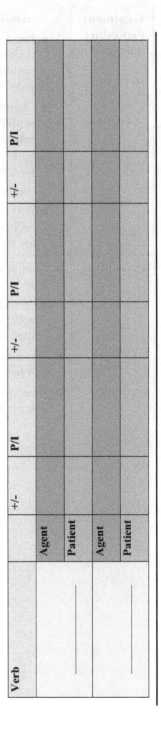

References | Edmonds, L. A., Nadeau, S. E., & Kiran, S. (2009). Effect of Verb Network Strengthening Treatment (VNeST) on lexical retrieval of content words in sentences in persons with aphasia, *Aphasiology, 23*(3), 402–424.

Appendix 9–3

Lesson Plan Example for Phonological Component Analysis (PCA)

(Created by Claire Small and Sarah Larsen)

Phonological Component Analysis (PCA)	
Objective	In 20 sessions, the client will name at least two phonological components per category and the target word with 80% accuracy with minimal cues, as measured by clinician data.
Therapy Materials	■ Laminated PCA chart ■ Photo cards that depict target words (8-12 targets)
Treatment Procedure	■ Present the client with a picture depicting the target word and ask the client to name the picture. ■ If the client can name the target, continue filling out the chart for/with the client. ■ If the client cannot name the target, the clinician can provide choices aloud and fill in the chart with the client's response. ■ After the chart is completed, ask the client to name the picture again. If they are incorrect or don't respond, provide them with the target and prompt them to repeat it. ■ Review all phonological components and prompt the client to name the target a final time.
Prompting	If the client responds with **the wrong initial sound** For example, if the picture is of a soda can and the client says that it starts with a /p/. ■ Instruct the client to use a different word to describe the object, such as using the word [pop] instead of [soda].

Data Collection

Key	
+/−	Correct/incorrect
P/I	Prompted/ Independent

Target Word		Rhyme Production		First Sound		First sound associate		Final Sound		# of Syllables				
+/−	I/P	+/−	I/P	+/−	I/P	+/−	I/P	+/−	I/P	+/−	I/P			

continues

Appendix 9–3. *continued*

| References | Leonard, C., Rochon, E., & Laird, L. (2008). Treating naming impairments in aphasia: Findings from a phonological components analysis treatment, *Aphasiology, 22*(9), 923–947. |

Appendix 9–4
Lesson Plan Example for Phonomotor Treatment (PMT)
(Created by Claire Small and Sarah Larsen)

Phonomotor Treatment (PMT)	
Objective	By _(date)_ , the client will accurately name the target word in 8/10 trials with minimal cues as measured by clinician data.
Therapy Materials	■ Small mirror ■ Letter tiles ■ Colored blocks ■ Line drawings/images of mouth positions for phonemes

Treatment Procedure	*Targets used in this session will include real and nonwords of the following structure: CCVC or CVCC
	
	Perception Tasks:
	The following targets are produced by the clinician: *mart, fims, clap, tasp, barb*
	
	1. Mouth pictures
	  ■ Have the client use the mouth pictures to represent the word dictated by the clinician (e.g., for *fims*, they would select the mouth pictures that reflect the 4 phonemes in the word).
	
	2. Colored blocks
	  ■ Have the client use the colored blocks to reflect the syllable structure of the word. All vowels should be reflected with the same color. If the same consonant is used twice in a word, that color should be consistent. (e.g., *mart*: red, white, orange, blue; *barb*: purple, white, orange, purple).
	
	3. Verbal
	  ■ Provide a verbal same/different task for the client. Either produce the target twice or create a minimal pair using the target. (e.g., *mart/ mart, mart/mark*).

continues

Appendix 9–4. *continued*

Treatment Procedure *continued*	4. <u>Letters</u> ■ Have the client spell the target using the letter blocks. **Production Tasks:** Targets: *ships, gump, wand, clun, star* 1. <u>Mouth pictures</u> ■ Lay the mouth pictures out to represent the target, have the client touch each picture and say the sound. Then have them blend all the sounds together to produce the word. 2. <u>Verbal</u> ■ Prompt the client to repeat a non-word and then identify each sound in the word (e.g., *gump: g-uh-m-p*) 3. <u>Letters</u> ■ Use the letter tiles to spell the target. Have the client produce each sound and then blending them together to produce the whole word.
Prompting	If the client struggles to identify a phoneme in the target word: ■ *Watch me make the sound. Now you try, what does the sound feel like? What are you moving in order to make that sound? Where are your lips and your tongue?* ■ Have them use the mirror to describe the placement of their articulators. ■ Have them put their hand on their throat and describe the sound as quiet or noisy. If the client struggles to match the mouth pictures to the correct phoneme or vice versa: ■ Have them use the mirror to match the placement of their articulators to the pictures to produce the correct sound.
References	Guide to Phonomotor Treatment (Silkes, J. P., Oelke, M., Allen, W., & Kendall, D., n.d.) https://canvas.uw.edu/courses/1166215/pages/ guide-to-phonomotor-therapy

Appendix 9–5

Lesson Plan Example for Anagram and Copy Treatment (ACT)

(Created by Claire Small and Sarah Larsen)

Anagram and Copy Therapy (ACT)	
Objective	In 20 sessions, the client will write target words with 80% accuracy given minimal cues.
Therapy Materials	■ Picture cards depicting target word (i.e., nouns, verbs) ■ Paper & pencil ■ Letter tiles (i.e., Scrabble, Bananagram)
Treatment Procedure	1. Present the photo card depicting the target and provide prompt that elicits target in writing. 2. If the client successfully wrote the target, provide positive reinforcement and begin at Step 1 with a new target. 3. If the client was not able to successfully write the target, present the letter tiles (i.e., only the letters in the word) in a random order and have the client arrange the letter tiles to aid in their written response. 4. If they successfully write the target word, have them copy the completed word 3 more times. 　■ If they are unsuccessful, arrange the letter tiles for the client while providing feedback. 　■ Ask the client to write the target word and copy 3 times. 5. Remove the previous written responses and present the picture again, while prompting the client to write the target word.
Prompting	Visual/gesture cues: Letter tiles 　■ Moderate cue: provide them a field of 2 　■ Maximal cue: direct them to the correct letter tile

continues

Appendix 9–5. *continued*

Prompting *continued*	Verbal cues: Sound letter correspondence ■ Minimal cue: What is the first sound in the word? What letter makes that sound? ■ Moderate cue: provide them a field of 2 ■ Maximal cues: the "d" makes the /d/ sound, can you find the "d"?
References	Beeson, P. M. (1999). Treating acquired writing impairments: Strengthening graphemic representations. *Aphasiology, 13,* 767–785.

Appendix 9–6

Lesson Plan Example for Copy and Recall Treatment (CART)

(Created by Claire Small and Sarah Larsen)

Copy and Recall Treatment (CART)	
Objective	In 20 sessions, the client will write target words with 80% accuracy given initial modeling and minimal cues.
Therapy Materials	■ Picture cards depicting target word (i.e., nouns, verbs) ■ Paper & pencil
Treatment Procedure	1. Present the photo card depicting the target and provide prompt that elicits target in writing. 2. If the client successfully writes the target, provide positive reinforcement and begin at Step 1 with a new target. 3. If the client was unable to successfully write the target, provide a written model for the client to copy at least 3 times. 4. Remove their written responses and prompt the client to write the target with only the picture stimulus as reference. 5. If the client is successful, provide feedback and begin at Step 1 with a new target. ■ If the client is unsuccessful, go back to Step 3 6. If the client continues to be unsuccessful, assign this target word as homework and move to the next target.
Prompting	Visual cues: Written model of target Verbal cues: Sound-letter correspondence ■ Minimal cues: What is the first sound in the word? What letter makes that sound? ■ Moderate cues: What letter makes the /d/ sound? Is it "p" or "d"?

continues

Appendix 9–6. *continued*

| References | Beeson, P. M., Rising, K., & Volk, J. (2003). Writing treatment for severe aphasia: Who benefits? *Journal of Speech, Language, and Hearing Research, 46,* 1038-1060. |

Appendix 9–7

Lesson Plan Example for Promoting Aphasics' Communication Effectiveness (PACE)

(Created by Claire Small and Sarah Larsen)

Promoting Aphasics' Communication Effectiveness (PACE)	
Objective	In 20 sessions, the client will successfully communicate their message using a multimodal approach (e.g., speech, writing, gestures, drawing) with 80% accuracy given minimal cues.
Therapy Materials	■ Picture cards depicting target word (i.e., nouns, verbs) ■ Paper & pencil
Treatment Procedure	1. The clinician and client should sit across from one another to keep the stimulus from view of the listener. 2. To begin, the first speaker (either the clinician or client) will draw a picture card and attempt to describe the picture without using the target word. The speaker may use any modality to communicate their message (e.g., speech, writing, gestures, drawing). 3. If the listener correctly guesses the target, the listener draws a new card and repeats Step 1 in the role of the speaker. ■ If the listener is incorrect, the speaker can continue to provide the listener with information in any modality to help them guess the target word. 4. The client and clinician continue to switch roles for each card until all targets have been attempted.

continues

Appendix 9–7. *continued*

Prompting	Feedback is embedded in the activity. For example, the speaker will know they've been successful if the listener is able to guess their intended message.
	■ Minimal cues: If needed, the clinician can remind the client of the potential modalities that can be used to convey their message.
	■ Moderate cues: If the client is the speaker and is having difficulty, the clinician can prompt them with questions to guide them. For example, *"I saw that you were stirring, are you thinking of something in the kitchen?"*
	■ Maximal cues: The clinician and the client can look at the card together and rehearse several ways of communicating it using different modalities.
References	Davis, G. A. (2005). PACE revisited. *Aphasiology*, *19*(1), 21–38.

10

SEMANTIC PROCESSING IN BILINGUALS

Belinda Daughrity

There Might Be a Language Difference, But All Kids Are
Generally the Same
Bilingual Children Can Exhibit Minimal Semantic Delays
in Comparison to Monolingual Children, So I Should
Refer Bilingual Children for Intervention Just to Be
Safe
Clinical Implications
Chapter Summary
Discussion Questions

Chapter Objectives

1. List at least three common misconceptions about bilingual language development.
2. Identify the key components of an appropriate semantic assessment for bilinguals.
3. Define the differences between simultaneous and successive bilinguals.

Introduction

As the prevalence of bilingualism continues to rise and our world becomes progressively more global and interconnected, understanding the complexity of semantic processing in bilinguals becomes increasingly important among speech-language pathologists, especially as professionals strive to be culturally competent while serving culturally and linguistically diverse (CLD) clients. Understanding semantic processing among bilinguals is essential to understanding linguistic diversity. This understanding of semantic processing in bilingual and multilingual clients becomes even more imperative as most practicing speech-language pathologists are monolingual and lack direct understanding of bilingual experiences and differences. According to the American Speech-Language Hearing Association (ASHA) Profile of Bilingual Clinicians, Year-End 2018 Review, about 6% of all speech-language pathologists and audiologists are bilingual or multilingual. The relative scarcity of bilingual and multilingual clinicians is startling when taking into account that expected speech and language caseloads will consist of increasing amounts of CLD populations (Crawford, 2013). Additionally, many SLPs report a lack of appropriate assessment tools for linguistically diverse clients, and developmental norms (Guiberson & Atkins, 2012). Thus, understanding semantic processing in bilinguals is an important step in providing appropriate services to diverse clients.

Theoretical Models

There has been extensive research investigating the differences between monolinguals and bilinguals in semantic processing. Kroll and Stewart's (1994) Revised Hierarchical Model asserts a distinction between the lexical and conceptual level among bilinguals, contending that initially, links are assumed to be stronger between L2 to L1 because many L2 words are first learned by correlating them with their L1 translation. Thus, what might initially appear as word finding difficulty may actually be the process of mental translation. This model accounts for differences in translation latency particularly for late bilinguals who acquire a second language distinctly after the acquisition of a first language and remain dominant in L1 (Kroll, van Hell, Tokowicz, & Green, 2010). Figure 10–1 illustrates the process of mental translation.

Concrete words with more direct conceptual images that prompt the speaker to visualize a clear mental picture may present with different translation features than abstract words and concepts. For example, the word "apple" typically prompts a clear mental representation that can be clearly mapped into a new language. However, an abstract concept like "trust" or "love" may be encoded differently and somewhat more

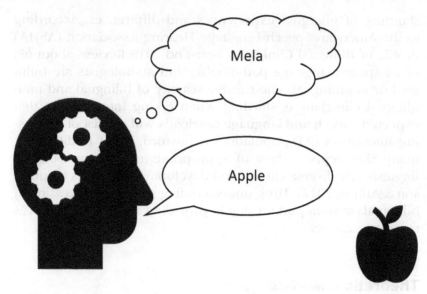

Figure 10–1. Illustration of mental translation.

challenging to retrieve. Such processing differences are outlined in the Distributed Feature Model (van Hell & de Groot, 1998), asserting faster translation of concrete words in comparison to abstract concepts. Figure 10–2 illustrates this concept of strong concrete connections in comparison to weaker, more abstract connections.

Other models of semantic learning among bilinguals highlight the dominance of words encompassing multiple meanings and thus evoking a variety of different senses when translated. The Sense Model introduced by Finkbeiner, Forster, Nicol, and Nakamura (2004) uses examples such as the Japanese word "kuroi" and its translation in English to "black." Whereas these words seemingly correlate on the basis of color, the English translation could have several different meanings in addition to color, such as "black coffee," "black humor," "black magic." The word in Japanese may also elicit a variety of different meanings other than a simple color translation. This model seems to support general principles of the Distributed Feature Model with both models overlapping in their acknowledgment of conceptual words with multiple meanings.

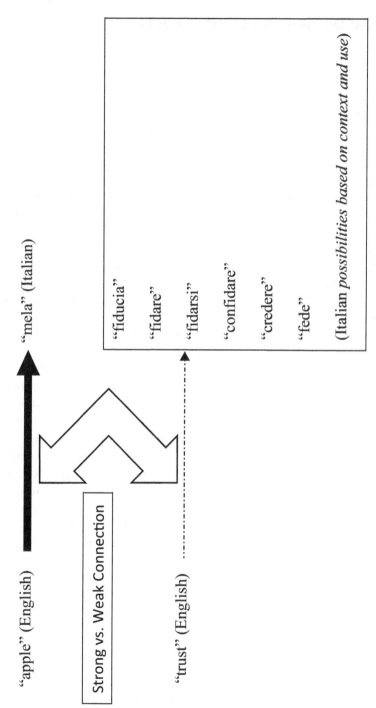

Figure 10–2. Illustration of strong concrete connections in comparison to weaker more abstract connections.

Lexical Development in Bilinguals

The period in language development at the time of second language exposure, in addition to frequency and context, have the most impact on semantic processing and lexical development in bilinguals. In considering lexical development, bilinguals may have basic interpersonal skills that include general conversation proficiency or cognitive academic language proficiency that includes more years of exposure resulting in near native skills (Cummins, 1984). Thus, learning a first language in early childhood and then having academic training in that language would result in both conversational and academic proficiency. This lexical environment differs from a bilingual who might speak one language at home and another at school or work. For example, bilingual children may develop some words in the home language, while developing other words in the language used at school (Paradis et al., 2011). This kind of context bound use of language is common especially for speech-language pathologists working in schools who may serve clients who are English language learners and present with speech and language delays. In such cases, SLPs might incorporate opportunities in intervention to support English vocabulary growth incidentally via strategies such as increasing comprehension and strengthening morphological awareness skills, while also leveraging the skills that are present in the native language (Fitton et al., 2016). Additionally, evidence suggests strategies like shared book reading tasks and repeated vocabulary exposure in both languages are helpful to encourage semantic development among English language learners (Davison & Qi, 2017; Fierro & Storkel, 2017).

Speech-language pathologists might consider semantic loss as a bilingual child can begin to show attrition of semantic skills in one language resulting from reduced exposure and growing language dominance. Evidence indicates language experience impacts receptive and expressive semantic skills (Gibson, Peña, & Bedore, 2012). Because experience is closely linked with semantic skills, clearly understanding a bilingual client's language experience is critical to diagnosing semantic disorders. Among bilingual children, omission of words and bound morphemes appear to predict language impairment (Jacobson &

Walden, 2013). Thus, in capturing a full picture of a client's semantic skills, accurately gathering linguistic background information on semantic development and language exposure is a vital element.

Clinical Implication

In a "real world" example, consider a typically developing African American male living and working in Japan. He was born in the United States and grew up exclusively speaking English before moving to Japan at age 30, where he became fluent in Japanese. He and his Japanese wife worked as translators and lived with her monolingual Japanese-speaking parents. After his stroke at age 55, the client demonstrated severe deficits in his use of Japanese and was left with significant limitations in his expressive output after more than 20 years of living and working in Japan as a late bilingual. His use of English remained relatively intact, although he did present with some residual semantic deficits, such as difficulty with word finding.

This example shows how bilingual clients can present with a linguistic advantage in cases of acquired brain injury and how lexical development can play a role in semantic loss following traumatic brain injury. In this case, the client demonstrated more semantic loss in his second language acquisition than with his first language. A speech-language pathologist only evaluating this client in Japanese might determine more severe semantic deficits than a speech-language pathologist accounting for both English and Japanese semantic skills and capturing abilities in both languages.

Semantic Access in Bilinguals

The "bilingual brain" is a fascinating thing. Bilinguals seem to use both languages in an integrated way, and evidence suggests the different languages can interact during processing (Desmet & Duyck, 2007). Among preschool children, evidence indicates there is an advantage among bilinguals in superior inhibitory control in comparison to monolingual peers (Bialystok & Martin, 2004). Research suggests a "bilingual advantage" with some actions, such as visual tasks of inhibition, but no significant differences in other performance areas such as visual and auditory inhibition of irrelevant information among early balanced bilinguals and their monolingual counterparts (Desjardins & Fernandez, 2018).

To understanding semantic access, we first need to understand the processes of bilingualism and second language acquisition. Paradis and colleagues (2011) clarify the terms sequential bilingualism, simultaneous bilingualism, and English language learners.

Sequential bilinguals learn a second language after age three when they have already achieved a level of proficiency in their primary language. Other terms for these individuals include **successive bilinguals**. At least initially, successive bilinguals can demonstrate better receptive skills of the secondary language before developing expressive skills in the secondary language.

In younger sequential bilinguals, language skills in L2 may become near native proficiency given the degree of exposure. This may be different for late successive bilinguals, such as individuals who learn a second language in early adulthood who might always demonstrate more dominance in their first language. **Simultaneous bilinguals** include individuals who develop two or more languages at the same time, typically in early childhood prior to age three. An example may be a child with bilingual parents who regularly speak two languages at home. The term **English language learners** often refers to students in schools for the sake of defining those students who may demonstrate limited English proficiency. Such students may benefit in school from additional support to access their academic curriculum, given reduced English language comprehension or expression.

Understanding your client's type of bilingualism is important in order to make appropriate decisions in assessment and intervention. For example, a child exposed exclusively to one language at home and then a secondary language at school may present with different semantic skills than a child exposed to both languages at home via fluent, bilingual parents. The first child would be labeled as a **successive bilingual**, having first learned one language followed by another. The second child would be labeled a **simultaneous bilingual** with concurrent exposure to both languages in early childhood. This information should impact how a clinician goes about assessment procedures. Prior to assessment, it is critical to ask about language exposure and dominance in order to select appropriate evaluation measures. This background knowledge helps to differentiate differences from disorders.

Word Retrieval in Bilingual Speakers

Although some clinicians caution bilingual families against speaking two languages in fear of "confusing" the child, this negative theory has been strongly refuted by evidence suggesting the absence of adverse effects and potential advantages of dual language exposure (Byers-Heinlein & Lew-Williams, 2013). Bilingual and multilingual speakers present with strong metalinguistic skills as they often conceptualize a term in one language and then translate it into another language depending upon the linguistic context (see Figure 10–1). As they do so, bilingual clients indicate an ability to consider the language dominance of their communication partners and an ability to adjust their linguistic output to match their environment. Clinically, in evaluation, interventionists should consider probing in the home language prior to using English to permit the child the opportunity to communicate in that language before the child attempts to code switch to English for the benefit of the evaluator.

Clinical Application

Consider a bilingual child attempting to code switch a word without a clear meaning. For example, a child hears the word "orange" without context. To translate the word into Spanish, does the child consider the word "naranja" for orange fruit or the word "anaranjado" for the color orange? Likely, the child would use context clues to discern which entity best fits the speaker's meaning. This mental process is one unique to bilingual and multilingual speakers.

Clinical Considerations in Evaluation

For speech-language pathologists, evaluations of bilingual or multilingual individuals must be carefully planned and strategized to ensure appropriate assessment and results that properly inform treatment planning and intervention. A frequent challenge in bilingual semantic evaluation may be the lack of appropriate dual language vocabulary tests, as evidence supports the importance of considering bilingual clients' cultural linguistic backgrounds when evaluating semantic abilities (Kan et. al., 2020). A key point in assessment of this population is that an evaluation must differentiate language differences from disorders. This means clinicians must use their clinical judgment to determine language dominance and administer appropriate assessments to assess semantic strengths and weaknesses. For clients who are bilingual in English and Spanish, a growing population within the United States, there are several standardized assessments for semantics that assess an individual's ability to name and comprehend objects, actions, and concepts in pictured illustrations such as the Expressive One-Word Picture Vocabulary Test Spanish-Bilingual Edition–4th Edition (EOWPVT-4: SBE; Martin, 2013) and the Receptive One-Word Picture Vocabulary Test Spanish-Bilingual Edition–4th Edition (ROWPVT-4: SBE; Martin, 2013). Both standardized assessments are based upon dual language scoring. If the client misses an item presented in the dominant language, the client is prompted to respond in the non-dominant language. If the client responds correctly to identify the target word in either language, then the item is counted as correct. Such assessments allow clinicians to note how many items the client identifies correctly and *in which language*. This scoring helps the clinician to collect evidence about language dominance by noting skills that may be present in one language, but not the other, while also noting skills that are absent across languages and may be indicative of a semantic disorder. Failure to consider semantic skills across both languages may falsely indicate semantic deficits and a language impairment (Peña et al., 2011).

Often, clients may demonstrate semantic strength differences between their expressive and receptive vocabulary skills, particularly as individuals age and exist within multiple contexts. For example, consider a child bilingual in English and Spanish who is exposed to one language at home (Spanish) and one language at school (English). More complex semantic knowledge may tend to be dominant in English as it is the language of academic instruction and more likely to be used in explicit teaching of higher order vocabulary. In contrast, words that may be more consistently heard in the home may be more dominant in Spanish. Consider a speech-language pathologist assessing a client's receptive knowledge of the concept "dangerous."

In Figure 10–3, the Spanish/English bilingual client was able to associate the target word with direct context and experience, which happened to occur more in the home environment where the dominant language is Spanish.

Figure 10–4 illustrates that, for bilinguals, context matters. By only assessing semantic knowledge in one language, a clinician fails to see the full scope of a client's abilities. In fact, assessment in only one language may create an illusion of a deficit that does not exist. Linguistic context may be most relevant among school-age bilingual children because these students are typically exposed to one language at home and then English

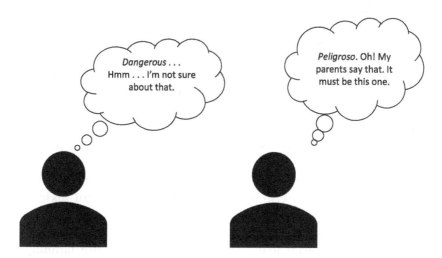

Figure 10–3. Illustration of Spanish/English bilinguals who are able to associate the target word with direct context and experience.

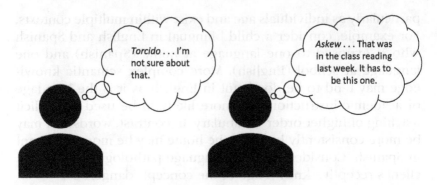

Figure 10–4. Illustration that shows that context matters for bilinguals.

at school. Thus, their semantic maps are even more strongly associated with context and can be language bound. Considering skills in all language exposures provides the opportunity to fully capture a client's semantic skills, a primary goal for clinicians probing for semantic deficits during language assessments.

As clinicians explore a client's semantic skills, it is important to get information on how and when languages were learned. This information would be critically important during assessment. A clinician cannot assume a client does not have semantic skills in a language simply because there is limited expressive output. To the contrary, depending on the exposure and stage of learning, the receptive skills may far exceed the level of expressive output.

Figure 10–5 demonstrates the typical development of L2 semantic skills among speakers who are first exposed exclusively to one language and then to another. It should be noted semantic skills in L1 are also maintained with continued use and exposure.

Evidence suggests bilingual children demonstrate distinct differences from their monolingual peers in regards to vocabulary learning. With two semantic systems, research suggests bilingual children can discriminate between their different lexicons for different communication partners and contexts (Petitto et al., 2001). This differentiation indicates complex metalinguistic skills as bilingual children learn early to hypothesize the language dominance of their communication partner and respond accordingly. Among bilingual speakers, the importance of context, age

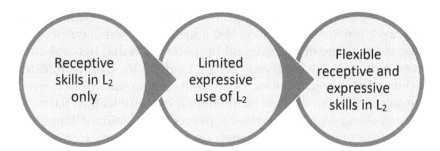

Figure 10–5. Semantic skill development in L2 in successive bilinguals.

of linguistic exposure, and models cannot be underestimated on their impact on semantic skills.

Issues in Bilingual Assessment

Clinical Example

Consider the case of Diego, a 5-year-old boy with a diagnosis of autism spectrum disorder. At the start of the academic year, he is undergoing an ASD assessment to confirm symptom presentation and severity to help inform his upcoming classroom placement, as his IEP team is deciding between a self-contained classroom with some inclusion and a mainstream classroom with resource supports. The evaluator administers evaluations in English only and determines his needs are better suited to a self-contained classroom after noting he produced limited flexible phrase speech and reduced semantic knowledge during the evaluation. Upon following up on Diego's case months later, it was discovered that he is regularly exposed to three languages. His mother is bilingual in English and Spanish, his father is bilingual in English and French, and he received early intervention services in English prior to transitioning to the school district. Every summer, he and his parents spend two consecutive months in Europe visiting family who are monolingual in Spanish and French, respectively. This example gives several items to consider.

First, it is likely that Diego needed a bilingual evaluator, or at least a translator, to help probe if his limited verbal output was due to language difference and his perception that his evaluator was only able to communicate in English. Research indicates bilingual children as young as two will compensate for perceived linguistic deficits of their monolingual communication partners by speaking in their partner's perceived dominant language even if that language limits their own communicative efficiency (Genesee et al., 1996). What the evaluator noted as jargon during the assessment, may have been true words in Spanish or French, unbeknownst to the monolingual evaluator. Because it was the start of the academic year and Diego had not been exposed to significant English for the last two months, this possibility is even more likely.

Additionally, the results of this speech and language evaluation helped to inform classroom placement for the year, which has implications for his academic curriculum, as well as access to peer models to impact his social interaction skills as a student with ASD. If he had been assessed bilingually to account for all of his linguistic skills, then his IEP team may have made different decisions regarding his total programming needs to better suit his skills.

As the example illustrates, appropriate assessment is critically important for bilingual clients to ensure their semantic skills are adequately identified. Appropriate bilingual assessment is also an ethical consideration because, without proper evaluation of semantic knowledge, students may receive inappropriate services that do not effectively respond to their needs.

Guidelines to Assess Bilingual Clients for Semantic Skills

■ Conduct a thorough caregiver intake: Directly ask (repeatedly) about language exposure even if "it's just a little bit!" Research is clear on the importance of collecting detailed information on bilingual children because their exposure to and use of both languages highly impacts semantic development (Hammer et al., 2012). For children, it is important to ask parents about languages used at home, at school, and by other caregivers. For adults, you might want to ask about languages used at home and at work. For both children and adults, you want to make sure to provide an intake form in the preferred language of the caregiver or person completing the form. Note that the caregiver's dominant language may not be the dominant language of the client.

- If another language is reported and the client is bilingual, the evaluation should be conducted with a bilingual clinician in that language if available. If a bilingual clinician is not available, a trained interpreter or translator may be employed. If available, a bilingual speech-language pathology assistant (SLPA) may be helpful to assist with evaluation.

- Appropriate standardized assessments should be used. If the standardization sample does not include your client, you might consider using the test to provide descriptive information, rather than reporting standardized scores if the test is not representative of your client. Collect a thorough language sample in all languages. A language sample analysis (LSA) will help to reveal semantic skills across languages in a natural context.

- Questionnaires to relevant informants: Appropriate input from primary caregivers, teachers, or other pertinent informants can help to determine if semantic deficits, and other linguistic deficits, are consistent across contexts or only environment specific.

- Do the background work! Collect norms on the non-English language. ASHA's Practice Portal offers a wealth of evidence for clinicians to help learn about evidence-based practices for working with bilingual populations.

Taken together, these approaches help to determine if the bilingual client is demonstrating a language disorder or just a language difference. There is no doubt that bilingual assessment is more challenging than monolingual assessment because it can require more research to differentiate between differences and disorders. Although possibly more time consuming, bilingual assessment is certainly interesting as clinicians are able to probe comprehensively and triangulate suspicions to make appropriate diagnosis and recommendations, while fulfilling their ethical responsibility to culturally and linguistically diverse clients.

Obtaining Key Information From Caregivers: Considering Child Language Exposure

Collecting a thorough case history is important with all clients. For bilingual clients, it is vital to gather information on language use, age of exposure, and sources of language models. Given that bilingual families often exhibit cultural diversity in addition to linguistic diversity, it is important that clinicians consider how data are collected from culturally, linguistically diverse caregivers. When collecting case history, it is important to ask a question at least twice in two different ways. For example, consider a clinician asking, *Are there any other languages spoken at home?* The parent may report only English is spoken to the child. Later in the interview, the clinician may ask who lives in the home with the child or who helps to care for the child when parents are at work. The parent may report grandparents help with child care. That is another opportunity to probe for language exposure and ask, *Do grandparents speak English only?* Upon considering the question posed in a different way, the parent may report grandparents speak in a different language even though parents provide English input. This is vital information because, although the child may be mostly around the parents, grandparents providing child care just 5 days per week for a few hours a day results in several hours of consistent input in another language. Many parents may initially dismiss this information, but clinicians know it matters! It's important to probe for details that caregivers may disregard to make sure you collect a complete picture of the client's background that can help to inform assessment procedures and semantic considerations.

Using Appropriate Assessments

At times, clinicians may falsely believe that there are no standardized assessments appropriate for bilingual clients; however, that assumption is incorrect. Evidence suggests English-only measures can indicate vocabulary delays in typical bilingual children, whereas measures allowing for conceptual scoring that give bilingual children the opportunity to respond to missed items in their other language can help to eliminate the bias in single-language standardized vocabulary tests and more accurately rule out semantic deficits (Core et. al., 2013; Gross et al., 2014). Additionally, standardized assessments are increasingly available in bilingual editions to help meet the needs of our increasingly linguistically diverse clients. If semantic tests are not available, consider applying dual language scoring to assess semantic knowledge. Although you may not be able to report standardized scores, such an approach may help to provide more accurate information about semantic knowledge and deficits.

Importance of Language Sampling

In nearly all cases of assessment, a thorough language sample analysis (LSA) in both languages would be appropriate. This critical context allows the clinician to determine how the client is applying semantic knowledge in an unstructured context, such as conversation, illustrating how their semantic processing is working within a natural environment. The LSA can allow the clinician to determine types of words used in both languages to assess semantic complexity. For example, does the bilingual client use more specific vocabulary in one language compared to more general vocabulary in the other (*thing, stuff*, etc.)? Does the client demonstrate more use of fillers in one language than another? In one language, does the bilingual client demonstrate more semantic density or age-appropriate vocabulary? Is the client frequently code mixing, using vocabulary from one language, while speaking in another, indicative of semantic gaps in one language in comparison to another? All such information is critical for the assessing speech-language pathologist in consideration of a two-tiered investigation. Figure 10–6 illustrates the need to distinguish a semantic difference from a disorder.

Determining Language Dominance

Distinguishing between semantic differences and disorders is a critical component of bilingual assessments. For clients

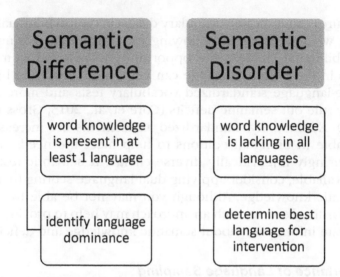

Figure 10–6. The illustration shows the need to distinguish a semantic difference from a disorder.

determined to have disorders, it is helpful to identify areas of strengths in each language to note semantic dominance in both receptive and expressive domains. This identification may help future clinicians and allied professionals who treat the client. Often, it may not be a question of simply one language or the other for intervention. Rather, it may be most appropriate to employ a bilingual approach to maximize the client's abilities to participate using their complete bilingual skill set. Whereas most people have a dominant hand, you still use the other hand to help perform critical functions such as the task of getting dressed. For individuals with semantic skills in both languages, forcing them to use just one language for intervention may add an additional barrier, making it even more challenging to address the semantic deficits. For adults, developing frameworks for assessing bilingual clients with aphasia is critical for clinicians to understand the connections between language proficiency, language loss, and semantic processing in bilingual aphasia (Gray & Kiran, 2013). In all cases, speech-language pathologists should consider the client's holistic needs to target increasing semantic skills to promote effective communication skills.

Typical Phenomena Among Bilinguals

Among adults, bilinguals seem to have several benefits in semantic processing and language. Studies examine the effect of bilingualism on delaying dementia symptoms and retaining cognitive function in older adults, which indicates bilinguals demonstrate later onset of cognitive decline than monolinguals (Bialystok et al., 2007). Studies of bilingual stroke patients indicate bilinguals demonstrate different neural activations during language processing of their native language in comparison to the second language (Sebastian et al., 2012). Evidence suggests differences in lexical retrieval skills among bilingual individuals with aphasia in comparison to their healthy bilingual peers (Calabria et al., 2019). Further, neuroimaging studies of bilinguals with aphasia indicate the need to consider language use, proficiency, production, and comprehension in both receptive and expressive domains in its influence on recovery in intervention with bilingual individuals with aphasia (Peñaloza & Kiran, 2017).

Misconceptions of Bilingual Clients

Clients With Any Bilingual Exposure Must Only Be Assessed by a Bilingual Clinician

Often, bilingual clinicians are not available, especially in consideration of the professional demographics of licensed, speech-language pathologists, who are overwhelmingly monolingual. With more than 90% of members of the American Speech-Language and Hearing Association (ASHA) identifying as monolingual English speakers, clinicians should consider alternatives to delaying assessment such as working collaboratively with bilingual speech-language pathology assistants, trained interpreters, or even an available bilingual helper such as a paraprofessional or client caregiver if no other alternatives are available.

When possible, monolingual clinicians should seek out a trained interpreter. Trained interpreters assist during evaluations by providing translation. Interpreters should be trained, either formally or informally, on professional practices such as making sure to effectively relay directions and instructions given by a speech-language pathologist to a client during test administration. Additionally, interpreters should be instructed to translate client responses exactly as stated, since speech-language pathologists are particularly interested in assessing semantic deficits, in addition to syntax and pragmatic deficits. Often it may be the responsibility of the SLP to effectively train bilingual interpreters because, while bilingual speakers available to assist might be present, such individuals may lack training to do the task appropriately (Langdon & Saenz, 2016).

If a trained interpreter is not available, other options may be employed, such as the use of a bilingual speech-language pathology assistant, paraprofessional, or even a family member who is available to help if that is appropriate. Bilingual speech-language pathology assistants may be particularly helpful because they hold an undergraduate degree in speech-language pathology and, thus, understand the fundamentals of the field and objectives in assessment. If utilizing a paraprofessional or family member as a last resort option, clinicians should be sure to remind the helper to avoid prompting the client in any way in order to reflect a true picture of the client's abilities. Clear instructions are helpful, such as "Say exactly what I say" or "I really want to see what the client can do independently so avoid giving any hints or rephrasing or repeating anything unless I ask you to."

There Might Be a Language Difference, But All Kids Are Generally the Same

Although this statement is often well intended, it is not completely accurate. Research of bilingual children in Mandarin and English found bilingual children demonstrate different organization of their semantic lexicon that differs in comparison to their monolingual peers (Sheng et al., 2006). Findings are consistent in research of Spanish and English bilingual children. Evidence shows assessing semantic knowledge in bilingual learners differs from monolingual peers due to variances in semantic networks regardless of vocabulary size (Sheng et al., 2012). With the vast variety of languages and intersection of time and quality of exposure, bilinguals are a highly heterogeneous population with drastically different presentations from case to case based upon a number of variables (Goldstein & Kohnert, 2005). Monolinguals and bilinguals do differ, but those differences do not equate to deficits and differences should not be assumed to be disorders.

Bilingual Children Can Exhibit Minimal Semantic Delays in Comparison to Monolingual Children, So I Should Refer Bilingual Children for Intervention Just to Be Safe

Although well intentioned, this perception is misinformed. Misidentifying a difference as a disorder ultimately does more harm than good. One may counter this statement by saying "Well speech therapy certainly can't hurt." However, if you have a caseload overburdened by clients exhibiting typical linguistic differences, this situation may prevent another child with a disorder from receiving timely and necessary services. The time the typical bilingual child spends in speech intervention is time the child is not spending in activities with peers or in the classroom receiving academic instruction, missing key opportunities for incidental and direct learning.

Clinical Implications

We all have bias. Becoming more aware of our preconceptions is often the first step to developing more cultural competence and allowing us to better serve culturally and linguistically diverse (CLD) clients. Clinicians need to first acknowledge their bias in order to properly address their misconceptions. The American Speech-Language Hearing Association (ASHA) offers several tools to help clinicians effectively serve diverse clients. Clinicians should take advantage of these free resources as a method of consistently improving clinical skills with culturally and linguistically diverse clients.

Chapter Summary

Semantic processing in bilingual speakers is complex and dynamic. Clinicians must consider issues such as type of bilingualism, language dominance, and language exposure to effectively assess and treat semantic disorders. Assessment should entail appropriate evaluation measures to determine client semantic knowledge. Intervention should focus on increasing communicative effectiveness, rather than only targeting one language domain. Finally, speech-language pathologists should readily utilize available resources such as translators, interpreters, and ASHA's Practice Portal for support in developing appropriate assessment and intervention plans.

Discussion Questions

1. What questions should a speech-language pathologist ask caregivers to probe for language exposure?
2. What assessment methods and/or tools can be used to gather information on semantic skills of bilingual individuals?
3. If a trained interpreter is not available, what resources can a monolingual speech-language pathologist utilize to serve the bilingual client in an effective and ethical way?
4. How might semantic processing differ between simultaneous and successive bilinguals?

References

Bialystok, E., Craik, F., & Freedman, M. (2007). Bilingualism as a protection against the onset of symptoms of dementia. *Neuropsychologia, 45*(2), 459–464.

Bialystok, E., & Martin, M. (2004). Attention and inhibition in bilingual children: Evidence for the dimensional change card sort task. *Developmental Science, 7*(3), 325–339.

Byers-Heinlein, K., & Lew-Williams, C. (2013). Bilingualism in the early years: What the science says. *LEARNing Landscapes, 7*(1), 95–112. https://doi.org/10.36510/learnland.v7i1.632

Calabria, M., Grunden, N., Serra, M., Garcia-Sanchez, C., & Costa, A. (2019). Semantic processing in bilingual aphasia: Evidence of language dependency. *Frontiers in Human Neuroscience, 13*, 205. https://doi.org/10.3389/fnhum.2019.00205

Core, C., Hoff, E., Rumiche, R., & Señor, M. (2013). Total and conceptual vocabulary in Spanish-English bilinguals from 22 to 30 months: Implications for assessment. *Journal of Speech, Language, and Hearing Research, 56*(5), 1637–1649.

Crawford, J. (2013). *At war with diversity: U.S. language policy in an age of anxiety.* Multilingual Matters

Cummins, J. (1984). *Bilingualism and special education: Issues in assessment and pedagogy.* College-Hill Press.

Davison, M., & Qi, C. (2017). Language teaching strategies for preschool English learners. *Perspectives of the ASHA Special Interest Groups, 2*(1), 170–178.

Desjardins, J., & Fernandez, F. (2018). Performance on auditory and visual tasks of inhibition in English monolingual and Spanish-English bilingual adults: Do bilinguals have a cognitive advantage? *Journal of Speech, Language, and Hearing Research, 61*(2), 410–419.

Desmet, T., & Duyck, W. (2007). Bilingual language processing. *Language and Linguistics Compass, 1*(3), 168–194.

Fierro, V., & Storkel, H. (2017). Interactive book reading to accelerate word learning in bilingual children with developmental language disorder: A preliminary intervention approach. *Perspectives of the ASHA Special Interest Groups, 2*(1), 194–202.

Finkbeiner, M., Forster, K., Nicol, J., & Nakamura, K. (2004). The role of polysemy in masked semantic and translation priming. *Journal of Memory and Language, 51*, 1–22.

Fitton, L., Bustamante, K., Wofford, M., Brown, D., Gabas, C., Hoge, R., & Wood, C. (2016). Intensifying English vocabulary instruction for English language learners. *Perspectives of the ASHA Special Interest Groups, 1*(16), 4–14.

Genesee, F., Boivin, I., & Nicoladis, E. (1996). Talking with strangers: A study of bilingual children's communicative competence. *Applied Psycholinguistics, 17* (4), 427–442.

Gibson, T., Peña, E., & Bedore, L. (2012). The relation between language experience and receptive-expressive semantic gaps in bilingual children. *International Journal of Bilingual Education and Bilingualism, 17*(1), 90–110. https://doi.org/10.1080/13670050.2012.743960

Goldstein, B., & Kohnert, K. (2005). Speech, language, and hearing in developing bilingual children: Current findings and future directions. *Language, Speech, and Hearing Services in Schools, 36*, 264–267.

Gray, T., & Kiran, S. (2013). A theoretical account of lexical and semantic naming deficits in bilingual aphasia. *Journal of Speech, Language, and Hearing Research, 56*(4), 1314 –1327.

Gross, M., Buac, M., & Kaushanskaya, M. (2014). Conceptual scoring of receptive and expressive vocabulary measures in simultaneous and sequential bilingual children. *American Journal of Speech-Language Pathology, 23*, 574–586.

Guiberson, M., & Atkins, J. (2012). Speech-language pathologists' preparation, practices, and perspectives on serving culturally and linguistically diverse children. *Communication Disorders Quarterly, 33*, 169–180. https://doi.org/10.1177/1525740110384132

Hammer, C., Komaroff, E., Rodriguez, B., Lopez, L, Scarpino, S., & Goldstein, B. (2012). Predicting Spanish-English bilingual children's language abilities. *Journal of Speech, Language and Hearning Research, 55*(5), 1251–1264.

Jacobson, P. & Walden, P. (2013). Lexical diversity and omission errors as predictors of language ability in the narratives of sequential Spanish-English bilinguals: A cross language comparison. *American Journal of Speech-Language Pathology, 22*(3), 554–565.

Kan, P., Huang, S., Winicour, E., & Yang, J. (2020). Vocabulary growth: Dual language learners at risk for language impairment. *American Journal of Speech-Language Pathology, 29*(3), 1178–1195.

Kroll, J. F., & Stewart, E. (1994). Category interference in translation and picture naming for asymmetric connection between bilingual memory representations. *Journal of Memory and Language, 33*, 149–174.

Kroll, J. F., van Hell, J. G., Tokowicz, N., & Green, D. W. (2010). The Revised Hierarchical Model: A critical review and assessment. *Bilingualism (Cambridge, England), 13*(3), 373–381. https://doi.org/10.1017/S136672891000009X

Langdon, H., & Saenz, T. (2016). Working with interpreters to support students who are English language learners. *Perspectives of the ASHA Special Interest Groups, 1*(16), 15–27.

Martin, N. A. (2013). *Expressive One-Word Picture Vocabulary Test–4: Spanish-Bilingual Edition (EOWPVT-4:SBE)*. Academic Therapy Publications.

Martin, N. A. (2013). *Receptive One-Word Picture Vocabulary Test–4: Spanish-Bilingual Edition (ROWPVT-4:SBE)*. Academic Therapy Publications.

Paradis, J., Genesee, F., & Crago, M.B. (2011). *Dual language development and disorders: A handbook on bilingualism & second language learning* (2nd ed.). Brookes.

Peña, E., Gilliam, R., Bedore, L., & Bohman, T. (2011). Risk for poor performance on a language screening measure for bilingual preschoolers and kindergarteners. *American Journal of Speech-Language Pathology, 20*(4), 302–314.

Peñaloza, C., & Kiran, S. (2017). Neuroimaging evidence in the treatment of bilingual/multilingual adults with aphasia. *Perspectives of the ASHA Special Interest Groups 2*(2), 126–131.

Petitto, L., Katerelos, M., Levy, B., Gauna, K., Tetreault, K., & Ferraro, V. (2001). Bilingual signed and spoken language acquisition from birth: Implications for the mechanisms underlying early bilingual language acquisition. *Journal of Child Language, 28*, 453–496.

Sebastian, R., Kiran, S., & Sandberg, C. (2012). Semantic processing in Spanish-English bilinguals with aphasia. *Journal of Neurolinguistics, 25*, 240–262.

Sheng, L., McGregor, K., & Marian, V. (2006). Lexical-semantic organization in bilingual children: Evidence from a repeated word association task. *Journal of Speech, Language, and Hearing Research, 49*, 572–587.

Sheng, L., Peña, E., Bedore, L., & Fiestas, C. (2012). Semantic deficits in Spanish-English bilingual children with language impairment. *Journal of Speech, Language, and Hearing Research, 55*, 1–15.

van Hell, J. G., & de Groot, A. M. B. (1998). Conceptual representation in bilingual memory: Effects of concreteness and cognate status in word association. *Bilingualism: Language and Cognition, 1*, 193–211.

INDEX

Note: Page numbers in **bold** reference non-text material.

A

AAC (Augmentative and alternative communication), 134
digital stimuli and, 154–156
Abstract
nouns, DLD (Developmental language disorders) and, 182
thinking, children, with language deficits and, 103
verbs, retrievability of, 134
words, emotionally charged, 148
Abundant linguistic input, 71–72
Academic Word List (AWL), 272
Access, lexical, 5
Acquired speech disorders, word production and, 224
ACRT (Anagram, Copy, and Recall Treatment), 369
ACT (Anagram and Copy Treatment), 369
lesson plan, 395–396
Additions morphological errors, 152
Adolescents
vocabulary expansion of, 98–106
Adult-child interaction, vocabulary development, 89
Adults
bilinguals, cognitive function of, 419

use of gestures, 64
WFD (Word finding difficulty)
age related, 195–199
dementia and, 199–202
error types, 186–192
in traumatic brain injury, 193–195
word finding difficulty and, 184–202
with aphasia, 186–192
word production framework, **185**
young, vocabulary size, 86
Age of acquisition (AoA)
word
familiarity and, 133
frequency and, 134–136
Alliteration words, 98
Alternative commination digital stimuli, 154–156
Alzheimer's disease, 200–203
Amazon Mechanical Turk, 136
Ambitransitive verbs, 139
American Psychiatric Association, autism spectrum disorders, defined by, 181
American Speech-Language and Hearing Association (ASHA)
CLD clients and, 421
client assessment, 419
Practice Portal, 194
Profiles of Bilingual Clinicians, 403